Osteoporosis and Related Bone Metabolic Disease

Osteoporosis and Related Bone Metabolic Disease

Editor

Heinrich Resch

MDPI • Basel • Beijing • Wuhan • Barcelona • Belgrade • Manchester • Tokyo • Cluj • Tianjin

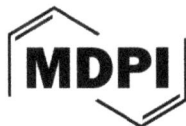

Editor
Heinrich Resch
Faculty of Medicine, Sigmund Freud
Universität Vienna
Austria

Editorial Office
MDPI
St. Alban-Anlage 66
4052 Basel, Switzerland

This is a reprint of articles from the Special Issue published online in the open access journal *Journal of Clinical Medicine* (ISSN 2077-0383) (available at: https://www.mdpi.com/journal/jcm/special_issues/Osteoporosis_Bone_Metabolic_Disease).

For citation purposes, cite each article independently as indicated on the article page online and as indicated below:

LastName, A.A.; LastName, B.B.; LastName, C.C. Article Title. *Journal Name* **Year**, *Volume Number*, Page Range.

ISBN 978-3-0365-6348-0 (Hbk)
ISBN 978-3-0365-6349-7 (PDF)

© 2023 by the authors. Articles in this book are Open Access and distributed under the Creative Commons Attribution (CC BY) license, which allows users to download, copy and build upon published articles, as long as the author and publisher are properly credited, which ensures maximum dissemination and a wider impact of our publications.

The book as a whole is distributed by MDPI under the terms and conditions of the Creative Commons license CC BY-NC-ND.

Contents

About the Editor vii

Heinrich Resch, Afrodite Zendeli and Roland Kocijan
Metabolic Bone Diseases—A Topic of Great Diversity
Reprinted from: J. Clin. Med. 2022, 11, 6447, doi:10.3390/jcm11216447 1

Meng-Huang Wu, Yu-Sheng Lin, Christopher Wu, Ching-Yu Lee, Yi-Chia Chen, Tsung-Jen Huang and Jur-Shan Cheng
Timing of Bisphosphonate (Alendronate) Initiation after Surgery for Fragility Fracture: A Population-Based Cohort Study
Reprinted from: J. Clin. Med. 2021, 10, 2541, doi:10.3390/jcm10122541 5

Margarita Ivanova, Julia Dao, Lauren Noll, Jacqueline Fikry and Ozlem Goker-Alpan
TRAP5b and RANKL/OPG Predict Bone Pathology in Patients with Gaucher Disease
Reprinted from: J. Clin. Med. 2021, 10, 2217, doi:10.3390/jcm10102217 17

Carlo Alfieri, Valentina Binda, Silvia Malvica, Donata Cresseri, Mariarosaria Campise, Maria Teresa Gandolfo, et al.
Bone Effect and Safety of One-Year Denosumab Therapy in a Cohort of Renal Transplanted Patients: An Observational Monocentric Study
Reprinted from: J. Clin. Med. 2021, 10, 1989, doi:10.3390/jcm10091989 31

Afrodite Zendeli, Minh Bui, Lukas Fischer, Ali Ghasem-Zadeh, Wolfgang Schima and Ego Seeman
High Cortico-Trabecular Transitional Zone Porosity and Reduced Trabecular Density in Men and Women with Stress Fractures
Reprinted from: J. Clin. Med. 2021, 10, 1123, doi:10.3390/jcm10051123 41

Maria-José Montoya-García, Mercè Giner, Rodrigo Marcos, David García-Romero, Francisco-Jesús Olmo-Montes, Mª José Miranda, et al.
Fragility Fractures and Imminent Fracture Risk in the Spanish Population: A Retrospective Observational Cohort Study
Reprinted from: J. Clin. Med. 2021, 10, 1082, doi:10.3390/jcm10051082 51

Judith Haschka, Daniel Arian Kraus, Martina Behanova, Stephanie Huber, Johann Bartko, Jakob E. Schanda, et al.
Fractal-Based Analysis of Bone Microstructure in Crohn's Disease: A Pilot Study
Reprinted from: J. Clin. Med. 2020, 9, 4116, doi:10.3390/jcm9124116 63

Agnieszka Podfigurna, Marzena Maciejewska-Jeske, Malgorzata Nadolna, Paula Mikolajska-Ptas, Anna Szeliga, Przemyslaw Bilinski, et al.
Impact of Hormonal Replacement Therapy on Bone Mineral Density in Premature Ovarian Insufficiency Patients
Reprinted from: J. Clin. Med. 2020, 9, 3961, doi:10.3390/jcm9123961 79

Chieh-Hua Lu, Chi-Hsiang Chung, Feng-Chih Kuo, Kuan-Chan Chen, Chia-Hao Chang, Chih-Chun Kuo, et al.
Metformin Attenuates Osteoporosis in Diabetic Patients with Carcinoma in Situ: A Nationwide, Retrospective, Matched-Cohort Study in Taiwan
Reprinted from: J. Clin. Med. 2020, 9, 2839, doi:10.3390/jcm9092839 89

Kazuyoshi Shigehara, Kouji Izumi, Yoshifumi Kadono and Atsushi Mizokami
Testosterone and Bone Health in Men: A Narrative Review
Reprinted from: *J. Clin. Med.* **2021**, *10*, 530, doi:10.3390/jcm10030530 . . . . **103**

Cosmin Iulian Codrea, Alexa-Maria Croitoru, Cosmin Constantin Baciu, Alina Melinescu, Denisa Ficai, Victor Fruth and Anton Ficai
Advances in Osteoporotic Bone Tissue Engineering
Reprinted from: *J. Clin. Med.* **2021**, *10*, 253, doi:10.3390/jcm10020253 . . . . **115**

Tai-Li Chen, Jing-Wun Lu, Yu-Wen Huang, Jen-Hung Wang and Kuei-Ying Su
Bone Mineral Density, Osteoporosis, and Fracture Risk in Adult Patients with Psoriasis or Psoriatic Arthritis: A Systematic Review and Meta-Analysis of Observational Studies
Reprinted from: *J. Clin. Med.* **2020**, *9*, 3712, doi:10.3390/jcm9113712 . . . . **143**

About the Editor

Heinrich Resch

Heinrich Resch, MD. Professor of Medicine, Medical University of Vienna. Head of the Department of Osteology/Rheumatology and Gastroenterology, KH Barmherzige Schwestern (St. Vincent Hospital) Vienna, Academic Teaching Hospital of the Medical University of Vienna. Chairman of the Metabolic Bone Disease Unit, Medical School, Sigmund Freud University of Vienna. Heinrich Resch is a gastroenterologist and rheumatologist and is a past President of the Austrian Society of Bone and Mineral Research. He is the Head of the Medical Department II at the KH Barmherzige Schwestern (St. Vincent Hospital Vienna), an Academic Teaching Hospital of the University Vienna, and is Chairman of the Metabolic Bone Disease Unit Medical School, Sigmund Freud University of Vienna. In addition, he served as the president of the German Society of Osteology in the past. Over the last 20 years, he has established one of the largest centers for the management of metabolic bone diseases in Austria. Being a clinician, he was able to combine his interest in basic research with routine clinical work, giving an example of patient-oriented and translational research. He used to serve as an IOF speaker worldwide, giving advanced educational courses regarding densitometry and the treatment of osteoporosis. For many years, he worked at the bone metabolic unit in Loma Linda University, CA, with David Baylink. His special interest is in performing and analyzing iliac crest bone biopsies, thus being the co-author of articles of top journals in the bone field. He serves as a reviewer for *JBMR*, *Bone*, *Maturitas*, *EJR*, and *Osteoporosis INT*, and he has published more than 250 articles and book chapters and given more than 300 invited lectures in the past.

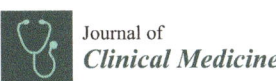

Editorial

Metabolic Bone Diseases—A Topic of Great Diversity

Heinrich Resch *, Afrodite Zendeli and Roland Kocijan

Faculty of Medicine, Sigmund Freud Universität Vienna, 1020 Wien, Austria
* Correspondence: heinrich.resch@bhs.at

The progress in research has improved the understanding of the epidemiology and pathogenesis of osteoporosis and bone disorders in general. Metabolic bone changes have advanced beyond the simple models of explanation of age-related loss in bone mass, combined with simple and easy assessment of fracture risk by the FRAX model. This was also shown in a Spanish retrospective population-based cohort study on patients suffering from a fragility fracture. The incidence rate of index fragility fractures and obtained information on the subsequent fractures and death during a follow-up of up to three years were assessed [1]. Beyond fracture risk assessment and bone mineral density (BMD) measurements using DEXA, invasive and noninvasive methods for the assessment of trabecular and cortical bone structure, strength and material properties have been developed. Bone microstructural deterioration at the distal radial and the unfractured distal tibia was quantified in a small but well-defined homogeneous group using high-resolution peripheral quantitative computed tomography [2]. It was shown that stress fractures were associated with compromised cortical and trabecular microstructure, changes which are not covered by standard BMD diagnostics.

In healthy people, peak bone mass and bone remodeling are stable for many years unless a secondary, stimulative cause of bone loss is present. In women, the decline in estrogen as early as in perimenopause results in an imbalance of bone remodeling, such that resorptive processes exceed formative processes and, as a consequence, bone mass decreases. Premature ovarian insufficiency as an example of hypergonadotropic hypogonadism caused by impaired ovarian function before the age of 40 is associated with an increased risk of BMD loss and development of osteopenia and osteoporosis which poses an important problem for public health [3]. At the same time, with these remodeling characteristics, a deterioration of bone architecture and disturbances in skeletal integrity occur. Thus, early initiation of full-dose hormone replacement therapy (HRT) has a significant and positive influence on bone mass in these patients.

Knowledge of bone relates primarily to primary osteoporosis in which bone loss can be attributed to aging per se or the known hormonal consequences of aging. A large number of heterogeneous causes (e.g., metabolic, inflammatory, autoimmune, vascular, renal diseases, genetic disorders and even drugs), defined as secondary causes of osteoporosis, may induce bone loss or structural deterioration through different mechanisms [4–6].

In a study on Gaucher disease (GD), standard biomarkers such as TRAP5b levels showed a positive correlation with GD biomarkers, including plasma glucosylsphingosine (lyso-Gb1) and macrophage activation markers, CCL18 as an example [7].

Secondary osteoporosis refers to those conditions that reflect adverse consequences of the primary disease itself which is not bone-related at first sight or caused by side-effects of pharmacotherapies being the standard treatment in those diseases. In this context, diabetic patients with carcinoma in situ under metformin therapy presented lower osteoporosis rates than those who were not receiving metformin therapy [8].

Although these secondary causes of osteoporosis are the most frequently observed causes of unexpected bone loss, they can only be diagnosed by a high degree of suspicion and clinical experience, performing the appropriate investigations. In inflammatory

Citation: Resch, H.; Zendeli, A.; Kocijan, R. Metabolic Bone Diseases—A Topic of Great Diversity. *J. Clin. Med.* **2022**, *11*, 6447. https://doi.org/10.3390/jcm11216447

Received: 16 October 2022
Accepted: 26 October 2022
Published: 31 October 2022

Publisher's Note: MDPI stays neutral with regard to jurisdictional claims in published maps and institutional affiliations.

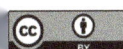

Copyright: © 2022 by the authors. Licensee MDPI, Basel, Switzerland. This article is an open access article distributed under the terms and conditions of the Creative Commons Attribution (CC BY) license (https://creativecommons.org/licenses/by/4.0/).

disorders such as rheumatoid arthritis or chronic inflammatory bowel diseases, but also vascular diseases, T-cell activation and consequently pro-inflammatory cascades trigger the increased expression of T-cell-derived RANKL [9,10]. In addition, there is a new biomarker signature of bone-related miRNAs which is promising in certain clinical features [11]. Glucocorticoids, often used to control disease activity, decrease the osteoblasts in number and function and additionally inhibit OPG expression. The ubiquitous occurrence of disease-related secondary changes in bone metabolism implies that numerous medical disciplines need to interact. Especially if surgical interventions and surgical fracture repair are necessary, initiation of specific osteoporosis medication such as bisphosphonates can avoid refractures after surgery [12,13].

Age-related bone loss occurs also in men; however, the mode of this process is still not as well-investigated, leading to an insufficient understanding of the development of the disease in comparison to females. Age-related declines in testosterone are important determinants of bone loss in males which can be reverted due to testosterone replacement [14].

The accelerated progress in bone research has resulted in the development of pharmacologic approaches to minimize or even reverse further bone loss in circumstances where changes in calcium and bone metabolism derive from kidney failure or transplanting the central organ in calcium regulation and homeostasis. In this context, denosumab is able to increase BMD in those patients [15].

Since bone remodeling depends on interactions between formative and resorptive processes, it makes sense to determine the most effective pharmacotherapy as well as the right timepoint to initiate treatment in the concept of sequential therapy [16–18]. Denosumab is already approved as an effective drug to reduce fracture risk with seemingly fewer adverse events than have been reported for other monoclonal antibodies used to treat diseases other than osteoporosis. Understanding the mechanisms by which sclerostin as a central regulator of bone formation can be manipulated by an antibody to permit excessive and fast formation of new bone, and molecules that interact with Wnt signaling and LRP5 are linked will finally lead to the development of other therapeutic drugs [19–23].

While this is highly exciting and represents significant progress in maintaining the integrity of bone, it remains to be seen whether this will lead to medications more effective in reducing fracture risk than those drugs currently available.

Screening for secondary causes of osteoporosis and the search for new modes of action should present a substantial part of osteoporosis management. With this Special Issue, we hope to encourage discussion of the current management of osteoporosis and related metabolic bone diseases.

Author Contributions: Conceptualization, H.R.; validation, H.R., R.K. and A.Z.; data curation, H.R. and A.Z.; writing—original draft preparation, H.R.; writing—review and editing, H.R., A.Z. and R.K.; supervision, H.R. All authors have read and agreed to the published version of the manuscript.

Funding: This research received no external funding.

Conflicts of Interest: The authors declare no conflict of interest.

References

1. Montoya-García, M.-J.; Giner, M.; Marcos, R.; García-Romero, D.; Olmo-Montes, F.-J.; Miranda, M.; Hernández-Cruz, B.; Colmenero, M.-A.; Vázquez-Gámez, M. Fragility Fractures and Imminent Fracture Risk in the Spanish Population: A Retrospective Observational Cohort Study. *J. Clin. Med.* **2021**, *10*, 1082. [CrossRef]
2. Zendeli, A.; Bui, M.; Fischer, L.; Ghasem-Zadeh, A.; Schima, W.; Seeman, E. High Cortico-Trabecular Transitional Zone Porosity and Reduced Trabecular Density in Men and Women with Stress Fractures. *J. Clin. Med.* **2021**, *10*, 1123. [CrossRef]
3. Podfigurna, A.; Maciejewska-Jeske, M.; Nadolna, M.; Mikolajska-Ptas, P.; Szeliga, A.; Bilinski, P.; Napierala, P.; Meczekalski, B. Impact of Hormonal Replacement Therapy on Bone Mineral Density in Premature Ovarian Insufficiency Patients. *J. Clin. Med.* **2020**, *9*, 3961. [CrossRef]
4. Kocijan, R.; Finzel, S.; Englbrecht, M.; Engelke, K.; Rech, J.; Schett, G. Decreased Quantity and Quality of the Periarticular and Nonperiarticular Bone in Patients with Rheumatoid Arthritis: A Cross-Sectional HR-pQCT Study. *J. Bone Miner. Res.* **2013**, *29*, 1005–1014. [CrossRef]

5. Chen, T.-L.; Lu, J.-W.; Huang, Y.-W.; Wang, J.-H.; Su, K.-Y. Bone Mineral Density, Osteoporosis, and Fracture Risk in Adult Patients with Psoriasis or Psoriatic Arthritis: A Systematic Review and Meta-Analysis of Observational Studies. *J. Clin. Med.* **2020**, *9*, 3712. [CrossRef]
6. Haschka, J.; Kraus, D.A.; Behanova, M.; Huber, S.; Bartko, J.; Schanda, J.E.; Meier, P.; Bahrami, A.; Zandieh, S.; Zwerina, J.; et al. Fractal-Based Analysis of Bone Microstructure in Crohn's Disease: A Pilot Study. *J. Clin. Med.* **2020**, *9*, 4116. [CrossRef]
7. Ivanova, M.; Dao, J.; Noll, L.; Fikry, J.; Goker-Alpan, O. TRAP5b and RANKL/OPG Predict Bone Pathology in Patients with Gaucher Disease. *J. Clin. Med.* **2021**, *10*, 2217. [CrossRef]
8. Lu, C.-H.; Chung, C.-H.; Kuo, F.-C.; Chen, K.-C.; Chang, C.-H.; Kuo, C.-C.; Lee, C.-H.; Su, S.-C.; Liu, J.-S.; Lin, F.-H.; et al. Metformin Attenuates Osteoporosis in Diabetic Patients with Carcinoma in Situ: A Nationwide, Retrospective, Matched-Cohort Study in Taiwan. *J. Clin. Med.* **2020**, *9*, 2839. [CrossRef]
9. Schett, G. Rheumatoid arthritis: Inflammation and bone loss. *Wien. Med. Wochenschr.* **2006**, *156*, 34–41. [CrossRef]
10. Schett, G.; Smolen, J. New Insights in the Mechanism of Bone Loss in Arthritis. *Curr. Pharm. Des.* **2005**, *11*, 3039–3049. [CrossRef]
11. Kocijan, R.; Muschitz, C.; Geiger, E.; Skalicky, S.; Baierl, A.; Dormann, R.; Plachel, F.; Feichtinger, X.; Heimel, P.; Fahrleitner-Pammer, A.; et al. Circulating microRNA Signatures in Patients with Idiopathic and Postmenopausal Osteoporosis and Fragility Fractures. *J. Clin. Endocrinol. Metab.* **2016**, *101*, 4125–4134. [CrossRef]
12. Codrea, C.I.; Croitoru, A.M.; Baciu, C.C.; Melinescu, A.; Ficai, D.; Fruth, V.; Ficai, A. Advances in Osteoporotic Bone Tissue Engineering. *J. Clin. Med.* **2021**, *10*, 253. [CrossRef]
13. Wu, M.-H.; Lin, Y.-S.; Wu, C.; Lee, C.-Y.; Chen, Y.-C.; Huang, T.-J.; Cheng, J.-S. Timing of Bisphosphonate (Alendronate) Initiation after Surgery for Fragility Fracture: A Population-Based Cohort Study. *J. Clin. Med.* **2021**, *10*, 2541. [CrossRef]
14. Shigehara, K.; Izumi, K.; Kadono, Y.; Mizokami, A. Testosterone and Bone Health in Men: A Narrative Review. *J. Clin. Med.* **2021**, *10*, 530. [CrossRef]
15. Alfieri, C.; Binda, V.; Malvica, S.; Cresseri, D.; Campise, M.; Gandolfo, M.; Regalia, A.; Mattinzoli, D.; Armelloni, S.; Favi, E.; et al. Bone Effect and Safety of One-Year Denosumab Therapy in a Cohort of Renal Transplanted Patients: An Observational Monocentric Study. *J. Clin. Med.* **2021**, *10*, 1989. [CrossRef]
16. Langdahl, B. Treatment of postmenopausal osteoporosis with bone-forming and antiresorptive treatments: Combined and sequential approaches. *Bone* **2020**, *139*, 115516. [CrossRef]
17. Kendler, D.; Chines, A.; Clark, P.; Ebeling, P.R.; McClung, M.; Rhee, Y.; Huang, S.; Stad, R.K. Bone Mineral Density After Transitioning From Denosumab to Alendronate. *J. Clin. Endocrinol. Metab.* **2019**, *105*, e255–e264. [CrossRef]
18. Cosman, F.; Nieves, J.W.; Dempster, D.W. Treatment Sequence Matters: Anabolic and Antiresorptive Therapy for Osteoporosis. *J. Bone Miner. Res.* **2017**, *32*, 198–202. [CrossRef]
19. Ke, H.Z.; Richards, W.G.; Li, X.; Ominsky, M.S. Sclerostin and Dickkopf-1 as Therapeutic Targets in Bone Diseases. *Endocr. Rev.* **2012**, *33*, 747–783. [CrossRef]
20. Chavassieux, P.; Chapurlat, R.; Portero-Muzy, N.; Roux, J.; Garcia, P.; Brown, J.P.; Libanati, C.; Boyce, R.W.; Wang, A.; Grauer, A. Bone-Forming and Antiresorptive Effects of Romosozumab in Postmenopausal Women with Osteoporosis: Bone Histomorphometry and Microcomputed Tomography Analysis After 2 and 12 Months of Treatment. *J. Bone Miner. Res.* **2019**, *34*, 1597–1608. [CrossRef]
21. Graeff, C.; Campbell, G.M.; Peña, J.; Borggrefe, J.; Padhi, D.; Kaufman, A.; Chang, S.; Libanati, C.; Glüer, C.-C. Administration of romosozumab improves vertebral trabecular and cortical bone as assessed with quantitative computed tomography and finite element analysis. *Bone* **2015**, *81*, 364–369. [CrossRef] [PubMed]
22. Genant, H.K.; Engelke, K.; Bolognese, M.A.; Mautalen, C.; Brown, J.P.; Recknor, C.; Goemaere, S.; Fuerst, T.; Yang, Y.-C.; Grauer, A.; et al. Effects of Romosozumab Compared with Teriparatide on Bone Density and Mass at the Spine and Hip in Postmenopausal Women with Low Bone Mass. *J. Bone Miner. Res.* **2016**, *32*, 181–187. [CrossRef] [PubMed]
23. Poole, K.E.S.; Treece, G.M.; Pearson, R.A.; Gee, A.H.; Bolognese, M.A.; Brown, J.P.; Goemaere, S.; Grauer, A.; Hanley, D.A.; Mautalen, C.; et al. Romosozumab Enhances Vertebral Bone Structure in Women with Low Bone Density. *J. Bone Miner. Res.* **2021**, *37*, 256–264. [CrossRef] [PubMed]

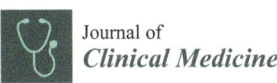

Article

Timing of Bisphosphonate (Alendronate) Initiation after Surgery for Fragility Fracture: A Population-Based Cohort Study

Meng-Huang Wu [1,2,†], Yu-Sheng Lin [3,4,†], Christopher Wu [5], Ching-Yu Lee [1,2], Yi-Chia Chen [6], Tsung-Jen Huang [1,2] and Jur-Shan Cheng [7,8,9,*]

1. Department of Orthopedics, Taipei Medical University Hospital, Taipei 110301, Taiwan; maxwutmu@gmail.com (M.-H.W.); ejaca22@gmail.com (C.-Y.L.); tjdhuang@tmu.edu.tw (T.-J.H.)
2. Department of Orthopaedics, School of Medicine, College of Medicine, Taipei Medical University, Taipei 110301, Taiwan
3. Department of Cardiology, Chang Gung Memorial Hospital, Chiayi 613016, Taiwan; dissert@cgmh.org.tw
4. College of Medicine, Chang Gung University, Taoyuan 333323, Taiwan
5. College of Medicine, Taipei Medical University, Taipei 110301, Taiwan; cjwuchris@gmail.com
6. Research Services Center for Health Information, Chang Gung University, Taoyuan 333323, Taiwan; chia0317@mail.cgu.edu.tw
7. Clinical Informatics and Medical Statistics Research Center, College of Medicine, Chang Gung University, Taoyuan 333323, Taiwan
8. Department of Biomedical Sciences, College of Medicine, Chang Gung University, Taoyuan 333323, Taiwan
9. Department of Emergency Medicine, Chang Gung Memorial Hospital, Keelung 204201, Taiwan
* Correspondence: jscheng@mail.cgu.edu.tw; Tel.: +886-3-211-8800 (ext. 3810)
† These authors contributed equally to this work.

Abstract: Bisphosphonates are used as first-line treatment for the prevention of fragility fracture (FF); they act by inhibiting osteoclast-mediated bone resorption. The timing of their administration after FF surgery is controversial; thus, we compared the incidence of second FF, surgery for second FF, and adverse events associated with early initiation of bisphosphonates (EIBP, within 3 months of FF surgery) and late initiation of bisphosphonates (LIBP, 3 months after FF surgery) in bisphosphonate-naïve patients. This retrospective population-based cohort study used data from Taiwan's Health and Welfare Data Science Center (2004–2012). A total of 298,377 patients received surgeries for FF between 2006 and 2010; of them, 1209 (937 EIBP and 272 LIBP) received first-time bisphosphonates (oral alendronate, 70 mg, once a week). The incidence of second FF (subdistribution hazard ratio (SHR) = 0.509; 95% confidence interval (CI): 0.352–0.735), second FF surgery (SHR = 0.452; 95% CI: 0.268–0.763), and adverse events (SHR = 0.728; 95% CI: 0.594–0.893) was significantly lower in the EIBP group than in the LIBP group. Our findings indicate that bisphosphonates should be initiated within 3 months after surgery for FF.

Keywords: fragility fracture; initiation timing; second fracture; adverse events

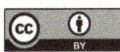

1. Introduction

Bisphosphonates are commonly used as first-line treatment for the prevention of primary and second fragility fractures (FFs). Bisphosphonates prevent FFs by inhibiting osteoclast-mediated bone resorption, thus increasing bone strength and preventing bone loss. They are endocytosed by osteoclasts and inhibit the activity of farnesyl pyrophosphate synthase, which is responsible for the production of cholesterol and intracellular localization of GTPase signaling proteins, which are essential for osteoclast functions [1]. However, osteoclasts play a vital role in callus formation and bone remodeling as well as remodeling of the callus into cortical bone [2,3]. Thus, bisphosphonates may exert adverse effects on fracture healing. However, animal studies have revealed dissimilar results: no effect on fracture healing [4,5], delayed fracture healing [6–8], and enhanced fracture healing [9–13].

In a case–control study, Li et al. stated that bisphosphonate use in the postfracture period was linked to increased likelihood of nonunion [14]. However, recent research in humans has indicated that early bisphosphonate administration does not affect the rate of healing of fractures, clinical outcomes, or the complications rate [15,16]. No whole-population-based study has examined this question.

We hypothesized that early bisphosphonate initiation has better outcomes than late bisphosphonate initiation. Therefore, we compared the incidence of second FF, surgery for second FF, and adverse events associated with early initiation of bisphosphonates (EIBP; within 3 months of FF surgery) and late initiation of bisphosphonates (LIBP; 3 months after FF surgery) used as an oral alendronate (70 mg once a week).

2. Materials and Methods

2.1. Data Sources and Study Samples

This retrospective cohort study used national data (2004–2012) including National Health Insurance (NHI) claims data, the Cancer Registry Database, and the Death Registry Database. More than 99% of the population is enrolled in the mandatory, single-payer NHI program, which provides comprehensive care, including outpatient and inpatient services, laboratory tests, and prescription drugs.

We include patients aged ≥ 50 years who underwent surgery for FF (spine, hip, upper limb, or lower limb fracture) during 2006–2010 (the index surgery and date) and received bisphosphonate monotherapy with medication possession ratio (MPR) ≥ 0.5 within the 1 year after the surgery (Figure 1, Table 1). We excluded patients with pathologic fracture, cancer history, traffic accident injury, multiple fractures, or history of taking antiosteoporotic medicine. In addition, patients with respiratory failure, pneumonia, an acute cardiac event, a cerebrovascular accident and spinal cord injury, nerve injury, renal failure, upper gastrointestinal (UGI) bleeding, acute postoperative hemorrhage, urinary tract infection, sepsis, osteomyelitis, postoperative infection, or nonunion or malunion within the 3 months before the index date were excluded. The index date was defined as the day of the first FF surgery. The selected participants were divided into EIBP and LIBP groups. To improve the comparability of the groups, the EIPB group was 1:1 matched with the LIBP group through propensity score matching by using a logistic model to estimate the probability of initiating the therapy more than 3 months after the index date. The covariates included in the model were age (<65 and ≥ 65 years), sex (male and female), Charlson comorbidity index (CCI; 0, 1, and ≥ 2), and FF surgery site (spine, hip, upper limb, and lower limb). All patients had a minimum 2-year follow-up.

2.2. Confounders and Bias

Registration and classification bias of fractures may be present in the NHI claims data of patients receiving FF surgery; patients may also have higher frequency of complications and reoperation following FFs, thus artificially inflating the fracture rate. To limit the possible biases, we introduced a 90-day "washout" period for each fracture and adverse event; thus, any new fracture with the same ICD-9 code or adverse event associated with surgery was ignored. However, the NHI claims data on fractures do not specify the side of appendicular fractures (i.e., left or right). Furthermore, fractures to the axial skeleton are classified only as lumbar, thoracic, or cervical. This may result in the exclusion of fractures to, for example, the left tibia, if a right tibial fracture was registered in the preceding 90 days. We risked underestimating the fracture rate. We could not correct for this possible bias.

Medications, including thyroxine, proton pump inhibitors, and steroids, affect the likelihood of FF and adverse events. The prescription of these medications for more than 3 months was recorded.

2.3. Statistical Analysis

All statistical analyses were conducted using SAS (version 9.4; SAS Institute, Cary, NC, USA). The incidence of outcomes in the EIBP and LIBP groups was estimated by calculating the number of cases per 100 person-years. Person-years were calculated using the time from the index date to the date of the event or the end of follow-up (31 December 2012), whichever occurred first. The cumulative incidence of the outcomes in the EIBP and LIBP groups was estimated using the modified Kaplan–Meier method and the Gray method, which considers death a competing risk event [17].

Subdistribution hazard models that accounted for competing mortality were used to estimate the adjusted subdistribution hazard ratio (SHR) of outcomes, with adjustments for age (<65 and ≥65 years old); sex (male and female); site of the index FF surgery (spine, upper limb, lower limb, and hip); CCI (0, 1, and ≥2); and comorbidities (cerebrovascular disease, chronic pulmonary disease, rheumatologic disease, peptic ulcer disease, diabetes, and renal disease). Risks of secondary FF, second FF surgery, and revision surgery in the EIBP and LIBP groups were also compared among the subgroups of the index FF surgery site and age [18].

If significant differences were noted in initial FF surgery and age between the groups (Table 1), we performed a subgroup analysis to evaluate the effect of initial FF surgery and age on the outcomes. Although the incidence of rheumatologic disease differed between the groups, we did not evaluate the effect of this disease because of the small number of patients.

This study was granted ethical approval by the Institutional Review Board of Chang Gung Memorial Hospital of Taiwan (104-3677B).

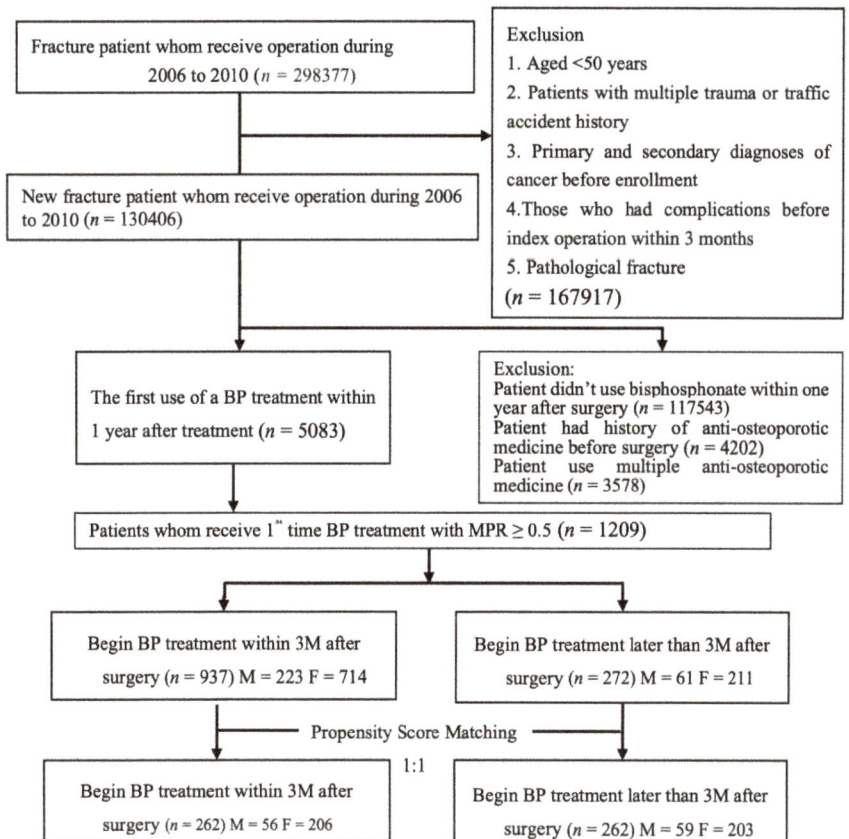

Figure 1. Study protocol. BP: bisphosphonate (alendronate); MPR: medication possession ratio.

Table 1. Clinicodemographic characteristics of the study population.

Variables		Total (n = 524)		EIBP (n = 262)		LIBP (n = 262)		p Value
		Count	%	Count	%	Count	%	
Sex								
	Male	115	21.946	56	21.374	59	22.519	0.752
	Female	409	78.053	206	78.626	203	77.481	
Age (years)								
	<65	129	24.618	65	24.809	64	24.427	0.919
	≥65	395	75.382	197	75.191	198	75.573	
CCI								
	0	327	62.405	163	62.214	164	62.595	
	1	123	23.473	61	23.282	62	23.664	0.968
	≥2	74	14.122	38	14.504	36	13.740	
Covariates								
	Cerebrovascular disease	14	2.672	11	4.198	3	1.145	0.030
	Chronic pulmonary disease	43	8.206	21	8.015	22	8.397	0.874
	Rheumatologic disease	21	4.008	8	3.053	13	4.962	0.265
	Peptic ulcer disease	20	3.817	10	3.817	10	3.817	1.000
	Diabetes	104	19.847	51	19.466	53	20.229	0.827
	Diabetes with chronic complications	26	4.962	13	4.962	13	4.962	1.000
	Renal disease	13	2.481	6	2.290	7	2.672	0.779
	Obesity	5	0.954	3	1.145	2	0.763	0.744
	History of fragility fracture	42	8.015	22	8.396	20	7.633	0.615
Fragility fracture surgery site								
	Spine	38	7.252	19	7.252	19	7.252	
	Hip	224	42.748	112	42.748	112	42.748	1.000
	Upper limb	188	35.878	94	35.878	94	35.878	
	Lower limb	74	14.122	37	14.122	37	14.122	
Concomitant drug								
	Proton pump inhibitor	4	0.331	3	0.320	1	0.368	0.905
	Steroid	30	2.481	19	2.028	11	4.044	0.059
	Antiepileptic	4	0.331	3	0.320	1	0.368	0.905
Follow-up time (mean years)		4.314		4.2456		4.3824		

CCI, Charlson comorbidity index; EIBP, early initiation of bisphosphonates (within 3 months of surgery); LIBP, late initiation of bisphosphonates (3 months after surgery).

3. Results

3.1. Baseline Characteristics

A total of 130,406 patients underwent FF surgery during 2006–2010. Among them, 12,863 received antiosteoporotic medicine. We identified 1209 patients who were first-time users of bisphosphonate (oral alendronate, 70 mg once a week) after FF surgery and who had an MPR of ≥0.5. Of these patients, 937 were included in the EIBP group and 272 in the LIBP group. After propensity score matching, both groups contained 262 patients (Table 1, Figure 1); these groups had similar sex distribution, CCIs, and medical history. More patients in the EIBP group had cerebrovascular disease than in the LIBP group (4.20% vs. 1.15%, $p = 0.030$).

Significant differences were observed in the incidence of second FF, second FF surgery, and adverse events between the EIBP and LIBP groups (Table 2). A higher incidence of second FF (32.44% vs. 19.08%, $p = 0.0005$) and second FF surgery (18.70% vs. 9.16%, $p = 0.0021$) was observed in the LIBP group.

Table 2. Incidence of second fragility fractures and surgeries, revision surgery, death, and complications.

Variables	EIBP (n = 262)			LIBP (n = 262)			Log-Rank p Value	Chi-Square p Value
	Count	%	Incidence *	Count	%	Incidence *		
Site of second fragility fracture	50	19.084	5.173	85	32.443	9.693	0.0005	0.0005
Trunk	<5	<5.000		<5	<5.000			
Spine	8	16.000		22	25.882			
Hip	22	44.000		31	36.471			
Upper Limb	16	32.000		23	27.059			
Lower Limb	<5	<5.000		<5	<5.000			
Site of second fracture surgery	24	9.160	2.323	49	18.702	4.943	0.0021	0.0016
Spine	<5	<5		5	10.204			
Hip	19	79.167		24	48.980			
Upper Limb	4	16.667		14	28.571			
Lower Limb	<5	<5		5	10.204			
Site of revision surgery	18	6.870	1.705	30	11.450	2.858	0.0789	0.0692
Spine	<5	<5.000		<5	<10.000			
Hip	15	83.333		11	36.667			
Upper Limb	<5	<15.000		14	46.667			
Lower Limb	<5	<5.000		<5	<5.000			
Death	35	13.359	3.146	51	19.466	4.442	0.1351	0.0591
Complication								
Respiratory failure	14	5.344	1.271	36	13.740	3.208	0.0025	0.0011
Pneumonia	81	30.916	8.577	93	35.496	9.974	0.3032	0.2657
Acute cardiac event	55	20.992	5.554	65	24.809	6.631	0.3111	0.2985
CVA and SCI, nerve injury	69	26.336	7.211	67	25.573	6.948	0.8965	0.842
Renal failure	6	2.290	0.543	18	6.870	1.597	0.0174	0.0122
UGI bleeding	170	64.885	11.738	199	75.954	35.809	0.0361	0.0055
Acute postoperative hemorrhage	11	4.198	0.989	12	4.580	1.045	0.8927	0.8311
Urinary tract infection	97	37.023	11.210	115	43.893	13.123	0.2457	0.1091
Sepsis	32	12.214	2.989	38	14.504	3.445	0.6182	0.441
Osteomyelitis	5	1.908	0.454	13	4.962	1.170	0.0604	0.055
Postoperative Infection	5	1.908	0.457	13	4.962	1.182	0.059	0.055
Nonunion/malunion	6	2.290	0.549	12	4.580	1.094	0.1581	0.1501

* per 100 person-years. EIBP, early initiation of bisphosphonates (within 3 months of surgery); LIBP, late initiation of bisphosphonates (3 months after surgery); CCI, Charlson comorbidity index; CVA, cerebrovascular accident; SCI, spinal cord injury; UGI, upper gastrointestinal.

A higher incidence of second FF surgery was detected in the LIBP group in patients with complications of respiratory failure (13.7% vs. 5.344%, $p = 0.0025$), renal failure (6.87% vs. 2.29%, $p = 0.0174$), and UGI bleeding (75.95% vs. 26.34%, $p = 0.0361$).

3.2. Second FF and Second FF Surgery

Multivariate subdistribution hazard regression analyses of factors associated with second FF, revision surgery, and second FF surgery were conducted (Figure 2). The findings indicated that the incidences of second FF (SHR = 0.509; 95% confidence interval (95% CI): 0.352–0.735, $p = 0.0003$) and second FF surgery (SHR = 0.452; 95% CI: 0.268–0.763, $p = 0.0029$) were significantly lower in the EIBP group than in the LIBP group (Figures 2 and 3). Patients aged <65 years (SHR = 1.632; 95% CI: 1.044–2.549, $p = 0.0315$), who had cerebrovascular disease (SHR = 3.182; 95% CI: 1.174–8.626, $p = 0.0229$), and who had renal disease (SHR = 5.259; 95% CI: 1.370–20.186, $p = 0.0156$) had significantly higher incidence of second FF. No significant difference was observed in any factor for incidence of revision surgery between the EIBP and LIBP groups (Figure 4).

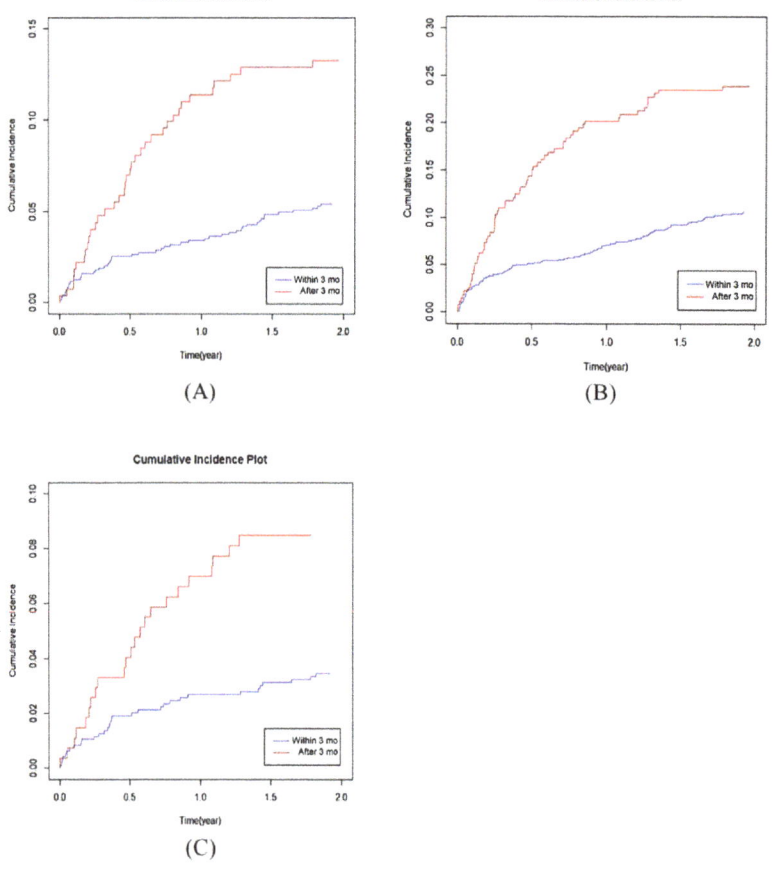

Figure 2. Risk factors and adjusted hazard ratio of fragility fractures stratified by bisphosphonate initiation time, sex, age, Charlson comorbidity index, and comorbidities, by using a proportional subdistribution hazards model. BP: bisphosphonate initiation; CCI: Charlson comorbidity index; CI: confidence interval.

Figure 3. Cumulative incidence of (**A**) second fragility fracture, (**B**) second fragility fracture surgery, and (**C**) revision surgery in patients with bisphosphonate initiation within 3 months after fragility fracture surgery versus more than 3 months after fragility fracture surgery.

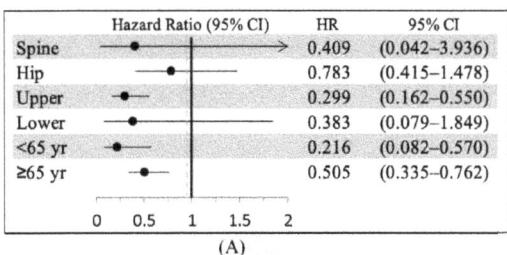

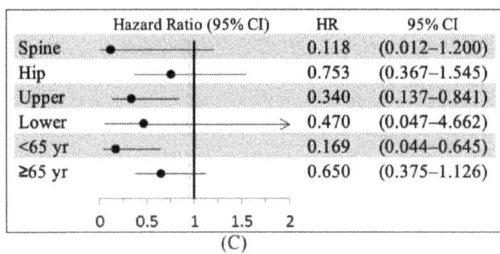

Figure 4. Forest plot of (**A**) second fragility fracture, (**B**) second fragility fracture surgery, and (**C**) revision surgery in patients with bisphosphonate initiation within 3 months after fragility fracture surgery versus more than 3 months after fragility fracture surgery for different fragility fracture types and age groups. SHR, subdistribution hazard ratio; CI, confidence interval; Upper, upper limb; Lower, lower limb.

3.3. Adverse Events after FFs

After initial FF surgery, the incidence of adverse events (Figure 4)—respiratory failure (SHR = 0.363; 95% CI: 0.189–0.697, p = 0.0024), renal failure (SHR = 0.346; 95% CI: 0.134–0.894, p = 0.0284), UGI bleeding (SHR = 0.76; 95% CI: 0.618–0.935, p = 0.0095), and overall complications (SHR = 0.7280; 95% CI: 0.5940–0.8930, p = 0.0023)—was lower in the EIBP group than in the LIBP group. The incidence of respiratory failure (SHR = 0.316; 95% CI: 0.174–0.572, p = 0.0001) and renal failure (SHR = 0.354; 95% CI: 0.140–0.895, p = 0.0282) was higher in women, but that of UGI bleeding (SHR = 1.508; 95% CI: 1.137–2.000, p = 0.004) and overall complications (SHR = 1.380; 95% CI: 1.051–1.810, p = 0.020) was higher in men.

A lower incidence of respiratory failure was noted in patients with upper limb FF surgery (SHR = 0.421; 95% CI: 0.196–0.904, p = 0.0024) and UGI bleeding (SHR = 0.79; 95% CI: 0.625–0.998, p = 0.0479), and a higher incidence in patients aged > 65 years (SHR = 7.281; 95% CI: 2.029–26.12, p = 0.0023). Peptic ulcer was associated with a higher incidence of complications (SHR = 1.85; 95% CI: 1.131–3.023, p = 0.0143).

4. Discussion

Osteoporosis is a common skeletal disorder and is associated with osteoporotic fractures, which lead to a considerable rise in the likelihood of morbidity and mortality as well as increased health care costs. Osteoporosis treatment can increase bone strength and decrease fracture risk. One of the drugs most commonly used to treat osteoporosis is bisphosphonate [19], especially alendronate due to its cost effectiveness and support from well-established evidence. Denosumab was popular, but it can cause rebound osteoporosis and increased risk of spine fracture after discontinuation, which has led to a decrease in use [20]. Therefore, recent studies have proposed a re-evaluation of bisphosphonate use. The most appropriate timing of bisphosphonate initiation remains debatable. Our data indicated that early initiation of oral alendronate was associated with lower incidence of second FF, second FF surgery, and adverse events than late initiation.

Several randomized clinical trials have investigated the effects of the early postoperative use of bisphosphonates (<3 months) on FFs. Eriksen et al. suggested bisphosphonate initiation (zoledronic acid) 2–12 weeks after surgery to decrease the incidence of clinical vertebral fracture, nonvertebral hip fracture, and mortality [21]. Lyles et al. found similar results when zoledronic acid was initiated within 90 days of hip fracture surgery [22]. Uchiyama et al. stated that early administration of alendronate did not delay fracture healing and decreased bone turnover [23]. A meta-analysis conducted by Li et al. included 253 individuals from four randomized clinical trials (RCTs) with measurements of healing time and 2365 participants from six RCTs with measurements of delayed or nonunion rates of fracture healing. The meta-analysis thus included 10 studies with 2888 patients. Four of the trials used alendronate, three used zoledronic, two used risedronate, and one used etidronate. No significant difference was observed in radiological fracture healing time between the bisphosphonate therapy group and control group (mean difference = 0.47, 95% CI: −2.75 to 3.69). In previous studies, early bisphosphonate administration resulted in higher bone mineral density (BMD). HORIZON recurrent fracture trials revealed that patients receiving bisphosphonate 6 weeks to 3 months after hip fracture had higher total hip and femoral neck BMD at 12 months than those receiving a bisphosphonate before 6 weeks [21]. This may be because bisphosphonates do not directly affect cells involved in the inflammatory phase (i.e., osteoblasts) or the formation of soft and hard callus; instead, bisphosphonates interrupt the remodeling of hard callus. Consequently, bisphosphonate initiation within 3 months after surgical treatment of FFs may be more effective timing for preventing second FFs and second FF surgeries.

Our cohort had lower incidence of respiratory failure, UGI bleeding, renal failure, and other complications. This may have been due to the faster bone integration or stabilization of implants, allowing early ambulation and preventing respiratory failure due to aspiration pneumonia.

Alendronate use has been demonstrated to decrease the risk of cardiovascular events. Sing et al. observed significantly lower risk of 1-year cardiovascular mortality (SHR 0.33; 95% CI: 0.17–0.65) and incident myocardial infarction (SHR 0.55; 95% CI: 0.34–0.89) following hip fracture [24]. This is due to nitrogen-containing bisphosphonates targeting the mevalonate pathway, specifically farnesyl pyrophosphate synthase, which has the same pathway as statins [25]. Alishiri et al. concluded that in patients with aortic stenosis and concurrent osteoporosis, alendronate treatment retarded stenosis progression and improved the outcome [26].

The lower risk of UGI bleeding may be related to the indication of bisphosphonate. Therefore, physicians should be cautious about using ulcer-inducing agents in patients with EIBP. Alendronate causes oxidative gastric damage by increasing myeloperoxidase activity and lipid peroxidation, which cause the formation of gastric ulcers and impair gastric ulcer healing [27]. In a population-based study, Peng et al. concluded that alendronate was a risk factor for UGI bleeding (SHR = 1.32; 95% CI: 1.02–1.71) [28]. This was inconsistent with our results, likely because EIBP may exacerbate certain symptoms in patients and is therefore usually avoided.

Bisphosphonate is contraindicated in patients with renal insufficiency because of the risk of renal function deterioration [29]. In our cohort, the risk of renal failure was lower in the EIBP group likely due to the avoidance of other medications causing renal toxicity due to shorter hospital stay. Moreover, improvement of function leads to lower nonsteroidal anti-inflammatory drug use, which may be another explanation for the finding.

Patients with EIBP have earlier physician attention and therefore have more awareness of their general condition because of programs such as the fracture liaison service (FLS). The FLS has improved the quality of care in patients with fracture and helped prevent secondary fractures [30]. This may be another reason for the fewer complications in the EIBP group. In a nationwide cohort study, Wang et al. reported that early initiation (15–84 days) of antiosteoporosis medicine reduced the risk of fracture-related hospitalization [31]. These findings also indicate the importance of the FLS in identifying patients suitable for ELBP.

The strengths of this study include the completeness of patient follow-up and high accuracy of coding in the national health database [32]. The study had some limitations. First, the NHI claims database lacks information on the Fracture Risk Assessment Tool score, BMD, smoking, compliance, vitamin D deficiency, and bone turnover markers. Second, we included only patients who received first-time alendronate. Third, we could not differentiate the causes of fractures, which may also have included atypical fractures. The incidence of atypical femoral fractures was found to be between 0.3 and 85.9 per 100,000 person-years [33,34]. Short- or long-term alendronate use is not significantly associated with higher risk of atypical femoral fractures [35]. Therefore, the low frequency of atypical fractures probably did not affect the study outcomes. Finally, we could only evaluate the associations of early and late bisphosphonate use with adverse events and could not follow up on the intergroup difference in perioperative complications that would have been attributable to bisphosphonate initiation. Prospective studies should be conducted to analyze this.

5. Conclusions

Bisphosphonate initiation within 3 months of FF surgery is associated with lower incidence of second FF, second fracture surgery, and adverse events and should therefore be considered over late initiation in these patients.

Author Contributions: Conceptualization: M.-H.W., Y.-S.L., C.W., C.-Y.L., Y.-C.C., T.-J.H. and J.-S.C. Interpretation of the results: M.-H.W., Y.-S.L., C.W., C.-Y.L., Y.-C.C., T.-J.H. and J.-S.C. Formal analysis: Y.-C.C. and J.-S.C. Writing—draft preparation: M.-H.W. and C.W. Writing—review and editing: M.-H.W., Y.-S.L., C.W., C.-Y.L., Y.-C.C., T.-J.H. and J.-S.C. All authors have read and agreed to the published version of the manuscript.

Funding: This research was funded by Research Services Center For Health Information, Chang Gung University, Taoyuan, Taiwan (J.-S.C. and Y.-S.L., CIRPD1D0031).

Institutional Review Board Statement: The study was approved by the Institutional Review Board of Chang Gung Memorial Hospital of Taiwan (104-3677B) and conducted in accordance with the Declaration of Helsinki.

Informed Consent Statement: The Institutional Review Board waived the requirement to obtain informed consent.

Data Availability Statement: The data presented in this study are available on request from the corresponding author.

Acknowledgments: The authors wish to thank Meng-Ling Tsai for assistance in the preparation of related documents. This manuscript was edited by Hannah Fox and Sudeep Agarwal.

Conflicts of Interest: The authors declare no conflict of interest.

References

1. Tsoumpra, M.K.; Muniz, J.R.; Barnett, B.L.; Kwaasi, A.A.; Pilka, E.S.; Kavanagh, K.L.; Evdokimov, A.; Walter, R.L.; Von Delft, F.; Ebetino, F.H.; et al. The inhibition of human farnesyl pyrophosphate synthase by nitrogen-containing bisphosphonates. Elucidating the role of active site threonine 201 and tyrosine 204 residues using enzyme mutants. *Bone* **2015**, *81*, 478–486. [CrossRef]

2. Cao, Y.; Mori, S.; Mashiba, T.; Westmore, M.S.; Ma, L.; Sato, M.; Akiyama, T.; Shi, L.; Komatsubara, S.; Miyamoto, K.; et al. Raloxifene, estrogen, and alendronate affect the processes of fracture repair differently in ovariectomized rats. *J. Bone Miner. Res.* **2002**, *17*, 2237–2246. [CrossRef] [PubMed]
3. Odvina, C.V.; Zerwekh, J.E.; Rao, D.S.; Maalouf, N.; Gottschalk, F.A.; Pak, C.Y. Severely suppressed bone turnover: A potential complication of alendronate therapy. *J. Clin. Endocrinol. Metab.* **2005**, *90*, 1294–1301. [CrossRef]
4. Bauss, F.; Schenk, R.K.; Hort, S.; Muller-Beckmann, B.; Sponer, G. New model for simulation of fracture repair in full-grown beagle dogs: Model characterization and results from a long-term study with ibandronate. *J. Pharmacol. Toxicol. Methods* **2004**, *50*, 25–34. [CrossRef] [PubMed]
5. Munns, C.F.; Rauch, F.; Zeitlin, L.; Fassier, F.; Glorieux, F.H. Delayed osteotomy but not fracture healing in pediatric osteogenesis imperfecta patients receiving pamidronate. *J. Bone Miner. Res.* **2004**, *19*, 1779–1786. [CrossRef] [PubMed]
6. Matos, M.A.; Tannuri, U.; Guarniero, R. The effect of zoledronate during bone healing. *J. Orthop. Traumatol.* **2010**, *11*, 7–12. [CrossRef]
7. Li, J.; Mori, S.; Kaji, Y.; Mashiba, T.; Kawanishi, J.; Norimatsu, H. Effect of bisphosphonate (incadronate) on fracture healing of long bones in rats. *J. Bone Miner. Res.* **1999**, *14*, 969–979. [CrossRef]
8. Li, C.; Mori, S.; Li, J.; Kaji, Y.; Akiyama, T.; Kawanishi, J.; Norimatsu, H. Long-term effect of incadronate disodium (YM-175) on fracture healing of femoral shaft in growing rats. *J. Bone Miner. Res.* **2001**, *16*, 429–436. [CrossRef]
9. Greiner, S.H.; Wildemann, B.; Back, D.A.; Alidoust, M.; Schwabe, P.; Haas, N.P.; Schmidmaier, G. Local application of zoledronic acid incorporated in a poly(D,L-lactide)-coated implant accelerates fracture healing in rats. *Acta Orthop.* **2008**, *79*, 717–725. [CrossRef]
10. Rozental, T.D.; Vazquez, M.A.; Chacko, A.T.; Ayogu, N.; Bouxsein, M.L. Comparison of radiographic fracture healing in the distal radius for patients on and off bisphosphonate therapy. *J. Hand Surg. Am.* **2009**, *34*, 595–602. [CrossRef]
11. Amanat, N.; Brown, R.; Bilston, L.E.; Little, D.G. A single systemic dose of pamidronate improves bone mineral content and accelerates restoration of strength in a rat model of fracture repair. *J. Orthop. Res.* **2005**, *23*, 1029–1034. [CrossRef]
12. Little, D.G.; McDonald, M.; Bransford, R.; Godfrey, C.B.; Amanat, N. Manipulation of the anabolic and catabolic responses with OP-1 and zoledronic acid in a rat critical defect model. *J. Bone Miner. Res.* **2005**, *20*, 2044–2052. [CrossRef]
13. Bransford, R.; Goergens, E.; Briody, J.; Amanat, N.; Cree, A.; Little, D. Effect of zoledronic acid in an L6-L7 rabbit spine fusion model. *Eur. Spine J.* **2007**, *16*, 557–562. [CrossRef]
14. Li, C.; Wang, H.R.; Li, X.L.; Zhou, X.G.; Dong, J. The relation between zoledronic acid infusion and interbody fusion in patients undergoing transforaminal lumbar interbody fusion surgery. *Acta Neurochir.* **2012**, *154*, 731–738. [CrossRef]
15. Kim, T.Y.; Ha, Y.C.; Kang, B.J.; Lee, Y.K.; Koo, K.H. Does early administration of bisphosphonate affect fracture healing in patients with intertrochanteric fractures? *J. Bone Jt. Surg. Br.* **2012**, *94*, 956–960. [CrossRef]
16. Gong, H.S.; Song, C.H.; Lee, Y.H.; Rhee, S.H.; Lee, H.J.; Baek, G.H. Early initiation of bisphosphonate does not affect healing and outcomes of volar plate fixation of osteoporotic distal radial fractures. *J. Bone Jt. Surg. Am.* **2012**, *94*, 1729–1736. [CrossRef]
17. Gray, R. A class of k-sample tests for comparing the cumulative incidence of a competing risk. *Ann. Stat.* **1998**, *1998*, 1141–1154. [CrossRef]
18. Fine, J.P.; Gray, R.J. A proportional hazards model for the subdistribution of a competing risk. *J. Am. Stat. Assoc.* **1999**, *94*, 496–509. [CrossRef]
19. Lewiecki, E.M. Bisphosphonates for the treatment of osteoporosis: Insights for clinicians. *Ther. Adv. Chronic. Dis.* **2010**, *1*, 115–128. [CrossRef] [PubMed]
20. Anastasilakis, A.D.; Polyzos, S.A.; Makras, P.; Aubry-Rozier, B.; Kaouri, S.; Lamy, O. Clinical Features of 24 Patients With Rebound-Associated Vertebral Fractures After Denosumab Discontinuation: Systematic Review and Additional Cases. *J. Bone Miner. Res.* **2017**, *32*, 1291–1296. [CrossRef] [PubMed]
21. Eriksen, E.F.; Lyles, K.W.; Colón-Emeric, C.S.; Pieper, C.F.; Magaziner, J.S.; Adachi, J.D.; Hyldstrup, L.; Recknor, C.; Nordsletten, L.; Lavecchia, C.; et al. Antifracture efficacy and reduction of mortality in relation to timing of the first dose of zoledronic acid after hip fracture. *J. Bone Miner. Res.* **2009**, *24*, 1308–1313. [CrossRef]
22. Lyles, K.W.; Colón-Emeric, C.S.; Magaziner, J.S.; Adachi, J.D.; Pieper, C.F.; Mautalen, C.; Hyldstrup, L.; Recknor, C.; Nordsletten, L.; Moore, K.A.; et al. Zoledronic acid and clinical fractures and mortality after hip fracture. *N. Engl. J. Med.* **2007**, *357*, 1799–1809. [CrossRef] [PubMed]
23. Uchiyama, S.; Itsubo, T.; Nakamura, K.; Fujinaga, Y.; Sato, N.; Imaeda, T.; Kadoya, M.; Kato, H. Effect of early administration of alendronate after surgery for distal radial fragility fracture on radiological fracture healing time. *Bone Jt. J.* **2013**, *95*, 1544–1550. [CrossRef]
24. Sing, C.-W.; Wong, A.Y.; Kiel, D.P.; Cheung, E.Y.; Lam, J.K.; Cheung, T.T.; Chan, E.W.; Kung, A.W.; Wong, I.C.; Cheung, C.-L. Association of Alendronate and Risk of Cardiovascular Events in Patients with Hip Fracture. *J. Bone Miner. Res.* **2018**, *33*, 1422–1434. [CrossRef]
25. Guney, E.; Kisakol, G.; Ozgen, A.G.; Yilmaz, C.; Kabalak, T. Effects of bisphosphonates on lipid metabolism. *Neuroendocrinol. Lett.* **2008**, *29*, 252–255.
26. Alishiri, G.; Heshmat-Ghahdarijani, K.; Hashemi, M.; Zavar, R.; Farahani, M.M. Alendronate slows down aortic stenosis progression in osteoporotic patients: An observational prospective study. *J. Res. Med. Sci.* **2020**, *25*, 65. [CrossRef]

27. Takeuchi, K.; Kato, S.; Amagase, K. Gastric ulcerogenic and healing impairment actions of alendronate, a nitrogen-containing bisphosphonate—Prophylactic effects of rebamipide. *Curr. Pharm. Des.* **2011**, *17*, 1602–1611. [CrossRef]
28. Peng, Y.L.; Hu, H.Y.; Luo, J.C.; Hou, M.C.; Lin, H.C.; Lee, F.Y. Alendronate, a bisphosphonate, increased upper and lower gastrointestinal bleeding: Risk factor analysis from a nationwide population-based study. *Osteoporos. Int.* **2014**, *25*, 1617–1623. [CrossRef]
29. Miller, P.D.; Jamal, S.A.; Evenepoel, P.; Eastell, R.; Boonen, S. Renal safety in patients treated with bisphosphonates for osteoporosis: A review. *J. Bone Miner. Res.* **2013**, *28*, 2049–2059. [CrossRef] [PubMed]
30. Chang, L.-Y.; Tsai, K.-S.; Peng, J.-K.; Chen, C.-H.; Lin, G.-T.; Lin, C.-H.; Tu, S.-T.; Mao, I.-C.; Gau, Y.-L.; Liu, H.-C.; et al. The development of Taiwan Fracture Liaison Service network. *Osteoporos. Sarcopenia* **2018**, *4*, 47–52. [CrossRef]
31. Wang, C.Y.; Fu, S.H.; Yang, R.S.; Chen, L.K.; Shen, L.J.; Hsiao, F.Y. Timing of anti-osteoporosis medications initiation after a hip fracture affects the risk of subsequent fracture: A nationwide cohort study. *Bone* **2020**, *138*, 115452. [CrossRef] [PubMed]
32. Lu, T.-H.; Lee, M.-C.; Chou, M.-C. Accuracy of cause-of-death coding in Taiwan: Types of miscoding and effects on mortality statistics. *Int. J. Epidemiol.* **2000**, *29*, 336–343. [CrossRef] [PubMed]
33. Saita, Y.; Ishijima, M.; Mogami, A.; Kubota, M.; Baba, T.; Kaketa, T.; Nagao, M.; Sakamoto, Y.; Sakai, K.; Homma, Y.; et al. The incidence of and risk factors for developing atypical femoral fractures in Japan. *J. Bone Miner. Metab.* **2015**, *33*, 311–318. [CrossRef]
34. Lee, Y.K.; Ahn, S.; Kim, K.M.; Suh, C.S.; Koo, K.H. Incidence Rate of Atypical Femoral Fracture after Bisphosphonates Treatment in Korea. *J. Korean Med. Sci.* **2018**, *33*, e38. [CrossRef] [PubMed]
35. Hsiao, F.-Y.; Huang, W.-F.; Chen, Y.-M.; Wen, Y.-W.; Kao, Y.-H.; Chen, L.-K.; Tsai, Y.-W. Hip and subtrochanteric or diaphyseal femoral fractures in alendronate users: A 10-year, nationwide retrospective cohort study in Taiwanese women. *Clin. Ther.* **2011**, *33*, 1659–1667. [CrossRef]

Article

TRAP5b and RANKL/OPG Predict Bone Pathology in Patients with Gaucher Disease

Margarita Ivanova *, Julia Dao, Lauren Noll, Jacqueline Fikry and Ozlem Goker-Alpan *

Lysosomal & Rare Disorders Research and Treatment Center, Fairfax, VA 22030, USA; jdaol@ldrtc.org (J.D.); lnoll@ldrtc.org (L.N.); jfikry@ldrtc.org (J.F.)
* Correspondence: mivanova@ldrtc.org (M.I.); ogoker-alpan@ldrtc.org (O.G.-A.)

Abstract: Background and objective: Bone involvement occurs in 75% of patients with Gaucher disease (GD), and comprises structural changes, debilitating pain, and bone density abnormalities. Osteoporosis is a silent manifestation of GD until a pathologic fracture occurs. Thus, early diagnosis is crucial for identifying high-risk patients in order to prevent irreversible complications. Methods: Thirty-three patients with GD were assessed prospectively to identify predictive markers associated with bone density abnormalities, osteopenia (OSN), and osteoporosis (OSR). Subjects were categorized into three cohorts based on T- or Z-scores of bone mineral density (BMD). The first GD cohort consisted of those with no bone complications (Z-score ≥ -0.9; T-scores ≥ -1), the second was the OSN group ($-1.8 \geq$ Z-score ≥ -1; $-2.5 \geq$ T-score ≥ -1), and the third was the OSR group (Z-score ≤ -1.9; T-scores ≤ -2.5). Serum levels of TRAP5b, RANKL, OPG, and RANK were quantified by enzyme-linked immunosorbent assays. Results: TRAP5b levels were increased in GD patients, and showed a positive correlation with GD biomarkers, including plasma glucosylsphingosine (lyso-Gb1) and macrophage activation markers CCL18 and chitotriosidase. The highest level of TRAP5b was measured in patients with osteoporosis. The elevation of RANKL and RANKL/OPG ratio correlated with osteopenia in GD. Conclusion: TRAP5b, RANKL, and RANKL/OPG elevation indicate osteoclast activation in GD. TRAP5b is a potential bone biomarker for GD with the ability to predict the progression of bone density abnormalities.

Keywords: Gaucher disease; osteoporosis; TRAP5b; OPG; RANKL; biomarker; lyso-Gb1; bone

1. Introduction

Gaucher disease (GD), the most common lysosomal storage disorder, is caused by a deficiency of the enzyme glucocerebrosidase (GCase) and the progressive accumulation of its substrate, glycosylceramide (GC), in various tissues and organs of the reticuloendothelial system [1]. GD affects monocyte lineage cells, primarily the macrophages, which play an essential role in bone metabolism, osteoclast differentiation, osteoclasts-osteoblasts interactions, and bone remodeling. Bone involvement in GD ranges from osteonecrosis to reduced bone density and developmental and structural bone abnormalities.

The progressive bone disease occurs in 75% of patients with type 1 GD, and signs and symptoms include structural bone changes, debilitating bone pain, and osteoporosis [2]. In addition to the extensive inflammatory response against GC and its toxic metabolite glucosylsphingosine (lyso-Gb1), GD bone pathology is possibly the result of the alterations in osteoclast function and osteoblast participation in bone remodeling and osteoclast differentiation [3]. Moreover, local GC accumulation affects osteoclast-osteoblast communication and mediates bone abnormalities [4–6].

Reduced bone density leads to progressive osteopenia and osteoporosis, and the aberrations in bone structure lead to abnormal vertebral remodeling and bone modeling, including Erlenmeyer flask deformity. Other bone structural abnormalities in GD include osteonecrosis and lytic lesions [3,7].

Tartrate-resistant acid phosphatase (TRAP) is an enzyme coded by *ACP5*, and is expressed in osteoclasts, macrophages, and dendritic cells. Two isoforms of TRAP circulate in the blood, TRAP5a secreted from macrophages and dendritic cells, and TRAP5b from osteoclasts. TRAP5b is a marker of osteoclast activity and indicators of bone resorption [8]. Moreover, the activator of TRAP5b expression, cathepsin K, is highly expressed in osteoclasts and has been shown to participate in bone resorption in GD [9]. Although elevated TRAP5b has previously been reported in GD, the limited number of patients included in this study prevented any further conclusions about its significance from being reached [10].

Among the essential factors that regulate bone turnover are the receptor activator of NF-kB (RANK), its ligand (RANKL), and osteoprotegerin (OPG), the receptor that binds to RANKL [9,11,12]. The cellular response to RANKL is contingent on the level of its receptor RANK and the presence of OPG [11]. RANKL and OPG are primarily involved in maintaining bone density. Given that bone is an organ with a slow turnover, and that bone mineral density (BMD) measurement in the short term does not provide enough information about prognosis, biomarkers will be valuable for the early assessment of bone density abnormalities.

2. Materials and Methods

2.1. Subjects

The study was conducted under an IRB approved protocol (NCT04055831) and included 33 subjects with GD (eight males and 25 females, age range 18 to 68 years, mean 41 ± 15) and 15 healthy controls (nine males and six females with an average age of 48 ± 11 years) (Supplemental Table S1). Ethics committees and data protection agencies approved the clinical protocol, and all subjects provided written informed consent for the collection of samples and analysis of their data. GD diagnosis was based on GCase residual activity and *GBA* molecular analysis. Participants were further categorized into three cohorts based on the T- or Z-score of BMD. The cohort designated 'normal' (N) included nine subjects without any bone complications and a normal BMD with a Z-score ≥ -0.9 or T-score ≥ -1. The osteopenia (OSN) group included 10 subjects with a Z score of -1 to -1.8 or a T-score of -1 to -2.5. The osteoporosis (OSR) group included 14 subjects with a Z score ≤ -1.9 or a T-score ≤ -2.5 (Table 1 and Supplemental Table S1).

Table 1. The clinical features of bone disease in GD (Gaucher disease) cohorts: no bone complications (N), osteopenia (OSN), and osteoporosis (OSR).

	N	OSN	OSR
T-score (average ± STDEV)	0.03 ± 0.2	-1.07 ± 0.2	-2.96 ± 0.8
Z-score (average ± STDEV)	-0.2	-1.6	-2.73 ± 0.4
Bone pain	4/9 (44%)	4/10 (40%)	10/14 (71%)
Bone surgery	0/9 (0%)	1/10 (10%)	6/14 (42%)
Pathologic fractures	0/9 (0%)	2/10 (20%)	3/14 (21%)
Bone marrow infiltration	7/9 (77%)	7/10 (67%)	8/14 (57%)
EM-flask deformity	5/9 (55%)	3/10 (30%)	8/14 (57%)
Cystic changes	0/9 (0%)	0/10 (0%)	1/14 (7%)
Osteonecrosis	3/9 (33%)	1/10 (10%)	4/14 (28%)

2.2. The Clinical Features of Bone Disease in GD Cohorts

Details of medical history with bone disease characteristics such as bone surgery, pathologic fractures, bone pain, bone marrow infiltration, EM-flask deformity, and osteonecrosis are listed in Table 1 and Supplemental Table S1. Demographic characteristics, genotypes, and relevant molecular analyses are summarized in Supplemental Tables S2 and S3.

2.3. Measurement of Biomarkers in Plasma Samples

Blood samples were collected in EDTA tubes. Plasma levels of bone markers were measured using commercially available ELISA kits. The concentration of TRAP5b was measured in 50 μL of plasma using TRAP5b ELISA kit (Quidel, San Diego, CA, USA). Recombinant TRAP5b was used for calibration, and the range of the assay was 0–16.5 U/L. The concentration of OPG and RANKL was measured in 100 μL of plasma using OPG and RANKL ELISA kits (Origene Technologies Inc., Rockville, MD, USA). Recombinant OPG was used as a standard, and the range of the assay was 0–6000 pg/mL. The RANKL range of the assay was 0–5000 pg/mL. The RANK concentration was measured in 100 μL of plasma using the RANK ELISA kit (Thermo Fisher Scientific, Waltham, MA, USA). Recombinant RANK was used as a standard, the range of the assay was 0–10 ng/mL, and the analytical sensitivity was 0.054 ng/mL.

2.4. Statistical Analysis

Statistical analysis was performed using Graph Prizm (GraphPad, San Diego, CA, USA). Differences between the two groups were tested by Student's *t*-test or F-test. The groups were compared using one-way analysis of variance (ANOVA), followed by Brown-Forsythe, Bartlett's multiple-comparison, and Kruskal-Wallis tests. Pearson's test, one or two tails, was used for correlation analysis. The value of $p < 0.05$ indicated a statistically significant result.

3. Results

3.1. Bone Pain Is Associated with Osteopenia and Osteoporosis in GD

Overall and individual characteristics of bone involvement in subjects with GD are given in Table 1 and Supplemental Table S1. Bone pain was more common in the OSR group (71%) compared to the N (44%) and OSN groups (40%) (Table 1). Increased frequency of pathological bone fractures and bone surgeries correlated with the progression of OSN and OSR (Table 1). However, the incidence of bone marrow infiltration, EM-flask deformity, and osteonecrosis were not associated with abnormal bone density, or with OSN or OSR pathology (Table 1).

3.2. TRAP5b Is Increased in GD and Correlates with Osteoporosis

TRAP5b is a marker of the number of active osteoclasts and an indicator of bone resorption. To examine the role of TRAP5b in GD, the peripheral levels of TRAP5b were measured. TRAP5b was significantly higher in the GD group than in the healthy controls (Figure 1A). Further analysis demonstrated that TRAP5b correlated with the progression of osteopenia towards osteoporosis (Figure 1B). TRAP5b was significantly higher in the OSR than in the OSN and N cohorts.

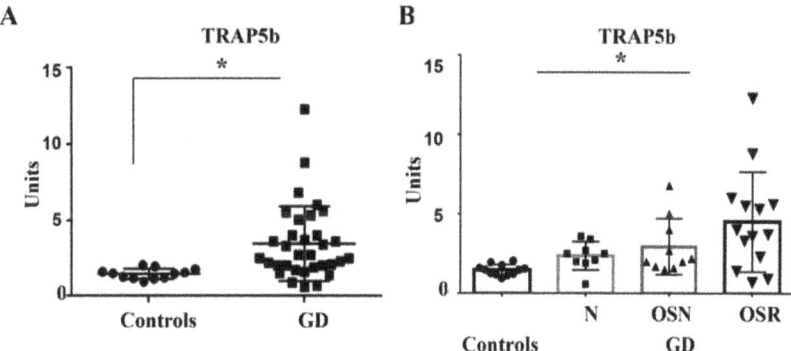

Figure 1. Plasma TRAP5b level. (**A**) TRAP5b level, GD (Gaucher disease) mean 3.4 ± 0.4, $n = 33$ vs. control mean 1.4 ± 0.1, $n = 10$, $p < 0.05$ unpaired *t*-test and F test. (**B**) TRAP5b concentrations in control and GD cohorts. GD and no bone complication (N, mean 2.6 ± 0.63), osteopenia (OSN, mean 3.1 ± 1.8), and osteoporosis (OSR, mean 4.2 ± 2.2). * $p < 0.05$; ANOVA, Brown-Forsythe, and Bartlett's multiple-comparison test. Data are means ± SEM. Measurements are in units/50 μL.

Furthermore, the finding that TRAP5b is elevated in GD patients remained unchanged after stratifying by gender (Supplemental Figure S1A). eight out of ten GD women and three out of four GD men with osteoporosis showed elevated levels of TRAP5b. (Supplemental Figure S1A). Taken together, these data indicate that plasma TRAP5b may be a clinically relevant marker for the evaluation of bone resorption in GD patients. There was no correlation between TRAP5b levels for different treatment modalities, enzyme replacement therapy (ERT), substrate reduction therapy (SRT), or treatment duration.

3.3. RANKL, Not RANK Is Elevated in GD and Correlates with Osteopenia

RANKL is highly expressed by osteoblasts and osteocytes. RANKL binds to its receptor (RANK) and activates osteoclasts' differentiation and maturation, favoring bone resorption [11,13]. Analysis of control plasma and plasma from GD subjects demonstrated that the level of RANKL was significantly higher in GD (Figure 2A). Comparing RANKL in controls and GD cohorts showed a significant increase in RANKL level in the OSN cohort compared with the N and OSR cohorts (Figure 2B). RANKL level was elevated in GD females with OSN (5/8) and in two women (2/10) with OSR (Supplemental Figure S1B). Three males with GD presented with the highest level of RANKL, one patient without bone complications and two patients with OSN. Five subjects with osteoporosis were treated with denosumab, a human monoclonal antibody against the RANK ligand. RANKL level was elevated in one of five patients treated with denosumab (Supplemental Figure S1B). Correlation between type or duration of Gaucher disease specific treatment and RANKL was not observed. Overall, these results show that plasma RANKL is a potential marker for OSN in GD.

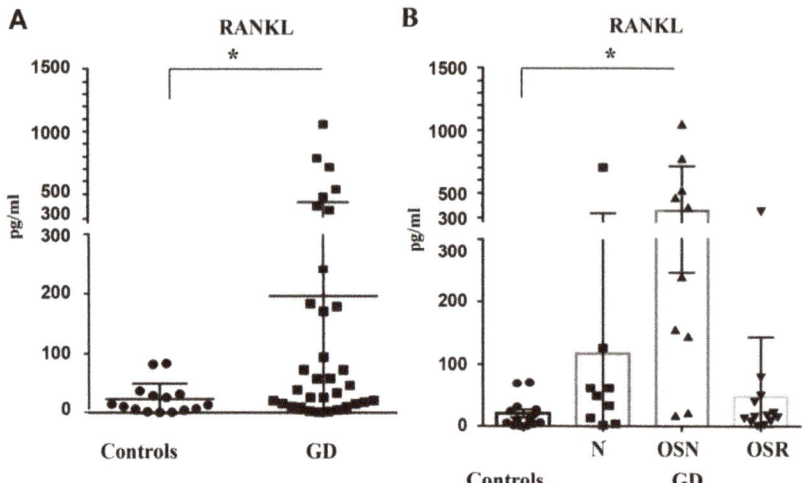

Figure 2. Plasma RANKL level. (A) RANKL levels, control vs. GD. Statistical analysis using unpaired t-test and F test to compare variance demonstrated a significant difference between control (mean 20 ± 5.8, $n = 15$) and GD cohorts (mean 166 ± 67.9, $n = 33$). * $p < 0.05$. (B) RANKL concentrations in control subjects and GD with no bone complication (N, mean 117 ± 74), osteopenia (OSN, mean 362 ± 118), and osteoporosis (OSR, mean 49 ± 26). * $p < 0.05$ ANOVA test, Tukey's multiple comparisons test control vs. OSN and control vs. OSR.

RANKL binds to the receptor activator of NF-kB (RANK) to induce osteoclastogenesis [11]. RANK is mainly expressed in osteoclast precursors, mature osteoclasts, dendritic cells, macrophages, and microglia. Surprisingly, despite being a membrane receptor, RANK was detectable in the serum of GD subjects. However, the measurement of plasma RANK showed no differences between the controls and GD patients (Figure 3A). Further analysis in three different GD cohorts did not show an association between RANK and the progression of bone density abnormalities (Figure 3B).

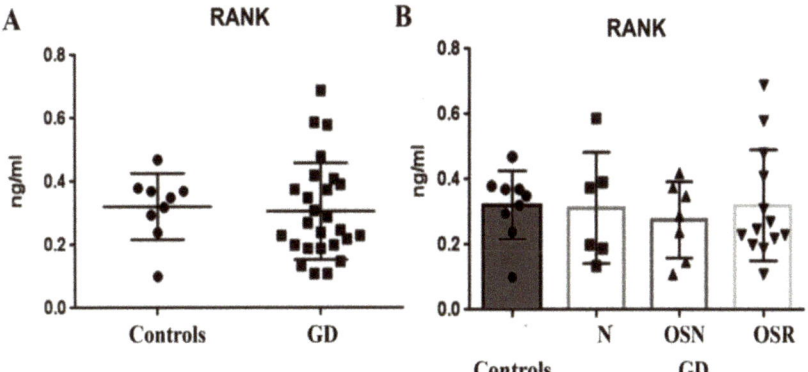

Figure 3. Circulating RANK levels in patients with GD. (**A**) RANK levels, control vs. GD group (mean 0.30 ± 0.02, $n = 30$). (**B**) RANK concentrations in control (mean 0.32 ± 0.03, $n = 10$) and GD groups N, OSN, and OSR. Data are means ± SEM. Measurements are in ng/mL.

3.4. Elevated OPG Does Not Correlate with OSN or OSR in GD

The decoy receptor for RANKL (OPG) is produced by osteoblasts. OPG binds RANKL and blocks RANKL activation, reducing the number of osteoclasts [14]. Plasma OPG was elevated in 15 out of 33 (46%) GD patients, and the average of OPG in GD was higher compared with healthy controls (Figure 4A). Further analysis, however, demonstrated that OPG did not correlate with osteopenia or osteoporosis (Figure 4B). The majority of patients with the highest level of OPG belonged to two cohorts: no bone complication (5 out of 8 patients) or OSN (5 out of 9 patients). After stratification for gender and treatment, there was no difference in OPG levels. (Supplemental Figure S1C).

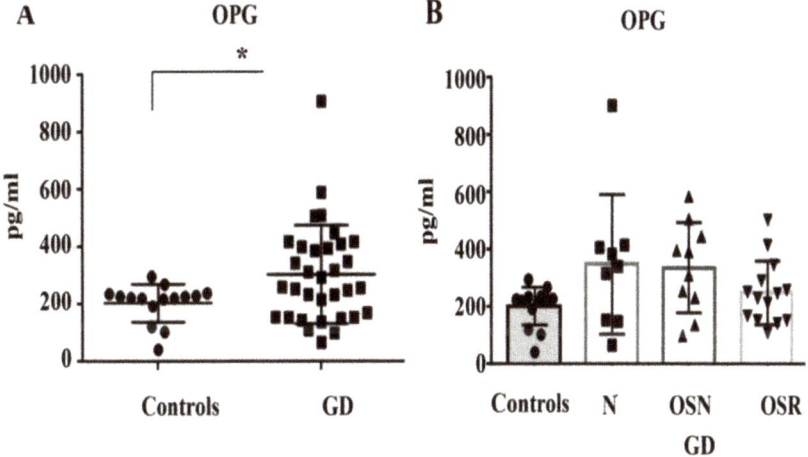

Figure 4. Plasma OPG (osteoprotegerin) concentrations. (**A**) OPG level, control (mean 206 ± 17, $n = 10$) vs. GD (mean 307 ± 30, $n = 33$). * $p < 0.05$ unpaired t test and F test. (**B**) OPG concentrations in control subjects and GD with no bone complication (N), osteopenia (OSN), and osteoporosis (OSR).

3.5. RANKL/OPG Ratio Is Higher in Patients with GD

Alterations of the RANKL/OPG balance have been characterized in a wide range of bone diseases, including osteoporosis [13]. Therefore, in addition to RANKL and OPG analysis, we calculated the RANKL/OPG ratio. Similar to RANKL and OPG, the RANKL/OPG ratio was higher in GD compared to controls (Figure 5A). Further analysis showed an increased RANKL/OPG ratio in the OSN cohort. Tukey's multiple-comparison test demonstrated significant differences between control vs. OSN groups (Figure 5B). The observation that RANKL/OPG ratio is higher in GD patients, especially in patients with osteopenia, remained the same for males and females (Supplemental Figure S1D).

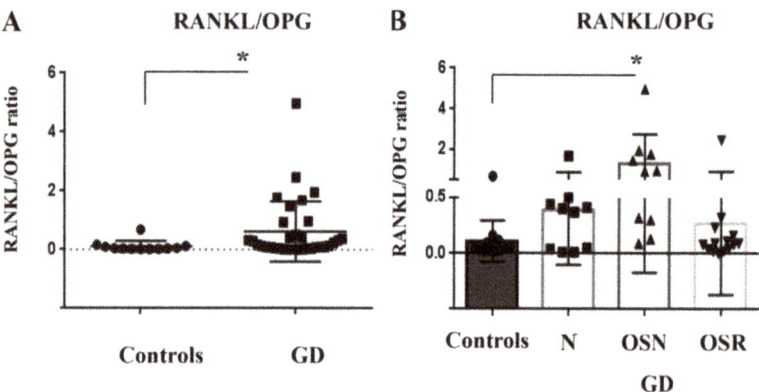

Figure 5. RANKL/OPG ratio. (**A**) Comparing RANKL/OPG ratio in control (mean 0.10 ± 0.06, $n = 10$) vs. GD cohorts (mean 0.60 ± 0.17, $n = 33$). F test significant $p < 0.05$ (**B**) RANKL/OPG ratio in control group (mean 0.11 ± 0.08, $n = 10$); GD-N (mean 0.39 ± 0.17, $n = 9$); GD-OSN (mean 1.3 ± 0.46, $n = 10$); and GD-OSR (mean 0.27 ± 0.170, $n = 14$) groups. Data are means $\pm$ SEM. ANOVA test, Bartlett's multiple-comparisons, and Kruskal–Wallis tests (* $p < 0.05$) showed significant differences between groups. Tukey's multiple-comparison test demonstrated significant differences between control vs. OSN groups.

3.6. The Relationship between TRAP5b, RANKL, and OPG in GD

Correlation analysis of RANKL/OPG/TRAP5b levels in GD patients with no bone complications (N) showed an increased level of TRAP5b and OPG, but not RANKL. From the GD-N cohort, only one patient had an elevated level of RANKL; however, this patient had a high level of OPG and a TRAP5b level comparable to the average control level (Figure 6A,B and Supplemental Figure S2).

Scatterplot analysis of the relationship between RANKL and OPG demonstrated that some samples from the OSN cohort with higher RANKL also showed increased OPG levels (Figure 6A and Supplemental Figure S2). Since RANKL promotes osteoclastogenesis, the elevated level of serum RANKL and the decreased level of OPG indicate accelerating osteoclast activation, resulting in osteoporosis progression. Scatterplot TRAP5b vs. RANKL demonstrates that TRAP5b is higher in the OSN cohort with an elevated RANKL and normal OPG (Figure 6B,C and Supplemental Figure S2). Thus, these data suggest that an increased level of OPG inhibits osteoclast activity in GD patients with osteopenia.

In the GD cohort with OSR, the RANKL and OPG levels were similar to control and GD-N cohorts, except for one patient with a high RANKL and three patients with high OPG only (Figure 6B and Supplemental Figure S2). There was no direct correlation between TRAP5b and RANKL or OPG levels in GD-OSR (Figure 6C,D). Because osteoclast activity is significantly greater than osteoblast activity in osteoporotic tissue [15], the significantly increased level of TRAP5b, but not RANKL or OPG, might be associated with a shift to osteoporosis in GD.

Among the five patients treated with denosumab, two (P6 and P10) had normal RANKL, OPG, and TRAP5b levels (Figure 6B–D). Three (P5, P7, P8), meanwhile, had an elevated TRAP5b, and two patients had increased OPG.

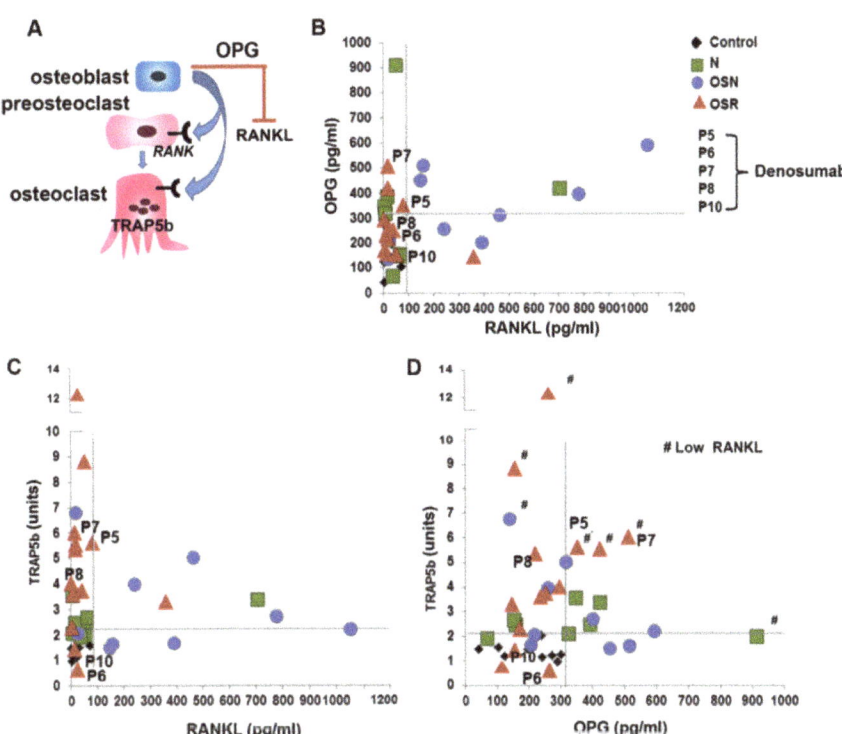

Figure 6. TRAP5b, RANKL, and OPG correlation in GD. (**A**) The RANKL-OPG-RANK pathway activates bone resorption and osteoclast differentiation. Osteoblasts express RANKL and OPG. Preosteoclasts express RANK, which is activated by RANKL. OPG neutralizes RANKL. TRAP5b, expressed by osteoclasts, is a marker of osteoclast activity. (**B–D**) Scatterplot analysis of correlation of OPG and RANKL (**B**), TRAP5n and RANKL (**C**), and TRAP5b and OPG (**D**). P5, P6, P7, P8, and P10 represent patients treated with denosumab. Healthy control (black diamond). GD cohorts: N (green), OSN (blue), and OSR (red). The graphs are divided into quadrants and demonstrate: left bottom (range of healthy controls), left top (higher than healthy control only in the vertical axis), right bottom (higher than healthy control only in the horizontal axis), and right top (higher than healthy control in both the vertical and the horizontal axis).

3.7. TRAP5b Positively Correlates with GD Biomarkers: CCL18, Chitotriosidase, and Lyso-Gb1

We next analyzed the correlation between circulating TRAP5b, RANKL, and OPG, and GD biomarkers chitotriosidase (CHITO), lyso-Gb1, and chemokine ligand 18 (CCL18) in all GD patients. CCL18 and CHITO are secreted by activated macrophages, and lyso-Gb1 represents the circulating metabolite derived from the deacylation of Gb1 [16–18]. A positive linear correlation was observed between CHITO, lyso-Gb1, and CCL18 (Supplemental Figure S3). TRAP5b showed a significant positive correlation with CCL18, lyso-Gb1, and CHITO (Figure 7 and Supplemental Figure S4). Furthermore, a negative correlation was observed between OPG and CHITO in the majority of GD patients with abnormal bone density (OSN and OSR) (Supplemental Figure S4), with the exception of two OSR patients who had incredibly high levels of CHITO and an elevated level of OPG (Supplemental Figure S4I). A negative correlation was observed between OPG and lyso-Gb1 in GD patients with OSN (Table 2). In comparison, there was no correlation between RANKL and GD biomarkers.

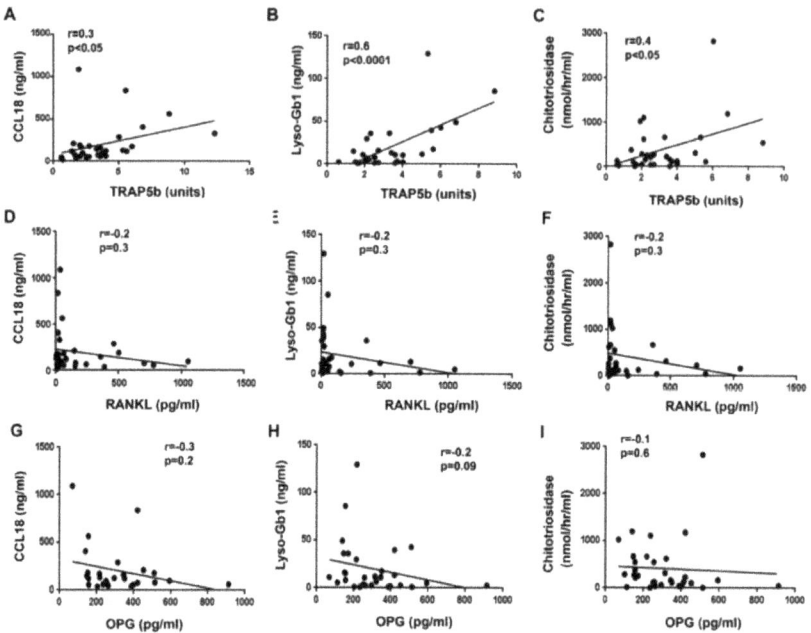

Figure 7. TRAP5b, RANKL, OPG correlation with biomarkers: CCL18, lyso-Gb1, and chitotriosidase in all GD patients. Scatterplot analysis of correlation of TRAP5b and CCL18 (**A**), TRAP5b and lyso-Gb1 (**B**), TRAP5b and chitotriosidase (**C**), RANKL and CCL18 (**D**), RANKL and lyso-Gb1 (**E**), RANKL and chitotriosidase (**F**), OPG and CCL18 (**G**), OPG and lyso-Gb1 (**H**), and OPG and chitotriosidase (**I**). p-values: statistical comparison was determined via Pearson's two tail linear regression correlation analysis.

Table 2. TRAP5b, RANKL, OPG correlation with CCL18, lyso-Gb1, and chitotriosidase (CHITO) in N, OSN, and OSR cohorts. Statistical comparisons were determined via Pearson's one tail linear correlation analysis. * Statistical analysis included GD patients with abnormal bone density (OSN and OSR), two OSR outliers were removed.

		TRAP5b	OPG	RANKL
CCL18	N	N	N	N
	OSN	positive correlation (R = 0.7; p = 0.02)	N	N
	OSR	positive correlation (R = 0.5, p = 0.03)	N	N
CHITO	N	N	N	N
	OSN	positive correlation (R = 0.8, p = 0.006)	negative correlation (R = −0.6, p = 0.03)	N
	OSR	positive correlation (R = 0.2, p = 0.05)	OSN + OSR (R = −0.4, p = 0.02 *)	N
Lyso-Gb1	N	N	N	N
	OSN	positive correlation (R = 0.7, p = 0.02)	negative correlation (R = −0.6, p = 0.03)	N
	OSR	positive correlation (R = 0.6, p = 0.02)	N	N

4. Discussion

Progressive bone disease is one of the primary untreated aspects of Gaucher disease. The majority of GD patients had structural bone involvement, and 43% had bone pain [19]. Bone metabolism, including turnover, remodeling, and mineralization, are affected in GD. One of GD's early signs involving bone pathology is the 'Erlenmeyer flask' deformity that affects long bones and abnormality of bone modeling. Later, the majority of GD patients develop skeletal complications, including osteopenia and osteoporosis [3]. GD patients with skeletal involvement could be asymptomatic or present symptoms such as pain, pathological fractures, cystic changes, or osteonecrosis. 'Erlenmeyer flask' deformity occurs during tubular and long bone growth [20], and can be the initial diagnostic sign in many patients. With GD, in our cohort, the 'Erlenmeyer flask' deformity did not correlate with OSN or OSR, suggesting different pathological pathways leading to abnormal bone remodeling and bone mineralization. However, in our study, an increasing number of GD patients with bone pain and bone fractures correlated with osteoporosis, suggesting similar underlying mechanisms for both. As is well known, multiple chronic immune and inflammatory disorders are associated with bone density abnormalities and accompanying pain [21].

While bone involvement is common in GD, there are no peripheral bone-related biomarkers in clinical use that could assist with therapeutic planning and clinical management. Our study's main conclusion is that TRAP5b is a biomarker that correlates with the progression of osteopenia to osteoporosis in GD. Excess osteoclastic bone resorption over osteoblastic bone formation leads to bone mineral loss and the development of osteopenia and osteoporosis [20]. The bone marker, TRAP5b, is a marker of osteoclast activation and reflects the number of active osteoclasts [8,22]. Two isoforms of TRAP circulate in the blood, TRAP5a and TRAP5b. TRAP5a is a biomarker of systemic inflammation [23], and TRAP5b is a biomarker of bone resorption. The development of specific TRAP5a and TRAP5b antibodies has made it possible to separate clinically relevant biomarkers for osteoclasts and inflammatory macrophages [24].

Interestingly, total TRAP, not TRAP5b, has been used as a biomarker for GD along with angiotensin-converting enzyme (ACE), CHITO, and ferritin, all of which are markers for activated macrophages [25]. Moreover, total TRAP, along with CHITO, ferritin, and ACE, is included in routine clinical monitoring of GD activity [26]. Our results demonstrate that higher TRAP5b levels correlate with OSN (3.1 ± 1.8) and OSR (4.2 ± 2.2) progression in GD. Similar to TRAP5b, cathepsin K is also secreted predominantly by activated osteoclasts [27,28]. Moreover, two studies demonstrated that cathepsin K increases in GD1 [29,30]. Thus, enhanced TRAP5b expression and cathepsin K activation confirm osteoclast activation in GD patients. Overall, our findings suggest that serum TRAP5b is a promising new biomarker with clinical relevance in GD, and evaluation of osteopenia–osteoporosis progression.

Circulating TRAP5b positively correlates with clinical biomarkers of GD pathology: CCL18, lyso-Gb1, and CHITO. We think that this finding is relevant to understanding the pattern of events that occurs in GD bones. Because the significant correlation was verified between TRAP5b and lyso-Gb1, and correlations between lyso-Gb1, CHITO are CCL18 have been observed in several clinical studies [18], we postulate that lyso-Gb1 is the primary contributor to TRAP5b activation, not CHITO or CCL18. A possible mechanism underlying activation expression of TRAP5 in osteoclasts is Gb1 accumulation in bone marrow cells, including monocytes/macrophages precursors cells, and osteoclasts. An analysis of osteoblasts differentiated from a GD1 patient's bone marrow demonstrated that exogenous lyso-Gb1 reduced mesenchymal cell viability for osteoblast differentiation and reduced osteoblast calcium deposition [6]. At the same time, an analysis of osteoclasts showed an increase in osteoclast generation of 37% in GD. Thus, increased osteoclast number and activity with reducing osteoblast activity lead to osteoclast/osteoblast disbalance in GD [6]. The alternative pathway of osteoclast activation is via inflammatory pathways that lead to an augmented and systemic loss of bone mineral density [31]. A wide range of in vitro studies have shown that lyso-Gb1 is a pro-inflammatory agent in immune cells, including chronic B-cell and T-cell activation and gammopathy [32–34]. We suggest that TRAP5b could be used along with other GD biomarkers to assess bone density abnormalities and response to therapy.

The level of RANKL and OPG are essential factors that determine the number and activity of osteoclasts [11,35,36]. RANKL binds to RANK on the surface of the osteoclast precursor or mononuclear osteoclast and promotes osteoclast differentiation and maturation. OPG binds to RANKL and inhibits osteoclast differentiation. RANK is expressed in osteoclast precursors, mature osteoclasts, dendritic cells, macrophages, and microglia. The RANKL is highly expressed by osteoblasts, and to a much lesser degree in osteocytes. OPG is mainly expressed by osteoblasts [35]. Mature monocytes and macrophages have the ability to differentiate into osteoclasts, but these cells also secrete factors that impact osteoblast activity [37–39]. Because cells of monocytes/macrophage lineage are primarily affected in GD, it is not unexpected that bone morphogenesis and remodeling are impaired [3,40]. GD patients with active bone disease formed more osteoclasts than GD patients without bone disease [6,40,41]. Moreover, an in vitro inhibitory GD model that demonstrated that PBMC differentiated into osteoclasts at a higher rate support the finding that GD patients with active bone disease formed more osteoclasts [41]. Thus, the altered RANKL/RANK/OPG triad plays an integral role in GD bone pathology [3,18].

In the present study, RANKL was elevated in 51% of the patients with GD. However, elevated plasma RANKL only correlates with osteopenia, and not osteoporosis, suggesting that the acceleration of osteoclast differentiation occurs before the onset of osteoporosis. This finding may also represent the activation of osteoclastic bone resorption in patients with osteopenia. Furthermore, the majority of GD patients had an average serum OPG level, and only 41% presented with an elevated OPG. Patients with a high level of OPG either belonged to the N or OSN cohorts. This finding suggests that in the early stages of bone disease, OPG is expressed and inhibits RANKL activity. Overall, our data fit with a previous study that demonstrated the normal values for OPG in GD type 1 [42]. Accumulated findings indicate that OPG-related osteoclast activity is not a major mechanism of bone pathology in GD patients with relatively mild form [42]. However, there is still controversy regarding RANKL/OPG and its effects on GD bone pathology [43]. The genetic variability of OPG and RANK genes in GD may also play a role in the GD bone pathology with its response to treatment. Similar to the RANKL data, RANKL/OPG level was mostly elevated in the OSN group and positively correlated with RANKL. The higher level of RANKL and RANKL/OPG in patients with osteopenia has been observed in postmenopausal women [44]. RANKL/OPG ratio is often used as a biomarker of bone pathology, which reflects a balance of bone formation and resorption.

The close relationship between osteoporosis and chronic inflammation has been studied for many years. The most detailed observations of osteoclast-mediated bone loss during chronic inflammation are described for autoimmune rheumatic diseases. Osteoclast-mediated resorption at the interface between synovium and bone is responsible for the joint erosion seen in patients suffering from inflammatory rheumatoid arthritis (RA) [45]. Inflammatory cytokines (tumor necrosis factor-alpha (TNFα) and interleukins (IL-1, and Il-6)) may drive osteoclastic bone loss [45,46]. Synovial macrophages in RA overexpress these inflammatory cytokines, including TNFα, which has particularly pervasive effects on osteoclastogenesis by promoting RANKL production [46,47]. RANKL, in turn, promotes differentiation of synovial macrophages into osteoclasts [48]. Because Gb1 and lyso-Gb1 induce expression of pro-inflammatory cytokines in macrophages, including TNFα, Il-6, and monocyte chemoattractant protein 1 (MCP-1) [18], we suggest that inflammatory cytokines contribute to RANKL/OPG imbalance and thus promote osteoclastic bone resorption. The bone pain that also correlates with bone density abnormalities suggests the contribution of a systemic inflammatory response to GD-related bone disease [49].

A relatively small number of subjects and small cohort numbers for each GD is one of the limitations of this study, and thus, the results of linear regression analysis should be interpreted with caution. Also, in this study, we did not take into account the age of disease onset, disease course, or duration of GD therapy, which could have contributed to current observations in OSN and OSR cohorts.

ERT leads to a substantial improvement of hematological manifestation in GD; however, bone involvement is refractory to therapy [50]. Limited studies have evaluated bone biomarkers in untreated vs. ERT treated patients with inconsistent results. The lack of differences in serum OPG levels between naïve and ERT-treated patients suggested that OPG-related osteoclast activity may not be a significant contributor to GD bone pathology [42]. However, in another study, there were decreased OPG and RANKL/OPG levels in GD [10]. Our group has previously demonstrated that plasma RANKL and OPG levels decreased in SRT-treated patients over time, but RANKL/OPG did not change with the treatment status [51].

There is no standard treatment for osteopenia–osteoporosis progression in GD. The most common medications for osteoporosis and others bone diseases, nitrogen-containing bisphosphonates (N-BPs), prevent bone mass loss by inhibiting osteoclast resorption via inhibition of farnesyl pyrophosphate synthase [52]. N-BPs, calcium, and vitamin D with a healthy lifestyle are standard recommendations for GD patients, especially for young patients [53,54]. Unfortunately, no clinical study using N-BPs in GD has been completed. While there are individual case reports, limited small patient series, and consensus statements on the use of N-BPs, there has not yet been a systemic study of this treatment modality in GD [53,55,56]. Emerging osteoporosis therapies utilize novel mechanisms, including monoclonal antibodies against RANKL, DKK1, and sclerostin [57]. The antibody against RANKL, denosumab, prevents osteoclast development through RANKL inhibition. In this study, five patients with OSR have been treated with denosumab; among those, four had normal RANKL, and one had borderline levels after receiving denosumab. Nevertheless, the majority of GD patients with elevated RANKL levels were patients with OSN. Currently, whether patients with osteopenia and an elevated RANKL but normal OPG levels have a higher risk of developing osteoporosis is not known. Similarly, the effects of denosumab in GD-related osteoporosis is yet to be studied [20].

This study furthers clinical knowledge regarding the circulating biomarkers (TRAP5, RANKL, RANK, and OPG), bone density, and osteoporosis progression in GD. We provide the first evidence that TRAP5b is a potential bone biomarker for GD with the ability to predict OSN and OSR progression. The pattern of elevation of RANKL and OPG provides additional evidence for the role of osteoclastic bone resorption in GD.

Supplementary Materials: The following are available online at https://www.mdpi.com/article/10.3390/jcm10102217/s1, Figure S1: TRAP5b and RANKL concentrations in controls and GD females vs. males, Figure S2: Scatterplots represent the correlation between RANKL, OPG, and TRAP5b, Figure S3: Scatterplots represent the correlation between Lyso-Gb1, CCL18, and chitotriosidase (CHITO) in all GD patients. Figure S4: Scatterplots represent the correlation between Lyso-Gb1, CCL18, chitotriosidase (CHITO) and bone biomarkers, Table S1: GD with bone pathology characteristics, Table S2: Demographic characteristics, Table S3: Genotype summary.

Author Contributions: Conceptualization, M.I. and O.G.-A.; methodology, J.D., L.N. and J.F.; validation, M.I. and J.D.; formal analysis, M.I. and O.G.-A.; investigation, M.I. and O.G.-A.; resources, M.I. and O.G.-A.; data curation, M.I. and O.G.-A.; writing—original draft preparation, M.I.; writing—review and editing, O.G.-A. and J.D.; visualization, M.I.; supervision, M.I.; project administration, M.I.; funding acquisition, M.I. All authors have read and agreed to the published version of the manuscript.

Funding: This work was supported by the Investigator-Initiated Award from Shire Pharmaceuticals USA, a member of the Takeda group of companies, IIR-US-002597 (to M.I.).

Institutional Review Board Statement: The study was conducted according to the guidelines of the Declaration of Helsinki, and approved by the Institutional Review Board of Western Institutional Review Board Inc, (protocol code NCT04055831, 15 May 2019).

Informed Consent Statement: Informed consent was obtained from all subjects involved in the study.

Data Availability Statement: Not applicable.

Acknowledgments: We would like to thank the treatment center of LDRTC for recruiting patients and their help with sample collection. We thank Elizabeth Barski for reviewing the manuscript. The authors are grateful to all participating patients and their families.

Conflicts of Interest: The authors declare no conflict of interest. The funders had no role in the design of the study, the collection, analyses, or interpretation of data, the writing of the manuscript, or the decision to publish the results.

References

1. Pandey, M.K.; Grabowski, G.A. Immunological cells and functions in Gaucher disease. *Crit. Rev. Oncog.* **2013**, *18*, 197–220. [CrossRef]
2. Masi, L.; Brandi, M.L. Gaucher disease: The role of the specialist on metabolic bone diseases. *Clin. Cases Min. Bone Metab.* **2015**, *12*, 165–169. [CrossRef]
3. Mucci, J.M.; Rozenfeld, P. Pathogenesis of Bone Alterations in Gaucher Disease: The Role of Immune System. *J. Immunol. Res.* **2015**, *2015*, 192761. [CrossRef] [PubMed]
4. Ersek, A.; Karadimitris, A.; Horwood, N.J. Effect of glycosphingolipids on osteoclastogenesis and osteolytic bone diseases. *Front. Endocrinol.* **2012**, *3*, 106. [CrossRef]
5. Mistry, P.K.; Liu, J.; Yang, M.; Nottoli, T.; McGrath, J.; Jain, D.; Zhang, K.; Keutzer, J.; Chuang, W.L.; Mehal, W.Z.; et al. Glucocerebrosidase gene-deficient mouse recapitulates Gaucher disease displaying cellular and molecular dysregulation beyond the macrophage. *Proc. Natl. Acad. Sci. USA* **2010**, *107*, 19473–19478. [CrossRef] [PubMed]
6. Reed, M.C.; Schiffer, C.; Heales, S.; Mehta, A.B.; Hughes, D.A. Impact of sphingolipids on osteoblast and osteoclast activity in Gaucher disease. *Mol. Genet. Metab.* **2018**, *124*, 278–286. [CrossRef] [PubMed]
7. Ivanova, M.; Limgala, R.P.; Changsila, E.; Kamath, R.; Ioanou, C.; Goker-Alpan, O. Gaucheromas: When macrophages promote tumor formation and dissemination. *Blood Cells Mol. Dis.* **2016**. [CrossRef] [PubMed]
8. Halleen, J.M.; Alatalo, S.L.; Suominen, H.; Cheng, S.; Janckila, A.J.; Vaananen, H.K. Tartrate-resistant acid phosphatase 5b: A novel serum marker of bone resorption. *J. Bone Miner. Res. Off. J. Am. Soc. Bone Miner. Res.* **2000**, *15*, 1337–1345. [CrossRef]
9. Kuo, T.R.; Chen, C.H. Bone biomarker for the clinical assessment of osteoporosis: Recent developments and future perspectives. *Biomark. Res.* **2017**, *5*, 18. [CrossRef]
10. Giuffrida, G.; Cingari, M.R.; Parrinello, N.; Romano, A.; Triolo, A.; Franceschino, M.; Di Raimondo, F. Bone turnover markers in patients with type 1 Gaucher disease. *Hematol. Rep.* **2012**, *4*, e21. [CrossRef]
11. Walsh, M.C.; Choi, Y. Biology of the RANKL-RANK-OPG System in Immunity, Bone, and Beyond. *Front. Immunol.* **2014**, *5*, 511. [CrossRef] [PubMed]
12. Pinzone, J.J.; Hall, B.M.; Thudi, N.K.; Vonau, M.; Qiang, Y.W.; Rosol, T.J.; Shaughnessy, J.D., Jr. The role of Dickkopf-1 in bone development, homeostasis, and disease. *Blood* **2009**, *113*, 517–525. [CrossRef]
13. Boyce, B.F.; Xing, L. Functions of RANKL/RANK/OPG in bone modeling and remodeling. *Arch. Biochem. Biophys.* **2008**, *473*, 139–146. [CrossRef] [PubMed]
14. Bi, H.; Chen, X.; Gao, S.; Yu, X.; Xiao, J.; Zhang, B.; Liu, X.; Dai, M. Key Triggers of Osteoclast-Related Diseases and Available Strategies for Targeted Therapies: A Review. *Front. Med.* **2017**, *4*, 234. [CrossRef]
15. Gruber, H.E.; Ivey, J.L.; Thompson, E.R.; Chesnut, C.H., 3rd; Baylink, D.J. Osteoblast and osteoclast cell number and cell activity in postmenopausal osteoporosis. *Miner. Electrolyte Metab.* **1986**, *12*, 246–254. [PubMed]
16. Schraufstatter, I.U.; Zhao, M.; Khaldoyanidi, S.K.; Discipio, R.G. The chemokine CCL18 causes maturation of cultured monocytes to macrophages in the M2 spectrum. *Immunology* **2012**, *135*, 287–298. [CrossRef] [PubMed]
17. Hollak, C.E.; van Weely, S.; van Oers, M.H.; Aerts, J.M. Marked elevation of plasma chitotriosidase activity. A novel hallmark of Gaucher disease. *J. Clin. Investig.* **1994**, *93*, 1288–1292. [CrossRef] [PubMed]
18. Revel-Vilk, S.; Fuller, M.; Zimran, A. Value of Glucosylsphingosine (Lyso-Gb1) as a Biomarker in Gaucher Disease: A Systematic Literature Review. *Int. J. Mol. Sci.* **2020**, *21*, 7159. [CrossRef] [PubMed]
19. Wenstrup, R.J.; Roca-Espiau, M.; Weinreb, N.J.; Bembi, B. Skeletal aspects of Gaucher disease: A review. *Br. J. Radiol.* **2002**, *75* (Suppl. 1), A2–A12. [CrossRef]
20. Hughes, D.; Mikosch, P.; Belmatoug, N.; Carubbi, F.; Cox, T.; Goker-Alpan, O.; Kindmark, A.; Mistry, P.; Poll, L.; Weinreb, N.; et al. Gaucher Disease in Bone: From Pathophysiology to Practice. *J. Bone Miner. Res. Off. J. Am. Soc. Bone Miner. Res.* **2019**, *34*, 996–1013. [CrossRef]
21. Iseme, R.A.; McEvoy, M.; Kelly, B.; Agnew, L.; Walker, F.R.; Attia, J. Is osteoporosis an autoimmune mediated disorder? *Bone Rep.* **2017**, *7*, 121–131. [CrossRef]
22. Lv, Y.; Wang, G.; Xu, W.; Tao, P.; Lv, X.; Wang, Y. Tartrate-resistant acid phosphatase 5b is a marker of osteoclast number and volume in RAW 264.7 cells treated with receptor-activated nuclear kappaB ligand. *Exp. Ther. Med.* **2015**, *9*, 143–146. [CrossRef]
23. Janckila, A.J.; Slone, S.P.; Lear, S.C.; Martin, A.; Yam, L.T. Tartrate-resistant acid phosphatase as an immunohistochemical marker for inflammatory macrophages. *Am. J. Clin. Pathol.* **2007**, *127*, 556–566. [CrossRef]

24. Pradella, S.D.; Slone, S.P.; Wu, Y.Y.; Chao, T.Y.; Parthasarathy, R.N.; Yam, L.T.; Janckila, A.J. Applications and performance of monoclonal antibodies to human tartrate resistant acid phosphatase. *J. Immunol. Methods* **2011**, *372*, 162–170. [CrossRef]
25. Troy, K.; Cuttner, J.; Reilly, M.; Grabowski, G.; Desnick, R. Tartrate-resistant acid phosphatase staining of monocytes in Gaucher disease. *Am. J. Hematol.* **1985**, *19*, 237–244. [CrossRef]
26. Stirnemann, J.; Belmatoug, N.; Vincent, C.; Fain, O.; Fantin, B.; Mentre, F. Bone events and evolution of biologic markers in Gaucher disease before and during treatment. *Arthritis Res. Ther.* **2010**, *12*, R156. [CrossRef]
27. Dai, R.; Wu, Z.; Chu, H.Y.; Lu, J.; Lyu, A.; Liu, J.; Zhang, G. Cathepsin K: The Action in and Beyond Bone. *Front. Cell Dev. Biol.* **2020**, *8*, 433. [CrossRef]
28. Goto, T.; Yamaza, T.; Tanaka, T. Cathepsins in the osteoclast. *J. Electron. Microsc.* **2003**, *52*, 551–558. [CrossRef]
29. Moran, M.T.; Schofield, J.P.; Hayman, A.R.; Shi, G.P.; Young, E.; Cox, T.M. Pathologic gene expression in Gaucher disease: Up-regulation of cysteine proteinases including osteoclastic cathepsin K. *Blood* **2000**, *96*, 1969–1978. [CrossRef]
30. Lobatoa, J.B.; Parejo, P.D.; Vázquez, R.J.; Jiménez, L.M. Cathepsin K as a biomarker of bone involvement in type 1 Gaucher disease. *Med. Clín.* **2015**, *145*, 6. [CrossRef]
31. Redlich, K.; Smolen, J.S. Inflammatory bone loss: Pathogenesis and therapeutic intervention. *Nat. Rev. Drug Discov.* **2012**, *11*, 234–250. [CrossRef]
32. Nair, S.; Boddupalli, C.S.; Verma, R.; Liu, J.; Yang, R.; Pastores, G.M.; Mistry, P.K.; Dhodapkar, M.V. Type II NKT-TFH cells against Gaucher lipids regulate B-cell immunity and inflammation. *Blood* **2015**, *125*, 1256–1271. [CrossRef]
33. Lukas, J.; Cozma, C.; Yang, F.; Kramp, G.; Meyer, A.; Nesslauer, A.M.; Eichler, S.; Bottcher, T.; Witt, M.; Brauer, A.U.; et al. Glucosylsphingosine Causes Hematological and Visceral Changes in Mice-Evidence for a Pathophysiological Role in Gaucher Disease. *Int. J. Mol. Sci.* **2017**, *18*, 2192. [CrossRef]
34. Nair, S.; Branagan, A.R.; Liu, J.; Boddupalli, C.S.; Mistry, P.K.; Dhodapkar, M.V. Clonal Immunoglobulin against Lysolipids in the Origin of Myeloma. *N. Engl. J. Med.* **2016**, *374*, 555–561. [CrossRef] [PubMed]
35. Cawley, K.M.; Bustamante-Gomez, N.C.; Guha, A.G.; MacLeod, R.S.; Xiong, J.; Gubrij, I.; Liu, Y.; Mulkey, R.; Palmieri, M.; Thostenson, J.D.; et al. Local Production of Osteoprotegerin by Osteoblasts Suppresses Bone Resorption. *Cell Rep.* **2020**, *32*, 108052. [CrossRef]
36. O'Brien, C.A. Control of RANKL gene expression. *Bone* **2010**, *46*, 911–919. [CrossRef]
37. Sinder, B.P.; Pettit, A.R.; McCauley, L.K. Macrophages: Their Emerging Roles in Bone. *J. Bone Miner. Res. Off. J. Am. Soc. Bone Miner. Res.* **2015**, *30*, 2140–2149. [CrossRef] [PubMed]
38. Pirraco, R.P.; Reis, R.L.; Marques, A.P. Effect of monocytes/macrophages on the early osteogenic differentiation of hBMSCs. *J. Tissue Eng. Regen. Med.* **2013**, *7*, 392–400. [CrossRef]
39. Pereira, M.; Petretto, E.; Gordon, S.; Bassett, J.H.D.; Williams, G.R.; Behmoaras, J. Common signalling pathways in macrophage and osteoclast multinucleation. *J. Cell Sci.* **2018**, *131*. [CrossRef] [PubMed]
40. Mucci, J.M.; Cuello, M.F.; Kisinovsky, I.; Larroude, M.; Delpino, M.V.; Rozenfeld, P.A. Proinflammatory and proosteoclastogenic potential of peripheral blood mononuclear cells from Gaucher patients: Implication for bone pathology. *Blood Cells Mol. Dis.* **2015**, *55*, 134–143. [CrossRef] [PubMed]
41. Reed, M.; Baker, R.J.; Mehta, A.B.; Hughes, D.A. Enhanced differentiation of osteoclasts from mononuclear precursors in patients with Gaucher disease. *Blood Cells Mol. Dis.* **2013**, *51*, 185–194. [CrossRef]
42. Magal, I.; Lebel, E.; Altarescu, G.; Itzchaki, M.; Rudensky, B.; Foldes, A.J.; Zimran, A.; Elstein, D. Serum levels of osteoprotegerin and osteoprotegerin polymorphisms in Gaucher disease. *Br. J. Haematol.* **2006**, *133*, 93–97. [CrossRef]
43. Zimmermann, A.; Popp, R.A.; Rossmann, H.; Bucerzan, S.; Nascu, I.; Leucuta, D.; Weber, M.M.; Grigorescu-Sido, P. Gene variants of osteoprotegerin, estrogen-, calcitonin- and vitamin D-receptor genes and serum markers of bone metabolism in patients with Gaucher disease type 1. *Ther. Clin. Risk Manag.* **2018**, *14*, 2069–2080. [CrossRef]
44. Azizieh, F.Y.; Shehab, D.; Jarallah, K.A.; Gupta, R.; Raghupathy, R. Circulatory Levels of RANKL, OPG, and Oxidative Stress Markers in Postmenopausal Women With Normal or Low Bone Mineral Density. *Biomark. Insights* **2019**, *14*. [CrossRef]
45. Coury, F.; Peyruchaud, O.; Machuca-Gayet, I. Osteoimmunology of Bone Loss in Inflammatory Rheumatic Diseases. *Front. Immunol.* **2019**, *10*, 679. [CrossRef]
46. Weitzmann, M.N. The Role of Inflammatory Cytokines, the RANKL/OPG Axis, and the Immunoskeletal Interface in Physiological Bone Turnover and Osteoporosis. *Science* **2013**, *2013*, 125705. [CrossRef]
47. Li, J.; Hsu, H.C.; Mountz, J.D. Managing macrophages in rheumatoid arthritis by reform or removal. *Curr. Rheumatol. Rep.* **2012**, *14*, 445–454. [CrossRef]
48. Takayanagi, H.; Oda, H.; Yamamoto, S.; Kawaguchi, H.; Tanaka, S.; Nishikawa, T.; Koshihara, Y. A new mechanism of bone destruction in rheumatoid arthritis: Synovial fibroblasts induce osteoclastogenesis. *Biochem. Biophys. Res. Commun.* **1997**, *240*, 279–286. [CrossRef]
49. Devigili, G.; De Filippo, M.; Ciana, G.; Dardis, A.; Lettieri, C.; Rinaldo, S.; Macor, D.; Moro, A.; Eleopra, R.; Bembi, B. Chronic pain in Gaucher disease: Skeletal or neuropathic origin? *Orphanet J. Rare Dis.* **2017**, *12*, 148. [CrossRef]
50. Goker-Alpan, O. Therapeutic approaches to bone pathology in Gaucher disease: Past, present and future. *Mol. Genet. Metab.* **2011**, *104*, 438–447. [CrossRef]
51. Limgala, R.P.; Goker-Alpan, O. Effect of Substrate Reduction Therapy in Comparison to Enzyme Replacement Therapy on Immune Aspects and Bone Involvement in Gaucher Disease. *Biomolecules* **2020**, *10*, 526. [CrossRef] [PubMed]

52. Kimmel, D.B. Mechanism of action, pharmacokinetic and pharmacodynamic profile, and clinical applications of nitrogen-containing bisphosphonates. *J. Dent. Res.* **2007**, *86*, 1022–1033. [CrossRef]
53. Cox, T.M.; Aerts, J.M.; Belmatoug, N.; Cappellini, M.D.; vom Dahl, S.; Goldblatt, J.; Grabowski, G.A.; Hollak, C.E.; Hwu, P.; Maas, M.; et al. Management of non-neuronopathic Gaucher disease with special reference to pregnancy, splenectomy, bisphosphonate therapy, use of biomarkers and bone disease monitoring. *J. Inherit. Metab. Dis.* **2008**, *31*, 319–336. [CrossRef]
54. Giuffrida, G.; Cappellini, M.D.; Carubbi, F.; Di Rocco, M.; Iolascon, G. Management of bone disease in Gaucher disease type 1: Clinical practice. *Adv. Ther.* **2014**, *31*, 1197–1212. [CrossRef] [PubMed]
55. Khan, A.; Hanley, D.A.; McNeil, C.; Boyd, S. Improvement in Bone Mineral Density and Architecture in a Patient with Gaucher Disease Using Teriparatide. *JIMD Rep.* **2015**, *22*, 23–28. [CrossRef] [PubMed]
56. Dekker, N.; van Dussen, L.; Hollak, C.E.; Overkleeft, H.; Scheij, S.; Ghauharali, K.; van Breemen, M.J.; Ferraz, M.J.; Groener, J.E.; Maas, M.; et al. Elevated plasma glucosylsphingosine in Gaucher disease: Relation to phenotype, storage cell markers, and therapeutic response. *Blood* **2011**, *118*, e118–e127. [CrossRef] [PubMed]
57. Tu, K.N.; Lie, J.D.; Wan, C.K.V.; Cameron, M.; Austel, A.G.; Nguyen, J.K.; Van, K.; Hyun, D. Osteoporosis: A Review of Treatment Options. *Pharm. Ther.* **2018**, *43*, 92–104.

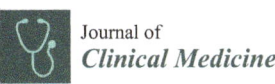

Article

Bone Effect and Safety of One-Year Denosumab Therapy in a Cohort of Renal Transplanted Patients: An Observational Monocentric Study

Carlo Alfieri [1,2,*], Valentina Binda [1], Silvia Malvica [1,3], Donata Cresseri [1], Mariarosaria Campise [1], Maria Teresa Gandolfo [1], Anna Regalia [1], Deborah Mattinzoli [1], Silvia Armelloni [1], Evaldo Favi [2,4], Paolo Molinari [1,3] and Piergiorgio Messa [1,2]

1. Unit of Nephrology, Dialysis and Renal Transplantation, Fondazione IRCCS Ca' Granda Ospedale Maggiore Policlinico, 20122 Milan, Italy; valentina.binda@policlinico.mi.it (V.B.); silvia.malvica@unimi.it (S.M.); donata.cresseri@policlinico.mi.it (D.C.); maria.campise@policlinico.mi.it (M.C.); mariateresa.gandolfo@policlinico.mi.it (M.T.G.); anna.regalia@policlinico.mi.it (A.R.); deborah.mattinzoli@policlinico.mi.it (D.M.); silvia.armelloni@policlinico.mi.it (S.A.); paolo.molinari1@unimi.it (P.M.); piergiorgio.messa@unimi.it (P.M.)
2. Department of Clinical Sciences and Community Health, University of Milan, 20122 Milan, Italy; evaldo.favi@unimi.it
3. Specialization School of Nephrology and Dialysis, University of Milan, 20122 Milan, Italy
4. Renal Transplantation Unit, Fondazione IRCCS Ca' Granda Ospedale Maggiore Policlinico, 20122 Milan, Italy
* Correspondence: carlo.alfieri1@gmail.com or carlo.alfieri@unimi.it; Tel.: +39-02-55034552; Fax: +39-02-55034550

Citation: Alfieri, C.; Binda, V.; Malvica, S.; Cresseri, D.; Campise, M.; Gandolfo, M.T.; Regalia, A.; Mattinzoli, D.; Armelloni, S.; Favi, E.; et al. Bone Effect and Safety of One-Year Denosumab Therapy in a Cohort of Renal Transplanted Patients: An Observational Monocentric Study. *J. Clin. Med.* **2021**, *10*, 1989. https://doi.org/10.3390/jcm10091989

Academic Editor: Heinrich Resch

Received: 1 April 2021
Accepted: 28 April 2021
Published: 6 May 2021

Publisher's Note: MDPI stays neutral with regard to jurisdictional claims in published maps and institutional affiliations.

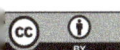

Copyright: © 2021 by the authors. Licensee MDPI, Basel, Switzerland. This article is an open access article distributed under the terms and conditions of the Creative Commons Attribution (CC BY) license (https://creativecommons.org/licenses/by/4.0/).

Abstract: In 32-kidney transplanted patients (KTxps), the safety and the effects on BMD and mineral metabolism (MM) of one-year treatment with denosumab (DB) were studied. Femoral and vertebral BMD and T-score, FRAX score and vertebral fractures (sVF) before (T0) and after 12 months (T12) of treatment were measured. MM, renal parameters, hypocalcemic episodes (HpCa), urinary tract infections (UTI), major graft and KTxps outcomes were monitored. The cohort was composed mainly of females, $n = 21$. We had 29 KTxps on steroid therapy and 22 KTxps on vitamin D supplementation. At T0, 25 and 7 KTxps had femoral osteoporosis (F-OPS) and osteopenia (F-OPS), respectively. Twenty-three and six KTxps had vertebral osteoporosis (V-OPS) and osteopenia (V-OPS), respectively. Seventeen KTxps had sVF. At T12, T-score increased at femoral and vertebral sites ($p = 0.05$, $p = 0.008$). The prevalence of F-OPS and V-OPS reduced from 78% to 69% and from 72% to 50%, respectively. Twenty-five KTxps ameliorated FRAX score and two KTxps had novel sVF. At T12, a slight reduction of Ca was present, without HpCa. Four KTxps had UTI. No graft rejections, loss of graft or deaths were reported. Our preliminary results show a good efficacy and safety of DB in KTxps. Longer and randomized studies involving more KTxps might elucidate the possible primary role of DB in the treatment of bone disorders in KTxps.

Keywords: denosumab; kidney transplantation; CKDMBD; vertebral fractures

1. Introduction

Chronic kidney disease (CKD) is now a serious problem because of the progressive rise of its incidence and prevalence worldwide [1]. Among the several complications present in CKD patients, the alterations of bone and mineral metabolism (MM) have a strong impact. Several changes in bone structure and progressive disarrangement in MM homeostasis occur progressively in CKD patients and cause the insurgence of vascular calcifications, cardiovascular events and bone fractures [2].

Kidney transplantation (KTx) is considered the best option for patients affected by CKD. Compared to dialyzed patients, KTx patients (KTxps) have globally better life expectancy and better cardiovascular and global outcomes [3]. Nevertheless, KTx is not able to completely solve the metabolic disorders developed during CKD. In addition, some specificities of KTxps exert additional effects on MM and bone homeostasis [4,5]. KTxps have, for these reasons, a higher fracture risk than the general population [6]. Post KTx bone loss and fractures incidence have their highest degree during the 12 months after KTx, but a progressive bone loss is reported during the entire life of the graft [7]. The principal therapeutic options for the treatment of bone anomalies in KTxps involve vitamin D, calcium supplements and, when indicated, bisphosphonates [8]. The concerns about bisphosphonate prescription in KTxps, mostly related to their potential nephrotoxicity and the limited data on their efficacy in preventing novel fractures, have limited the use of these drugs, making the management of bone disorders still unsatisfactory in KTxps [9]. Denosumab (DB) is a fully human monoclonal antibody directed against RANKL that inhibits the osteoclast activity resulting in a progressive decrease of bone resorption [10]. In the general population, DB is now used as a valid alternative to bisphosphonate in preventing osteoporosis and bone fractures [11]. Unfortunately, data concerning its role in KTxps are still limited. The aim of our study was to evaluate, in a cohort of KTxps who underwent a one-year treatment with DB: (1) the evolution of femoral and vertebral bone mineral bone density (BMD); (2) the effect on FRAX score and on the development of novel spontaneous vertebral fractures (sVF); (3) the modifications of the renal function and MM parameters; and (4) the safety of DB therapy.

2. Materials and Methods

2.1. Study Design

In our study, we evaluated prospectively, during the first year of treatment with DB, 32 KTxps ($M = 11$; median age 62 (58;69) years) followed up in our department. All patients studied were considered eligible to receive DB therapy by the presence of at least one of the following conditions: (1) sVF documented by X-ray; (2) femoral neck and/or vertebral osteoporosis; and (3) intolerance, long time treatment or contraindications to bisphosphonate therapy. In addition, only patients with basal Ca > 9.2 mg/dL and iPTH > 35 ng/dL were recruited.

After the initiation of DB, administered at the dosage of 60 mg every six months, all KTxps were followed regularly at our out-patient clinic for the whole period of observation and were treated in accordance with their clinical needs.

2.2. Instrumental Evaluations

Bone mass density was estimated at the proximal femur and at the lumbar spine (L1–L4) at T0 and T12 by means of dual energy X-ray absorptiometry (DEXA) as areal bone mineral density (BMD, g/cm^2). According to the World Health Organization (WHO) criteria, we defined BMD with a T-score above 1 SD as not pathologic. A T-score between -1.0 and -2.5 SD was classified as osteopenia, whereas a T-score below -2.5 SD was defined as osteoporosis [12].

Vertebral fractures were evaluated by means of complete lumbar X-ray at T0 and T12 by means of Genant classification [13].

2.3. FRAX Score Evaluation

The FRAX score (including age, sex, body weight, height, history of prior osteoporotic fracture, parental history of hip fragility fracture, current smoking, arthritis, alcohol consumption >3 units/day and T-score) was calculated at T0 and T12 using the tool for Italy provided on the FRAX website [14].

2.4. Biochemical Evaluations

Data about biochemical analyses were digitally recorded from the documents presented by each patient at the out-clinic visits.

Briefly, the following parameters were recorded at pre-determined timepoints:

Before DB initiation, not more than one month (T0): serum creatinine (sCr), urea, Calcium (Ca), Phosphorus (P), parathormone (PTH), native vitamin D (25OHD), active vitamin D (1-25OHD), alkaline phosphatase (ALP), Magnesium (Mg) and daily urinary protein excretion (Prot-U);

One month after the start of DB therapy (T1): sCr and Ca;

Three months after the start of DB therapy (T3): sCr, Ca, P and PTH;

Six months after the start of DB therapy (T6): sCr, urea, Ca, P, PTH, 25OHD, ALP and Prot-U;

Twelve months after the start of DB therapy (T12): serum creatinine (sCr), urea, Ca, P, PTH, 25OHD, 1-25OHD, ALP, Mg and Prot-U.

PTH was measured by DiaSorin LIAISON® kit. 25OHD levels were determined by enzyme-immunoassay (Kit EIA AC-57FI, immunodiagnostic system Boldon, UK), using a highly specific sheep 25OHD antibody and enzyme (horseradish peroxidase) labeled avidin. All other biochemical parameters were evaluated according to routine methodology used at the central laboratory of our Institution. All biochemical results were digitally recorded.

2.5. Clinical Events

During the follow up time, we evaluated the insurgence of the following clinical events:

- Hypocalcemia (HpCa): defined as a total serum Ca concentration < 8.0 mg/dl in the presence of normal plasma protein concentrations
- Urinary tract infections (UTI): defined by the presence of urinary symptoms associated to significative white blood cells (WBC > 50 m.f. 400×) and by the presence of positive urine-culture

In addition, biopsy proven graft rejection, graft failure and KTxps deaths were recorded.

2.6. Statistical Analyses

In statistical analyses, continuous variables were expressed as median value and interquartile range (25%;75%) and were log transformed if they had a skewed distribution.

Differences among groups were determined by Paired sign and Mann–Whitney, where indicated. Differences among percentages were determined by X_2 test.

Statistical analyses were performed using software SPSS version 20® and significance was set for *p* values < 0.05.

3. Results

3.1. Cohort Characteristics

Our cohort was composed mainly of females, and the median age of the overall cohort was 62 (58;69) years. As reported in Table 1, 24 KTxps underwent hemodialysis before KTx, and the median dialysis vintage was 53 (26;136). Glomerulonephritis was the main reason for end stage renal disease. Half of the patients received steroid therapy before KTx. Ninety-six percent of KTxps were transplanted by a deceased donor. Considering the overall cohort, DB was started after a median time of KTx of 144 (59;232) months.

In Table 2, the principal characteristics of the immunosuppressive and MM related therapies are reported. At both T0 and T12, the immunosuppressive therapy was composed principally by calcineurin inhibitors, mycophenolate and steroids, with no differences between the two timepoints considered. Steroid therapy was prescribed in 90% of KTxps, at a dosage of 5 (2.5;5) mg/day.

In 54% of KTxps, previous therapy with bisphosphonate was reported (Bisp+). The suspension of the drug was mainly related to the long-time course and/or the development of significant contraindications.

Table 1. Cohort characteristics.

Parameter	
Number of patients, n	32
Gender (M/F), n	11/21
Previous type of dialysis (HD/PD), n	24/8
Dialysis vintage (months)	53 (26;136)
Basal Nephropathy n (%)	
- Gnf	13 (40)
- ADPKD	6 (18)
- Secondary nephropathies	5 (15)
- Other	8 (27)
History of steroid therapy before KTx n (%)	16 (50)
Kind of transplant n (%) (deceased donor/living donor)	31/1 (96;4)
Age at Denosumab initiation (years)	62 (58;69)
Time of KTx at Denosumab initiation (months)	144 (59;232)

Footnotes: HD, hemodialysis; PD, peritoneal dialysis; Gnf, glomerulonephritis; ADPKD, autosomal dominant polycystic kidney disease; KTx, kidney transplantation.

Table 2. Immunosuppressive, mineral metabolism and anti-hypertensive therapies at T1 and T12.

Drug	T0	T12
CyA/Tac/MMF-MPA/AZA/mTor inhibitor N (%)	12/17/19/3/3 (37/53/58/9/9)	11/17/17/4/4 (34/53/50/12/12)
Steroid therapy N (%)	29 (90)	29 (90)
Daily steroids (mg)	5 (2.5;5)	5 (2.5;5)
Vitamin D therapy N (%)		
- No	10 (31)	8 (25)
- Native vitamin D	20 (63)	21 (66)
- Native + active vitamin D	2 (6)	3 (9)
Previous therapy with bisphosphonate n (%)	17 (54)	NA
Dosage of native vitamin D (µg/week)	75 (0;100)	75 (0;100)
Cinacalcet therapy N (%)	6 (18)	4 (12)
Calcium supplements N (%)	3 (9)	4 (12)

Footnotes: Cya, cyclosporine; Tac, Tacrolimus; MMF-MPA, mycophenolate: azathioprine.

More than half of KTxps were receiving at T0 25OHD supplementation. During the follow up time, in one patient, 25OHD supplementation was started, whereas, in another case, Calcitriol was added to 25OHD supplementation. The mean dosage/week of 25OHD supplementation was similar between T0 and T12.

3.2. DEXA and Lumbar X-ray Evaluations

In Table 3, the principal findings concerning femoral and vertebral DEXA and lumbar X-Ray examinations are summarized.

Table 3. Densitometry and X-ray evaluation at the two timepoints.

Parameters	T0	T12	p
F-BMD (g/cm^2)	0.53 (0.48;0.60)	0.56 (0.49;0.66)	**0.02**
F-T-score	−3.0 (−3.5;−2.5)	−2.8 (−3.5;−2.4)	**0.05**
V-BMD (g/cm^2)	0.72 (0.65;0.87)	0.79 (0.71;0.92)	**0.01**
V-T-score	−3.0 (−3.7;−1.9)	−2.6 (−3.0;−1.6)	**0.008**
Femoral bone density N (%)			
- Norman bone density	0 (0)	1 (4)	**0.001**
- Osteopenia	7 (22)	9 (28)	
- Osteoporosis	25 (78)	22 (69)	
Vertebral bone density N (%)			
- Normal bone density	3 (10)	4 (13)	**<0.001**
- Osteopenia	6 (18)	12 (37)	
- Osteoporosis	23 (72)	16 (50)	
FRAX score (%)	29 ± 15 *	26 ± 15 *	0.18
FRAX score amelioration n (%)	NA	25 (78)	NA
Patients with X-ray sVF N (%)	17 (53)	17 (53)	NA
Patients with novel X-ray sVF N (%)	NA	2 (6)	

Footnotes: BMD, bone mineral density; F-BMD, femoral BMD; V-BMD, vertebral BMD; F-T-score, T score measured at femoral level; V-T-score, T score measured at vertebral level; sVF, spontaneous vertebral fracture; bold format indicates statistical significance ($p < 0.05$); NA, not applicable; * mean ± standard deviation; X_2 square tests, paired sign tests were used.

At T0, normal bone density was found only in three KTxps, at vertebral level. The most prevalent finding was femoral osteoporosis (F-OPS), present in 78% of KTxps. At femoral level, F-BMD was 0.53 (0.48;0.60) g/cm^2 and median T-score was −3.0 (−3.5;−2.5). Vertebral osteoporosis (V-OPS) was found in 75% of KTxps, and V-BMD and T-score were, respectively, 0.72 (0.65;0.87) g/cm^2 and −3.0 (−3.7;−1.9). To investigate the possible effect on BMD improvement of a previous therapy with bisphosphonates, a sub-analysis considering Bisp+ and patients with no history of bisphosphonate before the DB treatment (Bisp−) separately was performed. No significant impact of previous bisphosphonate was evidenced at femoral and vertebral levels both at baseline and during the time of follow up.

After 12 months of DM therapy, global modifications in DEXA were found. At both femoral and vertebral level, the T-score significantly improved: femoral T-score reached −2.8 (−3.5;−2.4) ($p = 0.05$ vs. T0), whereas vertebral T-score −2.6 (−3.0;−1.6) ($p = 0.008$ vs. T0).

As reported in Figure 1A, the increase of T-scores also resulted in a re-distribution of the KTxps among the DEXA groups. At femoral level, a significant reduction of the prevalence of osteoporosis ($p = 0.001$) was found. Five patients moved from osteoporosis to osteopenia. One patient ameliorated his status from osteopenia to normal femoral T-score, whereas, in one patient, a worsening to osteoporosis was found.

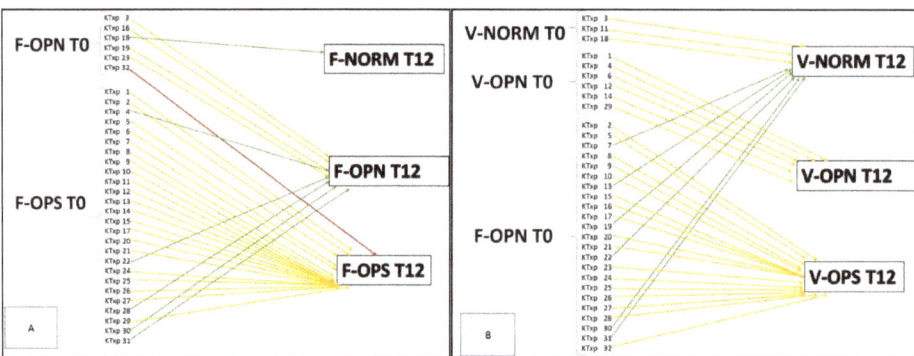

Figure 1. General distribution and DEXA class modifications at femoral (**A**) and vertebral (**B**) level during the time of observation. F-OPN, femoral osteopenia; F-OPS, femoral osteoporosis; F-norm, femoral normal DEXA; V-OPN, vertebral osteopenia; V-OPS, vertebral osteoporosis; V-norm, vertebral normal DEXA; red lines, worsening of DEXA category; yellow lines, stability of DEXA category; green lines, amelioration of DEXA category.

At vertebral level, a significant reduction of the prevalence of osteoporosis ($p < 0.0001$) was also found. In this case, six KTxps moved from osteoporosis, five KTxps to osteopenia and one case in the normal T-score values group. In addition, the three KTxps who showed normal T score values at T0 confirmed their result at T12 (Figure 1B).

A sub analysis considering 20 KTxps not included in the study (10 KTxps for femoral BMD and 10 other KTxps for vertebral BMD) who were treated with neither DB nor bisphosphonates was also performed.

Those patients were matched to those considered in the study for age, time of transplant, gender distribution and obviously femoral and lumbar BMD.

In femoral DEXA, we found not significant modifications at T0 and after one year in BMD (0.55 (0.54;0.58) vs. 0.55 (0.52;0.60), $p = 0.54$) and femoral T score (-2.8 (-3.1;-2.7) vs. -2.7 (-3.0;-2.4), $p = 0.13$). The same result was found at lumbar level for BMD (0.70 (0.65;0.77) vs. 0.70 (0.69;0.71), $p = 0.71$) and T score (-3.25 (-3.6;-2.5) vs. -3.15 (-3.4;-3.0), $p = 0.27$). Unfortunately, no data about sVF were available for those patients.

The treatment with DB resulted in a global modification of FRAX score in the overall cohort. In particular, a reduction of FRAX score was found in 78% of KTxps, with mean values of FRAX score at T0 of 29 ± 15 % and at T12 of 26 ± 15 % ($p = 0.18$). Accordingly, at the second vertebral X-ray evaluation, novel sVF were found only in 6% of KTxps. They already had sVF at T0.

3.3. Biochemical Evaluations

As reported in Table 4, renal functional parameters were similar between T0 and T12. Among MM evaluations, we found significant modifications only in Ca (9.60 (9.37;10.21) vs. 9.40 (8.98;9.83), $p = 0.01$), PTH (63 (36;86) vs. 115 (44;161), $p = 0.009$) and ALP (68 (61–90) vs. 51 (45;68), $p = 0.002$) levels. No significant differences were found in P, Mg, 25OHD and 1-25OH levels.

3.4. Clinical Outcomes

During the year of follow up, no symptomatic or asymptomatic HpCa episodes were reported. Four KTxps had UTI (mean time from DM initiation: 114 days) and required specific antibiotic treatments. Of note, those four KTxps (two of them symptomatic) had positive pathologic anamnesis for UTI, so a direct relation to DB therapy is not possible to demonstrate. In two KTxps, a hospitalization for UTI complications (sepsis) was required. No biopsy proven graft rejections were observed during the time of treatment and no graft loss or KTxps death was reported.

Table 4. Biochemical characteristics of the overall cohort at T1 and ad T12.

Parameters	T0	T1	T3	T6	T12	p *
s-Creatinine (mg/dL)	1.32 (0.96;1.78)	1.25 (1.0;1.80)	1.41 (1.13;1.80)	1.24 (0.92;1.60)	1.33 (0.97;1.72)	0.35
s-Urea (mg/dL)	62 (42;82)	NA	NA	57 (47;81)	61 (47;91)	0.15
Prot-U (g/24 h)	0.157 (0.12;0.31)	NA	NA	0.21 (0.13;0.35)	0.17 (0.11;0.34)	0.86
Ca (mg/dl)	9.60 (9.37;10.21)	9.60 (9.0;9.86)	9.79 (9.40;9.96)	9.53 (9.10;10.0)	9.40 (8.98;9.83)	**0.01**
P (mg/dL)	3.05 (2.60;3.40)	NA	2.70 (2.40;3.0)	2.90 (2.30;3.40)	2.85 (2.33;3.30)	0.06
PTH (ng/mL)	63 (36;86)	NA	119 (63;177)	101 (51;136)	115 (44;161)	**0.009**
ALP (U/dL)	68 (61;90)	NA	NA	53 (44;69)	51 (45;68)	**0.002**
25OHD (µg/dL)	26.7 (16.0;42.8)	NA	NA	31.5 (21.4;39.4)	32 (16;39.9)	0.35
1-25OHD (ng/L)	47.8 (36.1;61.1)	NA	NA	NA	37.9 (28.7;52.5)	0.69
Mg (mg/dL)	1.86 (1.70;2.09)	NA	NA	1.92 (1.75;2.08)	1.89 (1.68;2.07)	0.79

Footnotes: PTH, parathormone; Ca, calcium; P, phosphorus; ALP, alkaline phosphatase; Prot-U, daily urinary protein excretion; bold format indicates statistical significance ($p < 0.05$), where t-test, Mann–Whitney and Kruskal–Wallis test were used.; NA, not applicable; * T0 vs. T12.

4. Discussion

In this monocentric, observational, prospective study, 32 KTxps underwent, for clinical indications, DB therapy.

KTxps have a high risk of bone loss, initially related to pre-KTx clinical history. Steroid therapy before KTx, basal nephropathy and dialysis vintage are certainly impacting factors. In our cohort, similar to the data reported in the few investigations concerning DB therapy in KTxps, half of KTxps received steroids before KTx, and the most prevalent basal nephropathy was glomerulonephritis [15].

Even if most of the research present in the literature has focused their interests on the effect of DB in "early transplanted KTxps", osteopenia and osteoporosis are complications present also in long-term KTx [16]. For this reason, we decided to evaluate KTxps independently of their time of KTx.

Most of the KTxps evaluated in our study at baseline were receiving some MM specific therapies. In more than half of cases, native vitamin D was prescribed at baseline, and the levels of 25OHD were almost sufficient. Fifty-four percent of KTxps previously received bisphosphonate. In the few patients in which bisphosphonates were prescribed at T0, the principal reasons for the shift to DB were: (1) long-term bisphosphonate therapy (>3 years); and (2) presence of bisphosphonate related adverse events (gastrointestinal discomforts, suspected nephrotoxicity).

The initial aims of our study were to test the evolution of femoral and vertebral BMD and the incidence of novel sVF. At baseline, more than half of KTxps had F-OPS and V-OPS. Compared to the papers published by Brunova et al. in 2018 and by Bonani et al. in 2016, T0 F-Ts and V-Ts of our cohort were significantly worse [14,17]. This might be related to the longer time of transplant of our cohort. In addition, sVF were present in more than half of our cohort at T0. This result confirms the high prevalence of sVF in KTxps. Some data indicate a strong fracture risk, especially during the first 5–6 years after KTx, related to a higher need of steroids and stronger immunosuppressive therapy. In his paper, published in 2014, Sukumaran Nair indicated that fracture risk event rate is higher in the first year after KTx, but still present in the following years of KTx [18]. Some years before, Nikkel reported fracture events in 22.5% of the cohort of KTxps studied within five years of KTx [19]. Currently, however, the increasing attention to the fracture risk and the consequent use of immunosuppressive and MM schemes of therapy directed to prevent bone loss might have modified the fracture risk in KTxps.

After one year of therapy with DB, a global amelioration of BMD was observed at both femoral and vertebral levels. As shown in the results, the increase of BMD compared to the baseline was significant, especially at vertebral level. This result, after only one year of treatment, confirms the good effect of DB on osteoclastic resorption of trabecular structures already evidenced in the general population [20]. The beneficial effect of DB on BMD was confirmed also by the relative low incidence of novel sVF during the year of treatment. Of note, a global amelioration of FRAX score was also observed [21]. Novel sVF were found in only two KTxps at T12. The role of DB in preventing VF was explored by Cummings in the general population by means of the evaluation of DB effect on 7868 women affected by osteoporosis. In this study, DB reduced the risk of new radiographic vertebral and non-vertebral fractures compared to placebo [11]. Now, to our knowledge, our study is the first that evaluated the follow up of vertebral fractures in KTxps treated with DB. However, the beneficial effect of this therapy in CKD patients might assume a similar effect also in the presence of KTx [22]. Certainly, this point should be analyzed in greater depth by means of specific prospective trials. In any case, our results even if partially limited by the limited time of follow up might be a good prospect. Another point that should be analyzed in the future is the impact on sVF of DB discontinuation, potentially a burden in the general population by a severe bone turnover rebound and a rapid loss of BMD, resulting in a strong increase of sVF risk [23]. Some possible solutions both in the general population and in KTxps might be the administration of bisphosphonate, as proposed by some authors [24], or the increase of time between each DB administration, resulting in a permanent turnover of the bone metabolism (personal opinion).

In our study, we also evaluated the trend of renal functional and MM parameters. During the year of observation, all renal functional parameters remained stable, and no differences between T0 and T12 were found. A good level of renal safety has already been reported in the general population and in solid organ transplantation [25].

The baseline values of Ca showed a significant decrease during the year of treatment. However, despite Ca levels of our cohort being similar to those reported in other studies, in our cohort neither symptomatic nor asymptomatic hypocalcemic events were reported. This might reflect the effect of the strict monitoring scheduled in our cohort that permitted a prompt correction of Ca levels, needed in a small part of the cohort studied. This observation is substantially in line with previous findings [26]. The reduction in Ca levels, mostly related to the reduced osteoclast activity, might in part also explain the increase of PTH levels. A slight increase of PTH levels during one year of therapy is in line with previous reports. An increase of PTH in those patients might have some beneficial effects on bone structure, especially on cortical porosity, as already reported in general population [27,28]. However, a deeper evaluation of bone effects of this increase of PTH in KTx population might be the topic of future studies by means also of bone biopsies [29].

Infections are an important cause of mortality and morbidity during KTx [30]. In our study, we also evaluated the insurgence of UTI in KTxps treated with DB. Some experimental evidence reports a possible influence of DB, by means of the inhibition of RANK/RANKL pathways, in favoring UTI insurgence [30]. The relationship between infection risk and DB therapy in de novo KTxps was explored by Bonani et al. in 2017. In their work, with the aim to evaluate the incidence of infections (especially UTI and viral), the authors randomized 90 de novo KTxps to receive or standard therapy without DB or DB therapy. The incidence of UTI was higher in the DB group. Of note, the prevalence of severe infections (pyelonephritis and/or urosepsis) was not different in the two study arms. [31] The UTI observed in our cohort were reported during the follow up period only in patients with a previous positive anamnesis for UTI. The single arm design, the different definition of UTI and the longer time of KTx of our cohort make the comparison of our results with those presented by Bonani difficult. However, future studies, possibly multicentric and with a uniform definition of UTI, might better explore this important topic.

The impact of DB therapy was considered also in the prevalence of graft rejection and graft and KTxps survival. No biopsy proven KTx rejections were found in our cohort during the follow up time. All KTxps who started the DB therapy ended safely the first year of therapy. The safety of Denosumab on those outcomes has been explored recently [14]. In accordance with the evidence found in our study, a directly related higher risk of worse graft and KTxps outcomes in patients treated with DB is not reported in the literature.

The present paper presents some limitations. Undoubtedly, the monocentric design reduced significantly the size of the cohort studied, but it allowed a uniformity in the cohort identification and its follow up. In addition, unfortunately, it was not possible to perform some more specific dosages concerning bone remodeling markers that might have clarified better the efficacy of DB in our cohort. The absence of a control group might be considered a limit of the study. In any case, our study was designed to evaluate the efficacy and the potential adverse events of the drug therapy and can be considered an important starting point for future randomized research.

In conclusion, the experience of our center demonstrated a good bone efficacy and general safety of one-year DB therapy in KTxps.

Certainly, future longer and randomized studies, involving more KTxps, might elucidate the possible primary role of DB in the treatment of bone disorders in these patients.

Author Contributions: P.M. (Piergiorgio Messa) was responsible for study concept and design; C.A., D.M. and S.A. collected clinical and instrumental data; C.A., V.B., D.C., M.C., M.T.G., S.M., A.R. and E.F. wrote and corrected the main manuscript; C.A. and P.M. (Paolo Molinari) performed the statistical analyses. All authors have read and agreed to the published version of the manuscript.

Funding: This research received no external funding.

Institutional Review Board Statement: Ethical approval of all procedures performed in studies involving human participants were in accordance with the ethical standards of the institutional and/or national research committee and with the 1964 Helsinki declaration and of the Declaration of Istanbul and its later amendments or comparable ethical standards.The study was approved by the Institutional Review Board (or Ethics Committee) of Fondazione IRCCS Ca' Granda Ospedale Maggiore Policlinico, Milan (protocol code 4759—1837/19 19/11/2019).

Informed Consent Statement: We declare that no organs/tissues analyzed for this study were procured from prisoners. Informed consent was obtained from all individual participants included in the study.

Data Availability Statement: If needed, data are available in anonymous form.

Acknowledgments: The authors thank Marina Balderacchi for the kind collaboration in the health research and in the realization of this study.

Conflicts of Interest: The authors declare no conflict of interest.

References

1. Hill, N.R.; Fatoba, S.T.; Oke, J.L.; Hirst, J.A.; O'Callaghan, C.A.; Lasserson, D.S.; Hobbs, F.D.R. Global Prevalence of Chronic Kidney Disease—A Systematic Review and Meta-Analysis. *PLoS ONE* **2016**, *11*, e0158765. [CrossRef]
2. Messa, P.; Cerutti, R.; Brezzi, B.; Alfieri, C.; Cozzolino, M. Calcium and Phosphate Control by Dialysis Treatments. *Blood Purif.* **2009**, *27*, 360–368. [CrossRef]
3. Hariharan, S. Long-term kidney transplant survival. *Am. J. Kidney Dis.* **2001**, *38*, S44–S50. [CrossRef]
4. Messa, P.; Sindici, C.; Cannella, G.; Miotti, V.; Risaliti, A.; Gropuzzo, M.; Di Loreto, P.L.; Bresadola, F.; Mioni, G. Persistent secondary hyperparathyroidism after renal transplantation. *Kidney Int.* **1998**, *54*, 1704–1713. [CrossRef]
5. Messa, P.; Cafforio, C.; Alfieri, C. Calcium and phosphate changes after renal transplantation. *J. Nephrol.* **2010**, *23*, S175–S181.
6. Veenstra, D.L.; Best, J.H.; Hornberger, J.; Sullivan, S.D.; Hricik, D.E. Incidence and long-term cost of steroid-related side effects after renal transplantation. *Am. J. Kidney Dis.* **1999**, *33*, 829–839. [CrossRef]
7. Pichette, V.; Bonnardeaux, A.; Prudhomme, L.; Gagné, M.; Cardinal, J.; Ouimet, D. Long-term bone loss in kidney transplant recipients: A cross-sectional and longitudinal study. *Am. J. Kidney Dis.* **1996**, *28*, 105–114. [CrossRef]
8. Bouquegneau, A.; Salam, S.; Delanaye, P.; Eastell, R.; Khwaja, A. Bone Disease after Kidney Transplantation. *Clin. J. Am. Soc. Nephrol.* **2016**, *11*, 1282–1296. [CrossRef]
9. Conley, E.; Muth, B.; Samaniego, M.; Lotfi, M.; Voss, B.; Armbrust, M.; Pirsch, J.; Djamali, A. Bisphosphonates and Bone Fractures in Long-term Kidney Transplant Recipients. *Transplantation* **2008**, *86*, 231–237. [CrossRef] [PubMed]
10. Dore, R.K. The RANKL Pathway and Denosumab. *Rheum. Dis. Clin. N. Am.* **2011**, *37*, 433–452. [CrossRef] [PubMed]
11. Cummings, S.R.; San Martin, J.; McClung, M.R.; Siris, E.S.; Eastell, R.; Reid, I.R.; Delmas, P.; Zoog, H.B.; Austin, M.; Wang, A.; et al. Denosumab for prevention of fractures in postmenopausal women with osteoporosis. *N. Engl. J. Med.* **2009**, *361*, 756–765. [CrossRef]
12. Cosman, F.; De Beur, S.J.; LeBoff, M.S.; Lewiecki, E.M.; Tanner, B.; Randall, S.; Lindsay, R. Clinician's Guide to Prevention and Treatment of Osteoporosis. *Osteoporos. Int.* **2014**, *25*, 2359–2381. [CrossRef] [PubMed]
13. Genant, H.K.; Wu, C.Y.; Van Kuijk, C.; Nevitt, M.C. Vertebral fracture assessment using a semiquantitative technique. *J. Bone Miner. Res.* **2009**, *8*, 1137–1148. [CrossRef]

14. FRAX Score. Available online: https://www.sheffield.ac.uk/FRAX/index.aspx (accessed on 29 April 2021).
15. Bonani, M.; Frey, D.; Brockmann, J.; Fehr, T.; Mueller, T.; Saleh, L.; Von Eckardstein, A.; Graf, N.; Wuthrich, R.P. Effect of Twice-Yearly Denosumab on Prevention of Bone Mineral Density Loss in De Novo Kidney Transplant Recipients: A Randomized Controlled Trial. *Arab. Archaeol. Epigr.* **2016**, *16*, 1882–1891. [CrossRef]
16. Dounousi, E.; Leivaditis, K.; Eleftheriadis, T.; Liakopoulos, V. Osteoporosis after renal transplantation. *Int. Urol. Nephrol.* **2014**, *47*, 503–511. [CrossRef] [PubMed]
17. Brunova, J.; Kratochvilova, S.; Stepankova, J. Osteoporosis Therapy With Denosumab in Organ Transplant Recipients. *Front. Endocrinol.* **2018**, *9*, 162. [CrossRef]
18. Nair, S.S.; Lenihan, C.R.; Montez-Rath, M.E.; Lowenberg, D.W.; Chertow, G.M.; Winkelmayer, W.C. Temporal trends in the incidence, treatment and outcomes of hip fracture after first kidney transplantation in the United States. *Arab. Archaeol. Epigr.* **2014**, *14*, 943–951. [CrossRef]
19. Nikkel, L.E.; Hollenbeak, C.S.; Fox, E.J.; Uemura, T.; Ghahramani, N. Risk of Fractures After Renal Transplantation in the United States. *Transplantation* **2009**, *87*, 1846–1851. [CrossRef]
20. McClung, M.R.; Lippuner, K.; Brandi, M.L.; Zanchetta, J.R.; Bone, H.G.; Chapurlat, R.; Hans, D.; Wang, A.; Zapalowski, C.; Libanati, C. Effect of denosumab on trabecular bone score in postmenopausal women with osteoporosis. *Osteoporos. Int.* **2017**, *28*, 2967–2973. [CrossRef]
21. Siris, E.; McDermott, M.; Pannacciulli, N.; Miller, P.D.; Lewiecki, E.M.; Chapurlat, R.; Jódar-Gimeno, E.; Huang, S.; Kanis, J.A. Estimation of Long-Term Efficacy of Denosumab Treatment in Postmenopausal Women With Osteoporosis: A FRAX- and Virtual Twin-Based Post Hoc Analysis From the FREEDOM and FREEDOM Extension Trials. *JBMR Plus* **2020**, *4*, e10348. [CrossRef]
22. Jamal, S.A.; Ljunggren, Ö.; Stehman-Breen, C.; Cummings, S.R.; McClung, M.R.; Goemaere, S.; Ebeling, P.R.; Franek, E.; Yang, Y.-C.; Egbuna, I.O.; et al. Effects of denosumab on fracture and bone mineral density by level of kidney function. *J. Bone Miner. Res.* **2011**, *26*, 1829–1835. [CrossRef]
23. Lamy, O.; Gonzalez-Rodriguez, E.; Stoll, D.; Hans, D.; Aubry-Rozier, B. Severe Rebound-Associated Vertebral Fractures After Denosumab Discontinuation: 9 Clinical Cases Report. *J. Clin. Endocrinol. Metab.* **2017**, *102*, 354–358. [CrossRef] [PubMed]
24. Everts-Graber, J.; Reichenbach, S.; Ziswiler, H.R.; Studer, U.; Lehmann, T. A Single Infusion of Zoledronate in Postmenopausal Women Following Denosumab Discontinuation Results in Partial Conservation of Bone Mass Gains. *J. Bone Miner. Res.* **2020**, *35*, 1207–1215. [CrossRef]
25. Block, G.A.; Bone, H.G.; Fang, L.; Lee, E.; Padhi, D. A single-dose study of denosumab in patients with various degrees of renal impairment. *J. Bone Miner. Res.* **2012**, *27*, 1471–1479. [CrossRef]
26. Bekker, P.J.; Holloway, D.L.; Rasmussen, A.S.; Murphy, R.; Martin, S.W.; Leese, P.T.; Holmes, G.B.; Dunstan, C.R.; DePaoli, A.M. A Single-Dose Placebo-Controlled Study of AMG 162, a Fully Human Monoclonal Antibody to RANKL, in Postmenopausal Women. *J. Bone Miner. Res.* **2004**, *19*, 1059–1066. [CrossRef] [PubMed]
27. Zebaze, R.M.; Libanati, C.; Austin, M.; Ghasem-Zadeh, A.; Hanley, D.A.; Zanchetta, J.R.; Thomas, T.; Boutroy, S.; Bogado, C.E.; Bilezikian, J.P.; et al. Differing effects of denosumab and alendronate on cortical and trabecular bone. *Bone* **2014**, *59*, 173–179. [CrossRef] [PubMed]
28. Seeman, E.; Libanati, C.; Austin, M.; Chapurlat, R.; Boyd, S.K.; Zebaze, R.; Hanley, D.A. The Transitory increase in PTH Following Denosumab Administration is Associated with Reduced Intracortical Porosity: A Dinstictive Attribute of Denosumab Therapy. *J. Bone Miner. Res.* **2011**, *26* (Suppl. S1), S1.
29. Evenepoel, P.; Behets, G.J.S.; Laurent, M.R.; D'Haese, P.C. Update on the role of bone biopsy in the management of patients with CKD–MBD. *J. Nephrol.* **2017**, *30*, 645–652. [CrossRef]
30. Karuthu, S.; Blumberg, E.A. Common Infections in Kidney Transplant Recipients. *Clin. J. Am. Soc. Nephrol.* **2012**, *7*, 2058–2070. [CrossRef]
31. Bonani, M.; Frey, D.; De Rougemont, O.; Mueller, N.J.; Mueller, T.F.; Graf, N.; Wüthrich, R.P. Infections in De Novo Kidney Transplant Recipients Treated With the RANKL Inhibitor Denosumab. *Transplantation* **2017**, *101*, 2139–2145. [CrossRef]

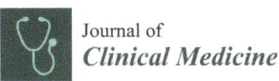

Article

High Cortico-Trabecular Transitional Zone Porosity and Reduced Trabecular Density in Men and Women with Stress Fractures

Afrodite Zendeli [1,*], Minh Bui [2], Lukas Fischer [3,4], Ali Ghasem-Zadeh [5], Wolfgang Schima [6] and Ego Seeman [5]

1. Medical Department of Internal Medicine, Rheumatology and Endocrinology at Krankenhaus Herz Jesu, 1030 Vienna, Austria
2. Centre for Epidemiology and Biostatistics, Melbourne School of Population and Global Health, University of Melbourne, Melbourne 3000, Australia; mbui@unimelb.edu.au
3. Computational Imaging Research Lab, Department of Biomedical Imaging and Image-Guided Therapy, Medical University of Vienna, 1090 Vienna, Austria; lukas.fischer@scch.at
4. Software Competence Center Hagenberg GmbH (SCCH), 4232 Hagenberg, Austria
5. Departments Medicine and Endocrinology, Austin Health, University of Melbourne, Melbourne 3084, Australia; alig@unimelb.edu.au (A.G.-Z.); egos@unimelb.edu.au (E.S.)
6. Department of Diagnostic and Interventional Radiology–Barmherzige Schwestern Krankenhaus, Goettlicher Heiland Krankenhaus und Sankt Josef Krankenhaus, 1060 Vienna, Austria; wolfgang.schima@khgh.at
* Correspondence: afrodite.zendeli@kh-herzjesu.at; Tel.: +43-664-1245621

Abstract: To determine whether stress fractures are associated with bone microstructural deterioration we quantified distal radial and the unfractured distal tibia using high resolution peripheral quantitative computed tomography in 26 cases with lower limb stress fractures (15 males, 11 females; mean age 37.1 ± 3.1 years) and 62 age-matched healthy controls (24 males, 38 females; mean age 35.0 ± 1.6 years). Relative to controls, in men, at the distal radius, cases had smaller cortical cross sectional area (CSA) ($p = 0.012$), higher porosity of the outer transitional zone (OTZ) ($p = 0.006$), inner transitional zone (ITZ) ($p = 0.043$) and the compact-appearing cortex (CC) ($p = 0.023$) while trabecular vBMD was lower ($p = 0.002$). At the distal tibia, cases also had a smaller cortical CSA ($p = 0.008$). Cortical porosity was not higher, but trabecular vBMD was lower ($p = 0.001$). Relative to controls, in women, cases had higher distal radial porosity of the OTZ ($p = 0.028$), ITZ ($p = 0.030$) not CC ($p = 0.054$). Trabecular vBMD was lower ($p = 0.041$). Distal tibial porosity was higher in the OTZ ($p = 0.035$), ITZ ($p = 0.009$), not CC. Stress fractures are associated with compromised cortical and trabecular microstructure.

Keywords: bone microstructural deterioration; cortical porosity; high resolution peripheral quantitative computed tomography; stress fracture

1. Introduction

Stress fractures are commonly the result of repetitive loading and are seen in athletes, military recruits and professional dancers, but stress fractures also occur in recreational athletic individuals as vigorous exercise increases the risk for injuries [1–5]. These fractures exist across a spectrum from low-grade stress reactions, bone marrow edema to complete fractures visible radiologically [6–8]. Despite there being little or no deficit in areal bone mineral density (aBMD) reported in most studies, there is evidence suggesting that abnormalities in bone microarchitecture are associated with these fractures and so may contribute to bone fragility [6,9–17].

As stress fractures are commonly reported in young adults abnormalities in bone morphology associated with these fractures are likely to be due, in part, to abnormalities in the growth and development of peak bone macro- and microstructure, not necessarily bone loss. In the diaphysis, a region composed virtually exclusively of cortical bone, growth in size and mass occurs by periosteal apposition with concurrent endocortical resorptive modeling producing a radial 'modeling drift' so the cortex becomes thinner relative to its increasing total cross-sectional area (CSA) [18,19].

By contrast, the metaphyseal region contains both cortical and trabecular bone. The cortical bone is formed by condensation or 'corticalization' of trabeculae as they arise from the periphery of the growth plate. Adjacent trabeculae coalesce by bone formation upon their surfaces while more centrally placed trabeculae form the metaphyseal trabecular compartment. The cortico-trabecular transitional region so formed between the cortical bone and the more centrally placed trabecular bone is composed of mineralized bone matrix that transitions from the more compact cortical configuration to a more open spongy trabecular configuration with more void volume (porosity) [20].

The purpose of this study was to quantify any association between bone microstructure and the presence of a stress fracture in the lower limb. We hypothesized that young adult individuals sustaining stress fractures have thinner and more porous cortices and reduced trabecular density characterised by reduced numbers and thinner trabeculae.

2. Materials and Methods

This was a cross sectional case control study. Thirty-four patients presenting with acute focal lower limb pain were assessed for possible stress fractures using magnetic resonance imaging (MRI) [21]. Participants were recruited from the osteoporosis out-patients department of the St. Vincent Hospital and the Austrian Military Hospital in Vienna/Austria.

Patients were included if they were above 18 years of age and sustained a recent MRI-diagnosed stress fracture within 14 days prior to inclusion. Patients receiving any medication affecting bone metabolism (parathyroid hormone, intravenous or oral bisphosphonate, strontium ranelate, raloxifene, hormonal replacement therapy or anabolic steroids) were excluded. Other exclusion criteria included the presence of metabolic bone disease, a history of malignancy, hypo- or hyperparathyroidism, pregnancy and lactation.

Of the 34 subjects, 26 were included (11 females, 15 males). The study group included five military recruits, three long distance runners, one sprinter and one professional tennis player, the other 16 patients were recreational sportsmen and women. We compared these results with data obtained from 62 healthy age- and sex matched Caucasian controls (42 Austrian subjects, 20 Australian subjects). The study was approved and supervised by an independent local ethics committee in Vienna/Austria.

2.1. Magnetic Resonance Imaging

Examinations were performed on 1.5 or 3.0 T scanners (Signa HDx, GE Healthcare, USA; Intera, Philips, The Netherlands, Avanto, Siemens, Germany) using a phased-array extremity coil. All MRI examinations included an axial T1-weighted spin-echo (SE) sequence and an axial fat-suppressed T2-weighted turbo spin-echo (TSE) or a short-tau inversion recovery (STIR) sequence. The presence of bone marrow edema and stress fracture was seen as decreased signal intensity on T1 weighted SE images, and markedly increased signal intensity on STIR images or T2 weighted fat-suppressed TSE images [22]. In 16 patients High Resolution Multi-Detector CT (HR-MDCT) scanning was performed with a 128-row MDCT scanner (Somatom AS+, Siemens, Forchheim, Germany). Images were acquired in ultrahigh resolution (UHR) mode covering the area of interest as defined by MRI. Slice thickness was 0.6 mm, field of view of 160–300 mm (x-axis) × 160–300 mm (y-axis), with a matrix of 512 × 512, which equates to a resolution of 0.3–0.6 mm (x-axis) × 0.3–0.6 mm (y-axis) × 0.6 mm slice thickness (z-axis). A linear stress fracture was visible in 16 of 26 cases (61.5%) [23]. In 8 patients the fracture was identified in the metatarsals, in 8 patients in the calcaneus and ankle, in 6 patients in the proximal tibia adjacent to the knee, in 2 patients in the femur condyle, and in 2 patients in the hip (one femoral head and one acetabulum).

2.2. Measurement of Bone Microarchitecture

Scans were obtained from the non-dominant distal radius and unfractured side of the distal tibia using by HR-pQCT scanner (XtremeCT; Scanco Medical AG, Brüttisellen, Switzerland) using the standard in vivo protocol (60 kVp, 900 µA, 100-ms integration time) [24]. StrAx1.0 is a new algorithm that segments bone from background, and then bone into its compact appearing cortex (CC), outer transitional zone (OTZ) and inner transitional zone (ITZ), and trabecular compartments (see Figure 1); and in so doing correctly confines the trabecularized cortex (i.e., cortical fragments) to the transitional zone rather than incorrectly allocating cortical fragments (which look like trabeculae) to the medullary compartment; a segmentation error which overestimates 'trabecular' density [25]. The OTZ is the trabecularized cortex adjacent to the CC whereas the ITZ is the trabecularized cortex adjacent to the medullary cavity. The latter also contains true trabecular bone (of growth plate origin).

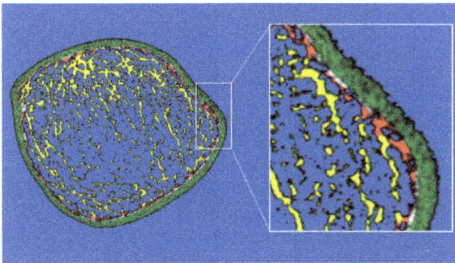

Figure 1. HR-pQCT image of the distal tibia of an 18-year-old male patient with a stress fracture. Compact appearing cortex (green); outer transitional zone (white); inner transitional zone (red); medullary area (yellow).

Of the 110 slices in the region of interest imaged by HR-pQCT the analysis is restricted to the 40 most proximal slices because the 70 distal slices often have very thin cortices, and hence are unsuitable for unambiguous quantification of cortical porosity. Porosity was quantified as previously reported. The coefficient of variation for segmentation and quantification of porosity ranges from 0.54 to 3.98% depending on the compartment [26,27].

2.3. Statistical Analysis

Testing for normality of distribution of a variable was conducted using Shapiro–Wilk test. Two sample t-test was used to test the difference in mean between cases and controls if the data was approximate normal, otherwise nonparametric Mann–Whitney test was used to test the difference in the medians. Post hoc power calculations were done. Initially, the statistical test was computed without adjustment for other covariates, and then adjustment for age and height was carried out. Spearman's correlations were used to assess relationships between porosity and medullary CSA/total CSA. Univariate logistic analysis was used to examine the association between porosity of CC, OTZ, ITZ and trabecular volumetric BMD and fracture risk. All variables were standardized to have mean of 0 and SD of 1 and were used to predict the odds ratio (OR). The analyses were performed on data at both tibia and radius site for males and females separately. We used statistical software STATA (StataCorp, 2009), version 11, to conduct all analyses. p-values were computed for two-sided tests and values less than 0.05 were considered as significant.

3. Results

Characteristics of the entire study population are described in Table 1.

Table 1. Characteristics of cases and controls.

	Males	Cases (15)	Controls (24)	p
	Age [ys]	29.2 ± 2.6	30.9 ± 1.7	0.450
	Weight [kg]	77.5 ± 3.5	84.1 ± 3.1	0.180
	Height [m]	1.81 ± 0.02	1.78 ± 0.02	0.140
	Females	Cases (11)	Controls (38)	p
	Age [ys]	47.8 ± 4.7	40.5 ± 2.3	0.140
	Weight [kg]	68.5 ± 5.4	61.8 ± 1.2	0.340
	Height [m]	1.67 ± 0.02	1.65 ± 0.01	0.290

Results are shown as mean ± SE (Standard error of mean); p-value comparing cases and controls ($p < 0.05$).

3.1. Males

As shown in Figure 1 and Table 2, relative to controls, at the distal radius, cases had smaller cortical CSA ($p = 0.012$) due to a smaller CC CSA ($p = 0.005$) and a smaller OTZ CSA ($p = 0.003$). Cases had higher porosity of the OTZ ($p = 0.006$), ITZ ($p = 0.043$) and CC ($p = 0.023$). Cortical vBMD was lower ($p = 0.002$). Trabecular vBMD was lower ($p = 0.002$). Trabecular thickness was reduced ($p = 0.001$), connectivity was reduced ($p = 0.012$) and separation increased ($p = 0.007$) (Figure 1, Table 2).

Table 2. Comparison of microarchitecture of the distal radius and distal tibia in cases and controls.

	Distal Radius						Distal Tibia					
	Males			Females			Males			Females		
	Cases (15)	Controls (24)	p	Cases (11)	Controls (38)	p	Cases (15)	Controls (24)	p	Cases (11)	Controls (38)	p
TCSA [mm^2]	314 ± 25	287 ± 14	0.418 **	225 ± 8.1	203 ± 5.9	0.878 *	820 ± 54	762 ± 34	0.841 **	625 ± 19	603 ± 16	0.768 *
Medullary CSA [mm^2]	215 ± 24	177 ± 11	0.685 **	149 ± 7.7	126 ± 5.3	0.655 *	629 ± 52	553 ± 32	0.714 **	467 ± 16	437 ± 15	0.941 *
Medullary CSA/TCSA	67.1 ± 1.7	60.9 ± 1.2	0.006 *	66.0 ± 1.7	61.4 ± 1.0	0.161 *	75.8 ± 1.4	71.8 ± 1.1	0.059 *	74.5 ± 0.8	71.9 ± 0.7	0.326 *
Cortical CSA [mm^2]	98.7 ± 2.4	110 ± 4.3	0.012 *	76.0 ± 3.8	76.6 ± 1.5	0.363 *	190.3 ± 6.4	208.7 ± 6.0	0.008 *	159 ± 5.9	166 ± 2.6	0.272 *
CC CSA [mm^2]	62.8 ± 1.8	73.4 ± 3.2	0.005 *	49.6 ± 3.0	49.7 ± 1.2	0.414 **	125 ± 5.9	139 ± 5.3	0.015 *	104 ± 5.2	108 ± 2.2	0.590 *
OTZ CSA [mm^2]	8.12 ± 0.2	9.86 ± 0.5	0.003 *	6.63 ± 0.5	6.47 ± 0.2	0.320 **	17.5 ± 0.9	20.9 ± 1.1	0.012 **	13.8 ± 0.8	14.9 ± 0.4	0.349 *
ITZ CSA [mm^2]	27.8 ± 1.4	26.4 ± 1.4	0.616 *	19.8 ± 0.9	20.4 ± 0.7	0.139 *	48.9 ± 2.9	49.0 ± 1.9	0.512 *	41.4 ± 1.8	43.5 ± 1.5	0.182 *
Cortical CSA/TCSA	32.9 ± 1.7	39.1 ± 1.2	0.006 *	34.0 ± 1.6	38.6 ± 0.9	0.161 *	24.2 ± 1.4	28.2 ± 1.1	0.059 *	25.5 ± 0.8	28.1 ± 0.7	0.326 *
Porosity CC [%]	37.3 ± 2.0	32.2 ± 1.5	0.023 *	33.4 ± 1.8	29.6 ± 0.7	0.054 *	36.4 ± 1.1	33.7 ± 0.9	0.090 *	38.4 ± 2.2	33.8 ± 1.1	0.295 **
Porosity OTZ [%]	55.9 ± 1.2	52.0 ± 0.9	0.006 *	55.2 ± 1.1	52.3 ± 0.4	0.028 **	52.2 ± 0.9	50.4 ± 0.7	0.058 *	54.0 ± 1.0	50.8 ± 0.5	0.035 **
Porosity ITZ [%]	66.0 ± 0.6	64.4 ± 0.6	0.043 *	65.8 ± 0.7	64.3 ± 0.3	0.030 *	61.8 ± 0.7	61.3 ± 0.5	0.245 *	63.5 ± 0.7	61.4 ± 0.3	0.009 *
Total vBMD [mgHA/cm^3]	332 ± 16	412 ± 13	0.001 *	309 ± 21	369 ± 12	0.061	310 ± 15	366 ± 11	0.002 *	266 ± 12	311 ± 8.5	0.104 *
Cortical vBMD [mg HA/cm^3]	657 ± 20	731 ± 16	0.002 *	684 ± 20	721 ± 9.9	0.175 *	674 ± 13	717 ± 11	0.016 *	630 ± 20	684 ± 12	0.106 *
Tr. vBMD [mg HA/cm^3]	168 ± 5.9	205 ± 8.9	0.002 *	113 ± 11	144 ± 5.4	0.041 *	192 ± 9.5	225 ± 8.7	0.001 *	141 ± 8.7	1612 ± 5.4	0.354 *
Tr. thickness [mm]	0.07 ± 0.003	0.10 ± 0.004	0.001 *	0.05 ± 0.006	0.06 ± 0.003	0.056 *	0.08 ± 0.005	0.1 ± 0.004	0.0004 *	0.06 ± 0.004	0.07 ± 0.003	0.332 *
Tr. connectivity density [1/mm^2]	2.89 ± 0.2	3.56 ± 0.2	0.012 *	1.65 ± 0.2	2.16 ± 0.1	0.127 *	3.47 ± 0.2	4.09 ± 0.3	0.006 *	2.27 ± 0.2	2.67 ± 0.1	0.570 *
Tr. separation [mm]	0.89 ± 0.04	0.80 ± 0.03	0.007 *	1.15 ± 0.09	0.96 ± 0.03	0.070 **	0.86 ± 0.04	0.78 ± 0.03	0.007 *	1.06 ± 0.05	1.00 ± 0.03	0.885 *
Tr. number [1/mm^2]	3.16 ± 0.1	3.25 ± 0.1	0.246 *	2.60 ± 0.2	2.87 ± 0.1	0.320 **	3.67 ± 0.1	3.70 ± 0.1	0.166 *	3.21 ± 0.1	3.29 ± 0.08	0.587 *

Results are shown as mean ± SE (standard error of mean); p-value comparing healthy controls and fracture patients, adjusted for age and height, using * two-sample t-test and ** nonparametric Mann–Whitney test on the residuals of regression of a variable on age and height ($p < 0.05$). TCSA = total cross sectional area, CSA = cross-sectional area; CC = compact-appearing cortex; OTZ = outer transitional zone; ITZ = inner transitional zone; vBMD = volumetric bone mineral density; Tr = trabecular; HA = hydroxyapatite.

At the distal tibia, relative to controls, cases had a smaller cortical CSA ($p = 0.008$) due to smaller CC CSA ($p = 0.015$) and a smaller OTZ CSA ($p = 0.012$). Porosity was not higher at this site. Cortical vBMD was lower ($p = 0.016$). Trabecular vBMD was lower ($p = 0.001$). Trabecular thickness was reduced ($p = 0.0004$), connectivity was reduced ($p = 0.006$) and separation increased ($p = 0.007$) (Table 2).

3.2. Females

The results were similar in females. Relative to controls, at the distal radius, cases had significant higher porosity of the OTZ ($p = 0.028$) and ITZ ($p = 0.030$), but porosity was not significantly higher at CC ($p = 0.054$). Cortical vBMD was not lower, but trabecular vBMD was lower ($p = 0.041$). At the distal tibia, porosity was higher in the OTZ ($p = 0.035$) and ITZ ($p = 0.009$) but not at the CC. Cortical and trabecular vBMD were not lower. No differences in trabecular morphology were detected at either site (Table 2).

In both sexes, at both sites, associations were detected between porosity of CC, OTZ and ITZ and medullary CSA/TCSA ($p < 0.001$, except for the distal radius ITZ in males with $p = 0.004$) (Figure 2). Cortical porosity was associated with an increased odds of stress fracture, with ORs ranging from 1.24 to 3.13 depending on the cortical compartment, though not all sites demonstrated a statistically significant increase in odds. Higher trabecular vBMD was protective, demonstrating a statistically significantly lower odds of fracture at the distal radius in males and females and the distal tibia in males (Figure 3).

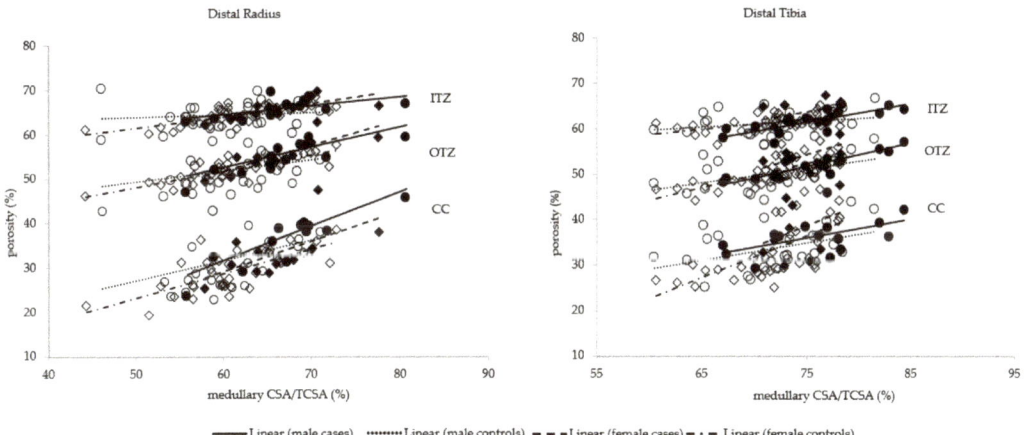

Figure 2. Porosity of the compact appearing cortex (CC), outer and inner transitional zones (OTZ, ITZ) as a function of medullary cross-sectional area (CSA)/total CSA at the distal radius and distal tibia in male cases (filled dots), male controls (open dots), female cases (filled squares) and female controls (open squares). All $p < 0.001$ except for the distal radius ITZ in males ($p = 0.004$).

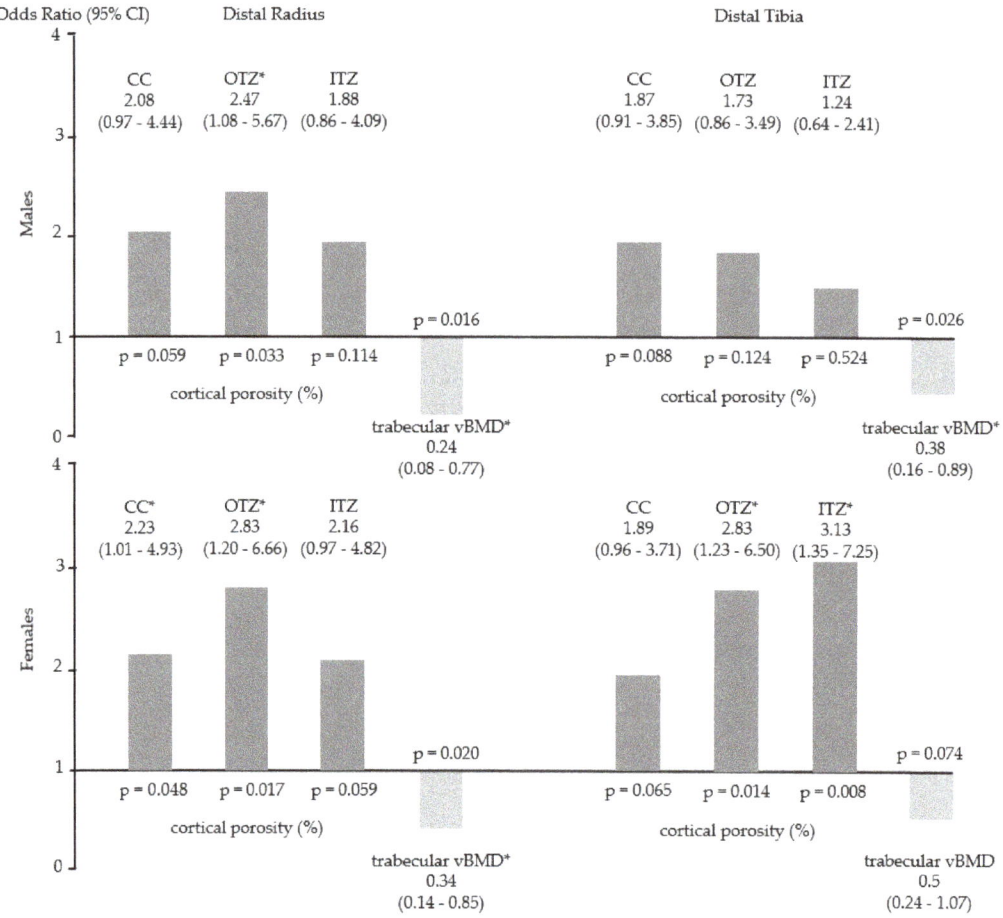

Figure 3. Odds ratio (OR) for fracture (mean and 95% Confidence Intervals, CI) for porosity of the compact appearing cortex (CC), outer and inner transitional zones (OTZ, ITZ) and trabecular volumetric bone mineral density (vBMD) at distal radius and distal tibia in males and females. * = significant *p*-values.

4. Discussion

We report that men and women with stress fractures had increased porosity, observed in the inner and outer cortico-trabecular transitional zones of the distal radius in both sexes and distal tibia in female cases. Porosity of the compact appearing cortex was increased only in males at the distal radius. Odds ratio for a stress fracture was associated with increased porosity of the outer cortico-trabecular transitional zone in three of four locations. Cortical vBMD, which in part, reflects porosity, was also reduced. Furthermore, trabecular vBMD was lower due to reduced trabecular thickness, not numbers. Males with stress fractures had thinner trabeculae with greater separation.

Stress fractures in military cadets and athletes have been subject of most studies using dual x-ray absorptiometry (DXA), x-ray and single photon absorptiometry or nuclear bone scanning [11–14,28]. Fewer studies have used peripheral quantitative computed tomography (pQCT), or HRpQCT to describe bone characteristics in association with stress fractures [10,17,29].

Our findings confirm some, not all previous studies. For example, Beck et al., reported thinner cortices in female cadets and narrower subperiosteal diameters in male cases [12].

Reduced cortical area was also reported by Popp et al., in runners with a stress fracture [30]. While the finding of greater total bone cross sectional was not statistically significant in our study, Weidauer et al., also reported greater periosteal circumference in athletes with a stress fracture [31]. Among military recruits and male runners, Giladi et al., and Popp et al., reported reduced tibial cross sectional area, while HRpQCT-analyses of our cases and work by Schanda et al., reported larger tibial and radial cross sectional area [14,17,29]. These subjects also had reduced cortical vBMD, reduced cortical CSA with increased cortical porosity. In both studies, and work by Schnackenburg et al., trabecular vBMD was found to be reduced [10].

While bone loss cannot be excluded as a cause of these deficits, 20 of the 26 subjects were under 50 years of age. Therefore, higher porosity in the cortico-trabecular junctional zone, with less consistently elevated porosity of the compact cortex, and deficits in trabecular bone may have their origin in the growth-related assembly of bone in some subjects rather than its age-related deterioration [18]. We cannot distinguish these alternatives in a cross sectional study.

We suggest that the thinner and more porous metaphyseal cortex in cases is, in part, the result of a reduction in bone formation upon trabeculae emerging from the periphery of the growth plate. These may fail to coalesce leaving a thinner and more porous cortex (failed corticalization of trabeculae). Reduced bone formation upon trabeculae emerging from the centre of the growth plate may result in the lower metaphyseal trabecular density [32]. This is supported by the presence of a smaller and more porous OTZ suggesting impairment of coalescence as thinner and more separated trabeculae fail to coalesce leaving larger pores adjacent to CC. The more porous cortex will also be thinner due to failure of cortical thickening taking place by adsorption of trabeculae upon the endocortical surface. The thinner cortices are unlikely to be due to reduced periosteal apposition because total CSA was not reduced. Less corticalization of trabeculae may also be partly responsible for the relatively larger medullary canal area as adsorption of trabecular bone upon the endocortical surface is partly responsible for reducing medullary canal area from the 'inside'.

The relatively larger medullary canal area, thinner cortices and higher porosity in the cases may also be due to greater growth related endocortical resorptive modeling excavating a larger medullary canal during growth and concurrent intracortical resorptive remodeling forming osteons, each with their central Haversian canal. The cases were slightly taller and had wider bones. Taller persons assemble their wider bones by excavation of a disproportionately larger medullary canal such that the wider bone has a thinner cortex relative to its total CSA [19]. Wider bones are assembled with less material relative to their size because resistance to bending is a fourth power function of their radius–less material is needed to achieve a given bending strength than is needed in a narrower bone [33,34].

Wider bones may also be more porous. The greater amount of modeling required to assemble a larger total and medullary CSA is accompanied by more intracortical remodeling forming secondary cortical osteons, each with their Haversian canal (which forms most 'porosity' as seen in cross section) [35]. This is suggested by the positive correlation between medullary canal area and porosity reported here, and elsewhere [19]. This correlation is consistent with the notion of coordinated assembly of the external size, shape and internal architecture of bone by periosteal, intracortical, endocortical surface dependent modeling and remodeling [36].

The increased risk for fracture reported in taller persons is inconsistent with greater resistance to bending observed in wider bones [19]. However, the greater porosity and relatively thinner cortices of wider bones may offset the advantage of greater width. Resistance to bending is a 4th power function of the distance a unit volume of bone is placed from the neutral axis of a long bone [33]. However, resistance to bending is a 7th power function of cortical porosity and a 3rd power function of trabecular density, so the deleterious effect of microstructural abnormalities may offset any benefit achieved by greater bone width [37]. The ability of bone to deform without cracking decreases as porosity increases [37,38]. The porosity may form stress concentrators predisposing a higher risk to fracture following repetitive loading [39]. Additionally, porosity may reduce compressive strength as the cross-sectional area of the cortex is less mineralized bone matrix and more void area [38].

Both deterioration in cortical and trabecular bone may result from impaired growth, particularly because cortical bone at metaphysis is partly formed by condensation of trabeculae in the periphery of the growth plate to form the cortex while trabeculae emerging from the center of the growth plate form metaphyseal trabecular bone.

Bone loss contributing to the deficits cannot be excluded but appears to be less likely given the age of the cases. Remodeling initiated upon Haversian canal surfaces excavate resorptive cavities enlarging the canal focally producing higher intracortical porosity and stress concentrators predisposing to micro cracks in cortical bone [39]. Even though remodeling may be still balanced in young adults, the refilling phase takes about 3 months, so resorption cavities upon trabeculae surfaces form stress concentrators which may predispose to microdamage in the face of repetitive strain [40]. The repetitive strains lead to accumulation of unrepaired microdamage ultimately producing a stress fracture [41–43].

This study has several limitations. First, it was a cross-sectional case control study. We cannot distinguish whether the porosity contributed to the stress fracture or whether the sequence of events was the reverse. However, measurements were performed within 14 days after injury on the contralateral side, which makes the latter less likely. Most of the cases were recreational sportsmen and women as were controls. We have no data concerning daily physical activity of the controls. Second, most of the male controls were from Australia. However, results were similar in females. Female cases and controls were Austrian. Third, the small number of cases, particularly in females, may have limited the power to achieve statistical significance of differences between cases and controls. Further investigation with a prospective study design and larger sample size are needed. The stress fractures in the cases were diagnosed in their lower limbs whereas differences in bone microstructure were measured at the distal tibia and the distal radius [26,44–46]. Despite this limitation Mikolajewicz et al., and others have reported fracture prediction using HRpQCT. [24,47,48]. Finally, the contribution of pore size and pore number to the reduction in total porosity was not evaluated.

5. Conclusions

In summary, stress fractures are common among young adults and are likely to be partly the result of deficits in cortical and trabecular bone microstructure. Whether these deficits have their origin established during growth, during advancing age or both requires further study.

Author Contributions: Study design: A.Z. Study conduct: A.Z. and E.S. Data collection: A.Z., L.F., A.G.-Z. and W.S. Data analysis and statistical calculations: A.Z., M.B. and E.S. Data interpretation: all authors; Drafting manuscript: A.Z. and E.S. All authors contributed to the development and critical revision of the manuscript and approved the final version for submission. A.Z. takes responsibility for integrity of the data analysis. All authors have read and agreed to the published version of the manuscript.

Funding: This study was not sponsored by any pharmaceutical company. Vinforce receives academic funding grants.

Institutional Review Board Statement: The study was approved by the local ethical committee (VINFORCE-013AZ) and conducted in accordance with the Declaration of Helsinki.

Informed Consent Statement: All patients agreed to participate to the study and signed an informed consent form.

Data Availability Statement: The data presented in this study are available on request from the corresponding author.

Acknowledgments: The authors thank Colonel Christian Rizzi (Van Swieten Kaserne-Austrian Military Hospital Vienna/Austria) for the help in recruitment of several cases with stress fracture. We further thank Christina Marterer and Rahbarnia Arastoo for HR-pQCT scanning of the participants.

Conflicts of Interest: A.G.-Z. is one of the inventors of the StrAx1.0 algorithm. E.S. is an inventor of the StrAx1.0 algorithm and Directors of Straxcorp. All other authors state that they have no conflicts of interest.

References

1. Saunier, J.; Chapurlat, R. Stress fracture in athletes. *Jt. Bone Spine* **2018**, *85*, 307–310. [CrossRef]
2. Waterman, B.R.; Gun, B.; Bader, J.O.; Orr, J.D.; Belmont, P.J.J. Epidemiology of Lower Extremity Stress Fractures in the United States Military. *Mil Med.* **2016**, *181*, 1308–1313. [CrossRef]
3. McInnis, K.C.; Ramey, L.N. High-Risk Stress Fractures: Diagnosis and Management. *PM&R* **2016**, *8*, S113–S124. [CrossRef]
4. Bennell, K.L.; Malcolm, S.A.; Thomas, S.A.; Reid, S.J.; Brukner, P.D.; Ebeling, P.R.; Wark, J.D. Risk Factors for Stress Fractures in Track and Field Athletes: A Twelve-Month Prospective Study. *Am. J. Sports Med.* **1996**, *24*, 810–818. [CrossRef] [PubMed]
5. Tschopp, M.; Brunner, F. Diseases and overuse injuries of the lower extremities in long distance runners. *Z. Rheumatol.* **2017**, *76*, 443–450. [CrossRef]
6. Burr, D.B.; Martin, R.B.; Schaffler, M.B.; Radin, E.L. Bone remodeling in response to in vivo fatigue microdamage. *J. Biomech.* **1985**, *18*, 189–200. [CrossRef]
7. Schaffler, M.B.; Jepsen, K.J. Fatigue and repair in bone. *Int. J. Fatigue* **2000**, *22*, 839–846. [CrossRef]
8. Rosenberg, Z.; Zanetti, M. Imaging of the Foot and Ankle. In *Musculoskeletal Diseases*; Springer: Berlin/Heidelberg, Germany, 2005; pp. 39–47.
9. Turner, C.H.; Burr, D.B. Basic biomechanical measurements of bone: A tutorial. *Bone* **1993**, *14*, 595–608. [CrossRef]
10. Schnackenburg, K.E.; Macdonald, H.M.; Ferber, R.; Wiley, J.P.; Boyd, S.K. Bone Quality and Muscle Strength in Female Athletes with Lower Limb Stress Fractures. *Med. Sci. Sports Exerc.* **2011**, *43*, 2110–2119. [CrossRef]
11. Beck, T.J.; Ruff, C.B.; Mourtada, F.A.; Shaffer, R.A.; Maxwell-Williams, K.; Kao, G.L.; Sartoris, D.J.; Brodine, S. Dual-energy X-ray absorptiometry derived structural geometry for stress fracture prediction in male U.S. marine corps recruits. *J. Bone Miner. Res.* **1996**, *11*, 645–653. [CrossRef] [PubMed]
12. Beck, T.J.; Ruff, C.B.; Shaffer, R.A.; Betsinger, K.; Trone, D.W.; Brodine, S.K. Stress fracture in military recruits: Gender differences in muscle and bone susceptibility factors. *Bone* **2000**, *27*, 437–444. [CrossRef]
13. Armstrong, D.W.; Rue, J.-P.H.; Wilckens, J.H.; Frassica, F.J. Stress fracture injury in young military men and women. *Bone* **2004**, *35*, 806–816. [CrossRef]
14. Giladi, M.; Milgrom, C.; Simkin, A.; Stein, M.; Kashtan, H.; Margulies, J.; Rand, N.; Chisin, R.; Steinberg, R.; Aharonson, Z. Stress fractures and tibial bone width. A risk factor. *J. Bone Jt. Surg. Ser. B* **1987**, *69*, 326–329. [CrossRef] [PubMed]
15. Jepsen, K.J.; Evans, R.; Negus, C.H.; Gagnier, J.J.; Centi, A.; Erlich, T.; Hadid, A.; Yanovich, R.; Moran, D.S. Variation in tibial functionality and fracture susceptibility among healthy, young adults arises from the acquisition of biologically distinct sets of traits. *J. Bone Miner. Res.* **2013**, *28*, 1290–1300. [CrossRef]
16. Cosman, F.; Ruffing, J.; Zion, M.; Uhorchak, J.; Ralston, S.; Tendy, S.; McGuigan, F.E.; Lindsay, R.; Nieves, J. Determinants of stress fracture risk in United States Military Academy cadets. *Bone* **2013**, *55*, 359–366. [CrossRef] [PubMed]
17. Schanda, J.E.; Kocijan, R.; Resch, H.; Baierl, A.; Feichtinger, X.; Mittermayr, R.; Plachel, F.; Wakolbinger, R.; Wolff, K.; Fialka, C.; et al. Bone Stress Injuries Are Associated with Differences in Bone Microarchitecture in Male Professional Soldiers. *J. Orthop. Res.* **2019**, *37*, 2516–2523. [CrossRef]
18. Seeman, E. From Density to Structure: Growing Up and Growing Old on the Surfaces of Bone. *J. Bone Miner. Res.* **1997**, *12*, 509–521. [CrossRef]
19. Bjørnerem, Å.; Bui, Q.M.; Ghasem-Zadeh, A.; Hopper, J.L.; Zebaze, R.; Seeman, E. Fracture risk and height: An association partly accounted for by cortical porosity of relatively thinner cortices. *J. Bone Miner. Res.* **2013**, *28*, 2017–2026. [CrossRef]
20. Cadet, E.R.; Gafni, R.I.; McCarthy, E.F.; McCray, D.R.; Bacher, J.D.; Barnes, K.M.; Baron, J. Mechanisms responsible for longitudinal growth of the cortex: Coalescence of trabecular bone into cortical bone. *J. Bone Jt. Surg. Am.* **2003**, *85*, 1739–1748. [CrossRef]
21. Matcuk, G.R.J.; Mahanty, S.R.; Skalski, M.R.; Patel, D.B.; White, E.A.; Gottsegen, C.J. Stress fractures: Pathophysiology, clinical presentation, imaging features, and treatment options. *Emerg. Radiol.* **2016**, *23*, 365–375. [CrossRef]
22. Boks, S.S.; Vroegindeweij, D.; Koes, B.W.; Bernsen, R.M.D.; Hunink, M.G.M.; Bierma-Zeinstra, S.M.A. MRI Follow-Up of Posttraumatic Bone Bruises of the Knee in General Practice. *Am. J. Roentgenol.* **2007**, *189*, 556–562. [CrossRef] [PubMed]
23. Kaeding, C.C.; Miller, T. The Comprehensive Description of Stress Fractures: A New Classification System. *J. Bone Jt. Surg.* **2013**, *95*, 1214–1220. [CrossRef] [PubMed]
24. Boutroy, S.; Bouxsein, M.L.; Munoz, F.; Delmas, P.D. In VivoAssessment of Trabecular Bone Microarchitecture by High-Resolution Peripheral Quantitative Computed Tomography. *J. Clin. Endocrinol. Metab.* **2005**, *90*, 6508–6515. [CrossRef] [PubMed]
25. Zebaze, R.; Ghasem-Zadeh, A.; Mbala, A.; Seeman, E. A new method of segmentation of compact-appearing, transitional and trabecular compartments and quantification of cortical porosity from high resolution peripheral quantitative computed tomographic images. *Bone* **2013**, *54*, 8–20. [CrossRef] [PubMed]

26. Bala, Y.; Zebaze, R.; Ghasem-Zadeh, A.; Atkinson, E.J.; Iuliano, S.; Peterson, J.M.; Amin, S.; Bjørnerem, Å.; Melton, L.J.; Johansson, H.; et al. Cortical Porosity Identifies Women with Osteopenia at Increased Risk for Forearm Fractures. *J. Bone Miner. Res.* **2014**, *29*, 1356–1362. [CrossRef]
27. Zebaze, R.M.; Libanati, C.; Austin, M.; Ghasem-Zadeh, A.; Hanley, D.A.; Zanchetta, J.R.; Thomas, T.; Boutroy, S.; Bogado, C.E.; Bilezikian, J.P.; et al. Differing effects of denosumab and alendronate on cortical and trabecular bone. *Bone* **2014**, *59*, 173–179. [CrossRef]
28. Giladi, M.; Milgrom, C.; Simkin, A.; Danon, Y. Stress fractures. Identifiable risk factors. *Am. J. Sports Med.* **1991**, *19*, 647–652. [CrossRef] [PubMed]
29. Popp, K.L.; Frye, A.C.; Stovitz, S.D.; Hughes, J.M. Bone geometry and lower extremity bone stress injuries in male runners. *J. Sci. Med. Sport* **2020**, *23*, 145–150. [CrossRef]
30. Popp, K.L.; Hughes, J.M.; Smock, A.J.; Novotny, S.A.; Stovitz, S.D.; Koehler, S.M.; Petit, M.A. Bone Geometry, Strength, and Muscle Size in Runners with a History of Stress Fracture. *Med. Sci. Sports Exerc.* **2009**, *41*, 2145–2150. [CrossRef] [PubMed]
31. Weidauer, L.A.; Binkley, T.; Vukovich, M.; Specker, B. Greater Polar Moment of Inertia at the Tibia in Athletes Who Develop Stress Fractures. *Orthop. J. Sports Med.* **2014**, *2*. [CrossRef]
32. Wang, Q.; Wang, X.-F.; Iuliano-Burns, S.; Ghasem-Zadeh, A.; Zebaze, R.; Seeman, E. Rapid growth produces transient cortical weakness: A risk factor for metaphyseal fractures during puberty. *J. Bone Miner. Res.* **2010**, *25*, 1521–1526. [CrossRef] [PubMed]
33. Ruff, C.B.; Hayes, W.C. Subperiosteal expansion and cortical remodeling of the human femur and tibia with aging. *Science* **1982**, *217*, 945–948. [CrossRef] [PubMed]
34. Zebaze, R.M.D.; Jones, A.; Welsh, F.; Knackstedt, M.; Seeman, E. Femoral neck shape and the spatial distribution of its mineral mass varies with its size: Clinical and biomechanical implications. *Bone* **2005**, *37*, 243–252. [CrossRef]
35. Thomas, C.D.L.; Feik, S.A.; Clement, J.G. Increase in pore area, and not pore density, is the main determinant in the development of porosity in human cortical bone. *J. Anat.* **2006**, *209*, 219–230. [CrossRef] [PubMed]
36. Seeman, E. Age- and Menopause-Related Bone Loss Compromise Cortical and Trabecular Microstructure. *J. Gerontol. Ser. A Boil. Sci. Med Sci.* **2013**, *68*, 1218–1225. [CrossRef] [PubMed]
37. Schaffler, M.B.; Burr, D.B. Stiffness of compact bone: Effects of porosity and density. *J. Biomech.* **1988**, *21*, 13–16. [CrossRef]
38. Yeni, Y.N.; Brown, C.U.; Wang, Z.; Norman, T.L. The influence of bone morphology on fracture toughness of the human femur and tibia. *Bone* **1997**, *21*, 453–459. [CrossRef]
39. Currey, J.D. The many adaptations of bone. *J. Biomech.* **2003**, *36*, 1487–1495. [CrossRef]
40. Parfitt, A.M. Targeted and nontargeted bone remodeling: Relationship to basic multicellular unit origination and progression. *Bone* **2002**, *30*, 5–7. [CrossRef]
41. Schaffler, M.B.; Radin, E.L.; Burr, D.B. Mechanical and morphological effects of strain rate on fatigue of compact bone. *Bone* **1989**, *10*, 207–214. [CrossRef]
42. Pattin, C.A.; Caler, W.E.; Carter, D.R. Cyclic mechanical property degradation during fatigue loading of cortical bone. *J. Biomech.* **1996**, *29*, 69–79. [CrossRef]
43. Hughes, J.M.; Popp, K.L.; Yanovich, R.; Bouxsein, M.L.; Matheny, J.R.W. The role of adaptive bone formation in the etiology of stress fracture. *Exp. Biol. Med.* **2017**, *242*, 897–906. [CrossRef]
44. Patsch, J.M.; Burghardt, A.J.; Kazakia, G.; Majumdar, S. Noninvasive imaging of bone microarchitecture. *Ann. N. Y. Acad. Sci.* **2011**, *1240*, 77–87. [CrossRef]
45. Szulc, P.; Boutroy, S.; Chapurlat, R. Prediction of Fractures in Men Using Bone Microarchitectural Parameters Assessed by High-Resolution Peripheral Quantitative Computed Tomography-The Prospective STRAMBO Study. *J. Bone Miner. Res.* **2018**, *33*, 1470–1479. [CrossRef]
46. Vilayphiou, N.; Boutroy, S.; Szulc, P.; Van Rietbergen, B.; Munoz, F.; Delmas, P.D.; Chapurlat, R. Finite element analysis performed on radius and tibia HR-pQCT images and fragility fractures at all sites in men. *J. Bone Miner. Res.* **2011**, *26*, 965–973. [CrossRef] [PubMed]
47. Mikolajewicz, N.; Bishop, N.; Burghardt, A.J.; Folkestad, L.; Hall, A.; Kozloff, K.M.; Lukey, P.T.; Molloy-Bland, M.; Morin, S.N.; Offiah, A.C.; et al. HR-pQCT Measures of Bone Microarchitecture Predict Fracture: Systematic Review and Meta-Analysis. *J. Bone Miner. Res.* **2020**, *35*, 446–459. [CrossRef]
48. Sornay-Rendu, E.; Boutroy, S.; Duboeuf, F.; Chapurlat, R.D. Bone Microarchitecture Assessed by HR-pQCT as Predictor of Fracture Risk in Postmenopausal Women: The OFELY Study. *J. Bone Miner. Res.* **2017**, *32*, 1243–1251. [CrossRef] [PubMed]

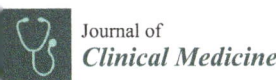

Article

Fragility Fractures and Imminent Fracture Risk in the Spanish Population: A Retrospective Observational Cohort Study

Maria-José Montoya-García [1], Mercè Giner [2,*], Rodrigo Marcos [3], David García-Romero [3], Francisco-Jesús Olmo-Montes [4], Mª José Miranda [4], Blanca Hernández-Cruz [5], Miguel-Angel Colmenero [4] and Mª Angeles Vázquez-Gámez [1]

1. Departamento de Medicina, Universidad de Sevilla, Avda. Dr. Fedriani s/n, 41009 Sevilla, Spain; pmontoya@us.es (M.-J.M.-G.); mavazquez@us.es (M.A.V.-G.)
2. Departamento de Citología e Histología Normal y Patológica, Universidad de Sevilla, Avda. Dr. Fedriani s/n, 41009 Sevilla, Spain
3. Orthopedic Surgery and Traumatology Service, Virgen Macarena University Hospital, Avda Sánchez Pizjuán s/n, 41009 Seville, Spain; rodri.marcos.rabanillo@gmail.com (R.M.); garciaromero5@hotmail.com (D.G.-R.)
4. Servicio de Medicina Interna, HUV Macarena, Avda Sánchez Pizjuán s/n, 41009 Sevilla, Spain; franciscoj.olmo.sspa@juntadeandalucia.es (F.-J.O.-M.); m.j.mir@telefonica.net (M.J.M.); mangel.colmenero.sspa@juntadeandalucia.es (M.-A.C.)
5. Rheumatology Service, Virgen Macarena University Hospital, Avda Sánchez Pizjuán s/n, 41009 Seville, Spain; blancahcruz@gmail.com
* Correspondence: mginer@us.es

Abstract: Fragility fractures constitute a major public health problem worldwide, causing important high morbidity and mortality rates. The aim was to present the epidemiology of fragility fractures and to assess the imminent risk of a subsequent fracture and mortality. This is a retrospective population-based cohort study (n = 1369) with a fragility fracture. We estimated the incidence rate of index fragility fractures and obtained information on the subsequent fractures and death during a follow-up of up to three years. We assessed the effect of age, sex, and skeletal site of index fracture as independent risk factors of further fractures and mortality. Incidence rate of index fragility fractures was 86.9/10,000 person-years, with highest rates for hip fractures in women aged ≥80 years. The risk of fracture was higher in subjects with a recent fracture (Relative Risk(RR), 1.80; $p < 0.01$). Higher age was an independent risk factor for further fracture events. Significant excess mortality was found in subjects aged ≥80 years and with a previous hip fracture (hazard ratio, 3.43 and 2.48, respectively). It is the first study in Spain to evaluate the incidence of major osteoporotic fractures, not only of the hip, and the rate of imminent fracture. Our results provide further evidence highlighting the need for early treatment.

Keywords: osteoporosis; fragility fracture; fracture risk; imminent fracture risk

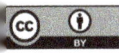

1. Introduction

Fragility fractures caused by osteoporosis constitute a major public health problem worldwide. The annual costs attributable to fragility fractures in the European Union (EU) currently equate to €37 billion, and these numbers are expected to rise due to population aging [1]. Fragility fractures are an important cause of disability, morbidity, and mortality in the population [2]. Such massive burden highlights the importance of risk assessment of fragility fractures and the need to adapt prevention strategies to individual risk patterns.

A large number of risk factors for fragility fracture have been identified [3]. Among them, a previous fragility fracture has been generally recognized as an assessment criteria of fracture risk in osteoporosis, regardless of bone mineral density (BMD) [4]. Although it is generally recognized that the risk of fracture increases throughout life with a previous fracture, a recent osteoporotic fracture increases even more the risk of an imminent fracture [5–7], and the magnitude of this risk and the contribution of other clinical risk factors still demand further research. Previous evidence suggests that the risk is not constant but rather fluctuates over time, being greatest within the first few years of the initial fracture [5,8–11]. The predictive importance of imminent (12 to 24 months) fracture risk is widely accepted. However, the significance of the early years after an index fracture need to be further explored. After a first fragility fracture, the skeletal location of the index fracture may also influence the magnitude of imminent fracture risk. However, only a few studies have measured its effect on the level of further fracture risk, and conclusions do not hold for solid generalization. [12–14]. Older age is also a well-defined clinical risk factor for fractures [15]. However, there is controversy between studies over its contribution on the risk of further fracture events. Some authors have observed a marked increase by age in the risk of a second major fragility fracture [11,16], whereas the association between age and subsequent fracture was not confirmed by other reports [3,17]. As with age, the predictive value of sex in the risk of further fracture events is also controversial. Originally, women were considered at higher risk of both initial and subsequent fracture and, indeed, some authors confirmed this hypothesis [11,16]. However, other studies have not reported differences in the risk of subsequent fracture events between men and women [18,19].

The primary objective of the present study was to explore the epidemiology of fragility fractures in southern Spain by using data from a population-based cohort of women and men, aged 50 or older, admitted to the emergency unit at Virgen Macarena University Hospital. Our study also provides an estimation of the incidence rate of subsequent fractures over 1–3 years following an index fracture. As secondary objectives, the study evaluated mortality over three years following an index fracture, analyzing the role of subsequent fractures as an independent risk factor.

2. Materials and Methods

This study was designed as a retrospective observational population-based cohort study involving men and women aged ≥50 years with an index fragility fracture (caused by an injury that would be insufficient to fracture normal bone; the result of a/or resistance to bone torsion [20]) occurring between 1 January 2014 and 31 December 2014.

Eligible study participants were followed until 31 December 2016, to obtain information on the outcomes: subsequent fragility fractures and deaths events. Age, sex, time from index fracture, and skeletal site were assessed as potential independent risk factors. Patients were identified using the emergency unit's medical records at Virgen Macarena University Hospital in Spain. Virgen Macarena University Hospital is a public tertiary hospital and its Emergency Unit serves up to 481,879 inhabitants, of whom 157,428 subjects are aged ≥ 50 years, within the healthcare area of North Seville. Furthermore, this is the single reference hospital of the healthcare area including emergency care attention. General medical records (Diraya) were also used to collect any relevant information on the study outcomes including demographic information, index fracture type, and causality as well as any relevant radiological confirmatory findings. Eligible incidental fragility fracture locations included axial (hip, pelvis, dorsal, and lumbar vertebrae) as well as appendicular bones (proximal humerus and wrist), according to the International Classification of Diseases, ICD-9 codes (Supplementary Table S1). Diagnosis was based on symptoms but must have included a radiologic confirmation of the fracture. Non-clinical radiographic vertebral fractures as well as other pathological or traumatic fractures were excluded. The identification of subsequent fractures required a similar main diagnosis of fracture. To distinguish subsequent fractures from previous events recorded at follow-up visits and/or patient history, the following criteria were applied: (1) Fractures in the same skeletal site of index fracture were only captured if a minimum of four months had elapsed since the index fracture; (2) hip fractures were only captured if an inpatient hospital admission was required; (3) all medical visits identified as follow-up examination of a previous fracture were excluded as further fracture events; (4) patients who died following a fracture were captured as having both outcomes; and (5) if the index fracture involved more than one skeletal sites, to avoid double counting, the fracture was assigned to the site of highest severity. Time at risk for subsequent fracture events began the day after the date of the index fracture and continued until outcome occurrence, either fracture or patient death.

We estimated the incidence rate over 12 months of (index) fragility fractures in the general population aged ≥ 50 years (based on a total estimated population of 157,428 individuals aged 50 or over served in Virgen Macarena Hospital catchment area on 1 January 2014). Then, we estimated the incidence rate of further fracture events during the study period among those who had a previous fragility fracture in 2014. Time at risk for subsequent fracture events began the day after the date of the index fracture and continued until outcome occurrence, either fracture or patient death. Fracture incidence rates per 10,000 person-years were calculated by age group, sex, and fracture type. The 95% confidence intervals (CIs) were calculated assuming a Poisson distribution. The excess risk of further fractures was compared to the general population using a Poisson regression model including age, sex, and location of previous fracture as covariates. Nelson–Aalen cumulative hazard estimates were plotted to analyze the time to a subsequent fracture event [21]. The risk of subsequent fracture was analyzed using a Cox proportional hazards regression model, as well as the model proposed by Fine and Gray [22], using death as a competing risk. All-cause mortality was also analyzed using the Cox hazard model. Furthermore, we included a time-dependent variable in this model to estimate the risk of all-cause death associated with the occurrence of subsequent fracture events during the study period. Estimates with p values < 0.05 were considered statistically significant. No imputation of missing data was necessary. All statistical analyses were performed using Stata software (STATA Corp., College Station, TX, USA).

3. Results

3.1. Patient Baseline Characteristics

Among a total population of 157,428 Caucasian individuals aged 50 or over served by Virgen Macarena University Hospital, 1068 women and 301 men (3.5 female/male ratio), with mean of age 75.1 and 72.1 years, respectively, registered eligible index fragility fractures in 2014 and were included in the analyses. Only 14 subjects were excluded due to miscoding of fractures (3/14) or traumatic (8/14) or pathological fractures (3/14), (Figure 1). The most frequent index fracture site in women was wrist (405 [37.9%]), whereas in men hip fractures were the most common (111 [36.9%]). Mean duration of follow-up was 2.3 years for all subjects, 2.2 years in males and 2.3 in females.

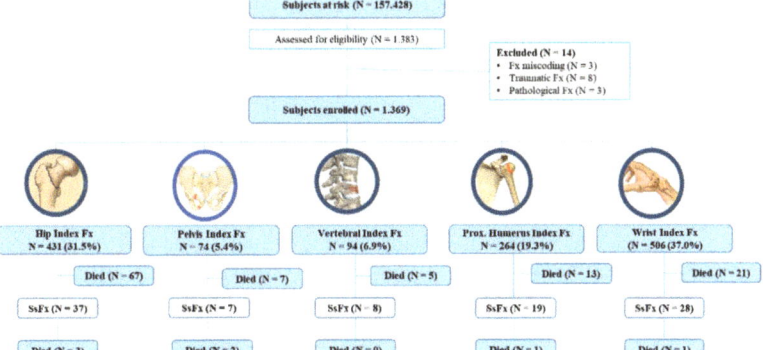

Figure 1. Flow diagram of study participants based on the Strobe statement. A total of 1383 subjects were assessed for eligibility, among a study population of 157,428 inhabitants. Fracture miscoding or traumatic or pathological causes of fractures were the causes for the exclusion of 14 subjects. Subjects were enrolled from January 2014 to December 2014 and followed up until December 2016. Mean duration of follow-up was 2.3 years for all subjects, 2.2 years in males and 2.3 in females. The most frequent types of index fracture were wrist (N = 506, 37.0%) and hip (N = 431, 31.5%), followed closely by proximal humerus (N = 264, 19.3%). Overall, 99 subjects registered a subsequent fracture, with 120 events of death occurring throughout follow-up. Fx: fracture. SsFx: subsequent fracture.

3.2. Incidence Rate of Index Fracture in the General Population

An overall incidence rate of 86.9 fractures/10,000 person-years was found in the general population aged ≥ 50 years (Table 1). The frequency of fragility fractures was significantly higher among women as compared to men: 123.9 (CI 95% 116.6–131.6) versus 42.3 (CI95% 37.7–47.4), respectively. Also, marked increase in the frequency was also observed with increasing age. The highest overall frequency was observed for wrist fractures. Despite this, hip fractures were the most frequent among women and men aged ≥ 80 years. On the other hand, the skeletal sites with the lowest incidence rate of fragility fractures were the pelvis and the spine.

Table 1. Incidence rate of index fracture in the general population aged ≥50 years, by index fracture site, sex, and age group. The total population values for males and females are marked in bold. The shading indicates that they are total values of the population, to differentiate them from the rest that are separated by gender and age.

			Index Fracture Site				
	Age *	All Sites	Hip	Pelvis	Vertebral	Prox. Humerus	Wrist
All subjects	50+ years	**86.9 (82.4–91.6)**	**27.5 (25.0–30.2)**	4.6 (3.6–5.8)	6.0 (4.8–7.3)	**16.8 (14.8–18.9)**	**32.1 (29.4–35.0)**
Males	All males	42.3 (37.7–47.4)	15.6 (12.8–18.8)	1.8 (0.0–3.1)	2.4 (1.4–3.8)	8.3 (6.3–10.7)	14.2 (11.6–17.3)
	50–59 years	23.4 (18.3–29.5)	2.3 (0.9–4.8)	0.0 (NA)	1.3 (0.4–3.4)	7.3 (4.5–11.0)	12.5 (8.9–17.2)
	60–69 years	24.7 (18.5–32.3)	4.7 (2.2–8.6)	0.9 (0.1–3.4)	0.9 (0.1–3.4)	6.1 (3.2–10.4)	12.1 (7.9–17.8)
	70–79 years	56.4 (44.1–71.0)	18.8 (12.1–28.0)	2.4 (0.5–6.9)	3.1 (0.9–8.0)	11.8 (6.6–19.4)	20.4 (13.3–29.8)
	80+ years	157.7 (129.0–190.9)	105.1 (82.0–132.8)	12.0 (5.2–23.7)	10.5 (4.2–21.7)	13.5 (6.2–25.7)	16.5 (8.25–29.6)
Females	All females	123.9 (116.6–131.6)	37.1 (33.2–41.4)	7.1 (5.4–9.1)	8.9 (7.1–11.2)	23.8 (20.6–27.3)	47.0 (42.5–51.8)
	50–59 years	48.3 (41.00–6.5)	3.7 (1.9–6.5)	0.6 (0.1 -2.3)	4.4 (2.4–7.3)	12.2 (8.6–16.6)	27.4 (22.0–33.8)
	60–69 years	77.9 (67.1–89.9)	5.8 (3.2–9.8)	2.5 (0.9–5.4)	2.9 (1.2–6.0)	19.6 (14.4–26.0)	47.1 (38.8–56.6)
	70–79 years	150.2 (132.4–169.7)	38.0 (29.3–48.4)	8.2 (4.5–13.7)	13.4 (8.5–20.2)	31.6 (23.7–41.2)	59.0 (48.1–71.7)
	80+ years	359.5 (327.7–393.6)	175.5 (153.5–199.8)	29.9 (21.3–40.9)	25.3 (17.4–35.5)	49.8 (38.5–63.5)	79.0 (64.4–95.8)

Data are incidence rate per 10,000 person-years (95% confidence interval). * Age is described as of index date.

3.3. Incidence of Subsequent Fractures

The frequency of clinical subsequent fracture events was 318.2/10,000 person-years. Incidence rate of subsequent fractures was higher in women than in men. However, the overall differences did not reach statistical significance (Table 2). By contrast, the frequency of clinical fracture events increased with age, with markedly higher incidences rates in men and women aged 70 years or older (Table 2). Overall, no significant differences in the frequency of subsequent fracture events were observed by index fracture type. However, a slight trend was observed toward increased incidence among subjects with pelvis and hip index fractures (Table 2). The rate of further fracture events was highest within the ≥80 years' age group, in women with a previous fracture in the pelvis and men with a previous wrist index fracture. The most frequent skeletal locations of further fractures were hip and wrist. The incidence rate of further fracture events during the first year after the index fragility fracture was not higher than the rates observed during the following second and third years of follow-up, regardless of sex and age (Figure 2). Similarly, no marked differences among follow-up periods were observed by site of index fracture. However, a slight trend was observed for wrist fractures (Supplementary Table S2).

Table 2. Incidence rate of subsequent fractures (any site) among patients with an index fracture, by index fracture site, sex, and age group. The total population values for males and females are marked in bold. The shading indicates that they are total values of the population, to differentiate them from the rest that are separated by gender and age.

	Age *	All Sites	Hip	Pelvis	Vertebral	Prox. Humerus	Wrist
All subjects	**50+ years**	**318.2 (261.3–387.5)**	**406.8 (294.7–561.4)**	**425.8 (203.1–893.1)**	**364.5 (182.3–728.9)**	**306.0 (195.2–479.8)**	**234.0 (161.6–338.9)**
Males	**All males**	**180.4 (93.2–315.1)**	**228.8 (74.3–534.0)**	**0.0 (NA)**	**504.4 (61.1–1821.9)**	**69.7 (1.8–388.5)**	**171.4 (46.7–438.8)**
	50–59 years	56.4 (1.4–314.2)	0.0 (NA)	0.0 (NA)	1014.3 (25.7–5651.3)	0.0 (NA)	0.0 (NA)
	60–69 years	0.0 (NA)	0.0 (NA)	0.0 (NA)	0.0 (NA)	0.0 (NA)	0.0 (NA)
	70–79 years	259.4 (70.7–664.1)	464.9 (56.3–1679.4)	0.0 (NA)	0.0 (NA)	0.0 (NA)	359.8 (43.6–1299.5)
	80+ years	333.0 (133.9–686.2)	218.9 (45.2–639.8)	0.0 (NA)	665.4 (16.9–3707.5)	473.4 (12.0–2637.8)	1048.8 (127.0–3788.7)
Females	**All females**	**355.7 (284.9–438.8)**	**463.0 (316.7–653.6)**	**521.8 (209.8–1075.1)**	**333.7 (122.4–726.2)**	**377.0 (223.4–595.8)**	**249.1 (159.6–370.7)**
	50–59 years	131.2 (42.6–306.3)	0.0 (NA)	0.0 (NA)	275.8 (7.0–1536.8)	107.0 (2.7–596.1)	137.7 (28.4–402.4)
	60–69 years	131.5 (48.3–286.2)	0.0 (NA)	0.0 (NA)	0.0 (NA)	0.0 (NA)	217.8 (79.9–474.0)
	70–79 years	352.4 (218.1–538.6)	414.11 (152.0–901.3)	0.0 (NA)	571.2 (117.8–1669.2)	658.4 (284.3–1297.3)	163.5 (44.5–418.6)
	80+ years	543.2 (409.2–707.0)	540.6 (353.1–792.1)	852.6 (342.8–1756.7)	262.7 (31.8–948.8)	607.8 (277.9–1153.8)	488.3 (243.8–873.7)

Data are incidence rate per 10,000 person-years (95% confidence interval). * Age is described as of index date.

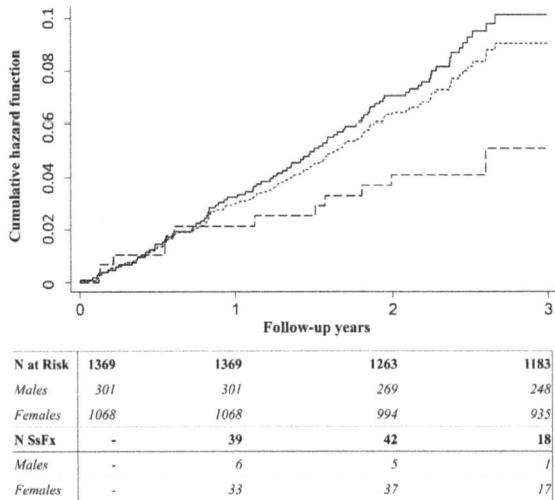

N at Risk	1369	1369	1263	1183
Males	301	301	269	248
Females	1068	1068	994	935
N SsFx	-	39	42	18
Males	-	6	5	1
Females	-	33	37	17

Figure 2. Nelson–Aalen cumulative hazard of subsequent fracture events after an index fracture in men and women aged ≥50 years over a period of three years of follow-up. Cumulative risk of subsequent fracture increased over the years following initial fracture. However, no significant differences were found in the incidence rate of subsequent fractures over 1, 2, and 3 years, regardless of sex and age. Dotted line represents the cumulative incidence of subsequent fractures in all subjects. Solid line represents the cumulative incidence of subsequent fracture events in females. Dashed line represents the cumulative incidence of subsequent fracture events in males. SsFx: subsequent fracture. The Y-axis represents the cumulative hazard function. The X-axis represents follow-up years after the first fracture.

3.4. Risk Factors of Subsequent Clinical Fracture

Overall, the incidence rate of fractures was higher for subjects with a previous index fragility fracture at any site compared with the general population (relative risk [RR] 1.80, $p < 0.01$) (Figure 3 and Supplementary Table S3). Independent risk factors for subsequent fracture, as identified by multivariate analysis using Cox as well as Fine and Gray regression models, Higher age ($\geq$70 years) was an independent risk factor for further fracture events, with a $\geq$1.5 increase in hazard risk (HR) observed for each decade from 60 years of age (Table 3). Multivariate analysis using Fine and Gray model revealed an increased risk of subsequent fractures in women. No effect of index fracture site on the level of risk of further fractures was observed (Table 3).

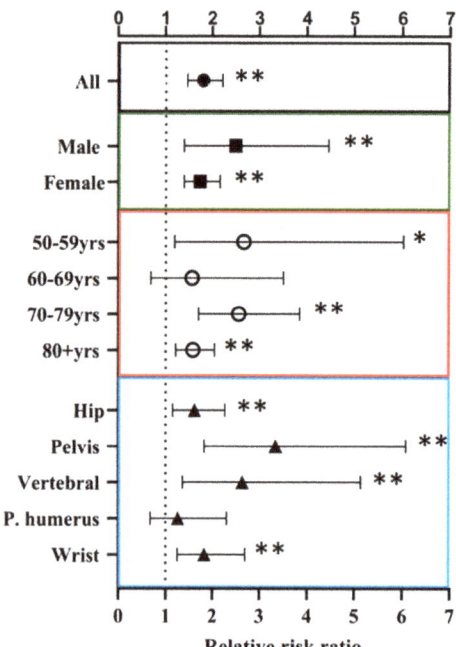

Figure 3. Relative risk of subsequent fractures among subjects with a previous fracture compared with the general population by sex (green box and square), age group (red box and circle), and index fracture site (blue box and triangle). Adjusted rate ratio estimated using Poisson regression models that included age, sex, and index fracture site as covariates. Corresponding data are presented in Supplementary Table S3. * $p < 0.05$, ** $p < 0.01$.

Table 3. Hazard ratio (Cox) and subhazard ratio (Fine and Gray) of subsequent fracture events associated to sex, age, and index fracture site.

Risk Factor	HR †	95% CI	$p > |z|$	SHR ‡	95% CI	$p > |z|$
Sex						
Male *	1			1		
Female	1.73	(0.94–3.17)	0.08	1.87	(1.01–3.46)	0.05
Age group						
50–59 years *	1			1		
60–69 years	0.92	(0.30–2.86)	0.88	0.91	(0.30–2.78)	0.87
70–79 years	2.94	(1.20–7.22)	0.02	2.88	(1.18–7.05)	0.02
80+ years	4.41	(1.85–10.51)	<0.01	4.15	(1.74–9.89)	<0.01

Table 3. Cont.

Risk Factor	HR [†]	95% CI	p > |z|	SHR [‡]	95% CI	p > |z|
		Index fracture site				
Hip	1.05	(0.62–1.77)	0.85	0.98	(0.58–1.66)	0.94
Pelvis	1.14	(0.49–2.64)	0.77	1.12	(0.49–2.57)	0.79
Vertebral	1.14	(0.52–2.53)	0.74	1.14	(0.51–2.53)	0.75
Prox. humerus	1.20	(0.67–2.15)	0.54	1.22	(0.68–2.18)	0.51
Wrist *	1			1		
Index fracture type [+]						
Appendicular	1			1		
Central	1	(0.66–1.53)	0.99	0.95	(0.61–1.46)	0.80

* Baseline category; [†] hazard ratio (HR) and 95% confidence interval (CI) estimates adjusted for all variables in the table using a Cox proportional hazards model. [‡] Subhazard ratio (SHR) and 95% confidence interval (CI) estimates adjusted for all variables in the table using a Fine and Gray competing risks model using death as competing risk. [+] Appendicular fractures: wrist and proximal humerus. Central fractures: vertebral, pelvis, and hip fractures.

3.5. Risk of Death Following Initial Fracture

A total of 120 deaths occurred during the study follow-up period in patients aged ≥50 years with an index fragility fracture, with overall mortality rates reaching 37.20/1000 person-years (29.09 and 67.42 per 1000 person-years in women and men, respectively). Mortality rates were higher among men as compared to women (HR, 0.41; $p < 0.01$) (Table 4). Age was the strongest determinant of mortality with significant excess risk for subjects aged 80 or older (HR, 3.43 $p < 0.01$). Mortality risk was also significantly higher among patients presenting an index fragility fracture in the hip (HR, 2.48; $p < 0.01$). Lower mortality rates were observed in subjects with index fractures located in peripheral bone positions (wrist and proximal humerus). Mortality risk also increased after a subsequent fracture occurred, although this association did not reach statistical significance (HR, 2.14; $p = 0.06$) (Table 4).

Table 4. Mortality hazard ratio associated to sex, age, type of index fracture, and presence of subsequent fracture events.

Risk Factor	MR × 1000 PY [‡]	HR [†]	95% CI	p > |z|
Sex				
Male *	67.42	1		
Female	29.09	0.41	(0.28–0.60)	<0.01
Age group				
50–59 years *	12.42	1		
60–69 years	17.04	1.43	(0.54–3.77)	0.47
70–79 years	29.30	2.00	(0.84–4.73)	0.12
80+ years	62.00	3.43	(1.51–7.77)	<0.01
Index fracture site				
Hip	73.50	2.48	(1.47–4.19)	<0.01
Pelvis	52.60	1.95	(0.88–4.35)	0.10
Vertebral *	22.07	1.01	(0.38–2.68)	0.99
Proximal humerus	21.83	1.13	(0.58–2.21)	0.73
Wrist	17.82	1		
Presence of SsFX				
no SsFX *	36.32	1		
SsFX	60.89	2.14	(0.97–4.70)	0.06

* Baseline category. [†] Mortality hazard ratio (HR) and 95% confidence interval (CI) estimates adjusted for all variables in the table using a Cox proportional hazards model. [‡] Mortality rate (MR) per 1000 person-years (PY). SsFx: subsequent fracture.

4. Discussion

This study presents the first report of the incidence rate of index of major fragility fractures and the risk of imminent fractures in a Spanish cohort of 1369 subjects (1068 women and 301 men) aged ≥50 years, by age group and fracture site. Our study confirmed markedly higher rates in women, as well as an age-related increase in the risk, with highest frequency rates found in women aged ≥80 years. The prevalence of osteoporosis and osteoporosis fracture rates is higher in women compared to men. This is due to differences in BMD, bone size, bone geometry, and bone strength [23,24]. Estrogen deprivation after menopause is a major contributing factor, which could be the reason for the observed gender-related differences [25]. Age, on the other hand, is a well-studied risk factor of index fragility fractures, contributing to risk independently of bone mass density [26]. Previous information on the incidence rate of fragility fractures in Spain is scarce. As a first approach, using the Q-FRACTURE tool, González López-Valcárcel et al. [27] estimated a level of risk ranging from 1.8–21.5% in women and 0.7–10.8% in men. According to our findings, the frequency of osteoporotic fractures in Spain may be sensitively higher than reported. Conversely, our numbers underestimate the crude rates published by the International Osteoporosis Foundation for Spain as well as for other EU countries [28]. This discrepancy may be partly explained by the exclusion of non-clinical vertebral fractures and other fracture sites less commonly associated with osteoporosis. Overall, the most frequent index fracture type was wrist. However, the rate of hip fractures exceeds that of wrist in older aged groups. Similar age-related trends in the frequency of fragility fractures were reported previously [29].

Estimated incidence rate of subsequent fractures was 318.2/10,000 person-years in all subjects during the three years that followed index fracture (i.e., 3.2% of patients with a previous fracture experienced a new fracture every year). To date, no other studies have been published that measure the risk of imminent fractures after a sentinel fracture in Spain. Only Azagra et al. have published 10-year fracture data in a population cohort in Catalonia that presented clinical risk factors for osteoporotic fractures, with the aim of validating the Frax tool in the Spanish population [30].

Overall, the incidence of fracture was higher for subjects with a previous index fragility fracture at any site, compared with the frequency in the general population aged 50 or older (RR, 1.80). According to our findings, Kanis et al. [17] observed that, for any type of previous fracture, the RR of any further fracture ranged from 1.83 to 2.03 depending upon age. The effect of gender as a predictor of the risk was only significant when the analysis considered death as a competing risk. Previous reports observed similar risks in men and women, except among subjects over 85 years of age [31]. Our data also, however, proved the well-known independent effect of aging on the risk of further fracture events, [11,14], with significant differences in the HR among older age (≥70 years). They also found a marked age-related increase in the risk but did not observe any differences in the risk among women and men.

Noticeable differences in the frequency of subsequent fractures were found depending upon site, with highest rates found in subjects with a previous pelvis or hip fracture. Our findings, however, could not confirm the effect of the skeletal site on the risk of further fractures. Previous reports on the associations between prior and subsequent fractures are not consistent [7]. The time that follows initial fracture is key with regard to the risk and prevention of subsequent fracture events. Several previous studies report that the highest risk of further fracture events occurs within the first year after the index fracture [8–11] and that the incidence decreases thereafter. In the current study, however, the incidence of subsequent fracture events during the first year after the index fracture was not higher than the rates observed during the following second and third years of follow-up, regardless of sex and age. Despite this, a slight trend was observed for wrist index fractures. Authors reporting higher levels of risk during the first year after the index fracture have assessed longer timescales than our study [9]. Like in our study, Banefelt et al. [11] focused only in the early years following the index fracture and found the highest incidence during the second year (12%), rather than the first (7.1%).

Overall mortality rate reached 37.20/1000 person-years, which showed an up-to-2-fold excess mortality due to osteoporotic fractures among the younger-aged groups [32]. The risk of death was significantly higher in patients with a previous hip index fracture

(HR, 2.48; $p < 0.01$), with an estimated rate of 73.50/1000 person-years. No significant excess mortality was found for index fractures in other skeletal locations or for the event of subsequent fractures ($p = 0.06$). As expected, our data also confirmed a higher age-specific death risk ($p < 0.01$, in subjects aged ≥ 80 years) as well as lower death risk in women ($p < 0.01$). In fact, 58.3% of all deaths occurred in patients with a previous hip index fracture and a mean age of 83.3 years. The observed death rate after a hip fracture was sensitively lower than previously reported [33,34], which could be explained by the longer observation period of this study, as mortality is highest during the six months that follow the event [35].

The main limitation of our study is the lack of data from other clinical factors that could have contributed to in-depth understanding of the risk of subsequent fractures (bone mass density, previous record of falls, history of prior fractures, use of drugs affecting bone metabolism). One of the strengths of our study is that, as opposed to database studies, we manually reviewed clinical records of all 1369 cases to confirm eligibility as well as outcomes' information.

5. Conclusions

In summary, this report provides information on the magnitude and consequences of fragility fractures in the as-yet unexplored Spanish population aged ≥ 50 years, involving both genders, as well as major skeletal sites associated with osteoporosis, not limited to hip. This is the first study to report on the incidence rate of imminent fractures after an osteoporotic sentinel fracture in Spain, with age, sex, and skeletal location of the index fractures as possible risk factors. Our results support the increased risk of imminent fracture after a recent fracture and provide key elements for early identification of risk and the application of targeted strategies aimed at preventing future fractures and mortality, such as the interventions recommended by the Fracture Liaison Services [36].

Supplementary Materials: The following are available online at https://www.mdpi.com/2077-0383/10/5/1082/s1. Table S1: Fracture codes according to ICD-9, Table S2: Incidence rate of subsequent fracture events by type of index fracture and follow-up period (years), and Table S3: Relative Risk of subsequent fracture events by age, sex and index fracture site.

Author Contributions: Conceptualization, M.G. and M.-J.M.-G.; methodology, M.-J.M.-G. and M.A.V.-G.; validation, F.-J.O.-M., M.-A.C., M.J.M. and B.H.-C.; formal analysis, M.G. and M.-J.M.-G.; investigation, all authors; resources, R.M. and D.G.-R.; writing—original draft preparation, M.G. and M.-J.M.-G.; writing—review and editing, M.-J.M.-G. and M.A.V.-G.; supervision, M.A.V.-G.; project administration, M.-J.M.-G.; funding acquisition, M.-J.M.-G. and M.-A.C. All authors have read and agreed to the published version of the manuscript.

Funding: This work was funded by Consejería de Salud de la Junta de Andalucía, Proyecto de Innovación PIN-0092-2016, which had no role in the design or conduct of the study; in the collection, analyses, and interpretation of the data; or in the preparation, review, or approval of the manuscript.

Institutional Review Board Statement: The study was approved by the Ethical Review Board of Seville (protocol code: CI#2147, 09/02/2013) and was performed in accordance with the ethical standards as laid down in the 1964 Declaration of Helsinki and its later amendments. For this type of study, individual formal consent was not required.

Informed Consent Statement: Informed consent was obtained from all subjects involved in the study.

Data Availability Statement: The data presented in this study are available on request from the corresponding author. The data are not publicly available due to privacy.

Acknowledgments: We thank the participants in this study for their valuable contribution. Writing assistance was provided by Juliana Martinez.

Conflicts of Interest: The authors declare no conflict of interest.

References

1. Hernlund, E.; Svedbom, A.; Ivergard, M.; Compston, J.; Cooper, C.; Stenmark, J.; McCloskey, E.V.; Jonsson, B.; Kanis, J.A. Osteoporosis in the European Union: Medical management, epidemiology and economic Burden: A report prepared in collaboration with the International Osteoporosis Foundation (IOF) and the European Federation of Pharmaceutical Industry Associations (EFPIA). *Arch. Osteoporos.* **2013**, *8*, 136. [CrossRef]
2. Shuid, A.N.; Khaithir, T.M.N.; Mokhtar, S.A.; Mohamed, I.N.; Nazrun, A.S.; Tzar, M.N. A systematic review of the outcomes of osteoporotic fracture patients after hospital discharge: Morbidity, subsequent fractures, and mortality. *Ther. Clin. Risk Manag.* **2014**, *10*, 937–948. [CrossRef]
3. Kanis, J.A. *Assessment of Osteoporosis at the Primary Health Care Level*; WHO Scientific Group Technical Report; WHO Collaborating Centre for Metabolic Bone Diseases, University of Sheffield Medical School: Sheffield, UK, 2007; pp. 1–339.
4. Papaioannou, A.; Kennedy, C. Diagnostic criteria for osteoporosis should be expanded. *Lancet Diabetes Endocrinol.* **2015**, *3*, 234–236. [CrossRef]
5. Roux, C.; Briot, K. Imminent fracture risk. *Osteoporos. Int.* **2017**, *28*, 1765–1769. [CrossRef] [PubMed]
6. Van Geel, T.A.C.M.; Huntjens, K.M.B.; Bergh, J.P.W.V.D.; Dinant, G.-J.; Geusens, P.P. Timing of Subsequent Fractures after an Initial Fracture. *Curr. Osteoporos. Rep.* **2010**, *8*, 118–122. [CrossRef]
7. Klotzbuecher, C.M.; Ross, P.D.; Landsman, P.B.; Abbott, T.A.; Berger, M. Patients with Prior Fractures Have an Increased Risk of Future Fractures: A Summary of the Literature and Statistical Synthesis. *J. Bone Miner. Res.* **2010**, *15*, 721–739. [CrossRef]
8. Schnell, A.D.; Curtis, J.R.; Saag, K.G. Importance of Recent Fracture as Predictor of Imminent Fracture Risk. *Curr. Osteoporos. Rep.* **2018**, *16*, 738–745. [CrossRef]
9. A Kanis, J.; Johansson, H.; Odén, A.; Harvey, N.C.; Gudnason, V.; Sanders, K.M.; Sigurdsson, G.; Siggeirsdottir, K.; A Fitzpatrick, L.; Borgström, F.; et al. Characteristics of recurrent fractures. *Osteoporos. Int.* **2018**, *29*, 1747–1757. [CrossRef] [PubMed]
10. Balasubramanian, A.; Zhang, J.; Chen, L.; Wenkert, D.; Daigle, S.G.; Grauer, A.; Curtis, J.R. Risk of subsequent fracture after prior fracture among older women. *Osteoporos. Int.* **2019**, *30*, 79–92. [CrossRef]
11. Banefelt, J.; Åkesson, K.; Spångéus, A.; Ljunggren, O.; Karlsson, L.; Ström, O.; Ortsäter, G.; Libanati, C.; Toth, E. Risk of imminent fracture following a previous fracture in a Swedish database study. *Osteoporos. Int.* **2019**, *30*, 601–609. [CrossRef] [PubMed]
12. Borgen, T.T.; Bjørnerem, Å.; Solberg, L.B.; Andreasen, C.; Brunborg, C.; Stenbro, M.; Hübschle, L.M.; Froholdt, A.; Figved, W.; Apalset, E.M.; et al. Post-fracture Risk Assessment: Target the Centrally Sited Fractures First! A Substudy of NoFRACT. *J. Bone Miner. Res.* **2019**, *34*, 2036–2044. [CrossRef]
13. Cosman, F.; De Beur, S.J.; LeBoff, M.S.; Lewiecki, E.M.; Tanner, B.; Randall, S.; Lindsay, R. Clinician's Guide to Prevention and Treatment of Osteoporosis. *Osteoporos. Int.* **2014**, *25*, 2359–2381. [CrossRef]
14. Gehlbach, S.H.; Saag, K.G.; Adachi, J.D.; Hooven, F.H.; Flahive, J.; Boonen, S.; Chapurlat, R.D.; Compston, J.E.; Cooper, C.; Díez-Perez, A.; et al. Previous fractures at multiple sites increase the risk for subsequent fractures: The global longitudinal study of osteoporosis in women. *J. Bone Miner. Res.* **2012**, *27*, 645–653. [CrossRef]
15. Kanis, J.; Cooper, C.; Rizzoli, R.; Reginster, J.-Y.; on behalf of the Scientific Advisory Board of the European Society for Clinical and Economic Aspects of Osteoporosis (ESCEO) and the Committees of Scientific Advisors and National Societies of the International Osteoporosis Foundation (IOF). European guidance for the diagnosis and management of osteoporosis in postmenopausal women. *Osteoporos. Int.* **2019**, *30*, 3–44. [CrossRef]
16. Johansson, H.; Siggeirsdóttir, K.; Harvey, N.C.; Odén, A.; Gudnason, V.; McCloskey, E.; Sigurdsson, G.; A Kanis, J. Imminent risk of fracture after fracture. *Osteoporos. Int.* **2017**, *28*, 775–780. [CrossRef]
17. Kanis, J.; Johnell, O.; De Laet, C.; Johansson, H.; Oden, A.; Delmas, P.; Eisman, J.; Fujiwara, S.; Garnero, P.; Kroger, H.; et al. A meta-analysis of previous fracture and subsequent fracture risk. *Bone* **2004**, *35*, 375–382. [CrossRef]
18. Langsetmo, L.; Goltzman, D.; Kovacs, C.S.; Adachi, J.D.; Hanley, D.A.; Kreiger, N.; Josse, R.; Papaioannou, A.; Olszynski, W.P.; Jamal, S.A.; et al. Repeat low-trauma fractures occur frequently among men and women who have osteopenic BMD. *J. Bone Miner. Res.* **2009**, *24*, 1515–1522. [CrossRef]
19. De Laet, C.E.D.H.; Van Der Klift, M.; Hofman, A.; Pols, H.A.P. Osteoporosis in Men and Women: A Story About Bone Mineral Density Thresholds and Hip Fracture Risk. *J. Bone Miner. Res.* **2002**, *17*, 2231–2236. [CrossRef] [PubMed]
20. World Health Organization. *Guidelines for Preclinical Evaluation and Clinical Trials in Osteoporosis Geneva*; World Health Organization: Geneva, Switzerland, 1998; pp. 1–59.
21. García-Gavilán, J.; Bulló, M.; Canudas, S.; Martínez-González, M.; Estruch, R.; Giardina, S.; Fitó, M.; Corella, D.; Ros, E.; Salas-Salvadó, J. Extra virgin olive oil consumption reduces the risk of osteoporotic fractures in the PREDIMED trial. *Clin. Nutr.* **2018**, *37*, 329–335. [CrossRef] [PubMed]
22. Fine, J.P.; Gray, R.J. A Proportional Hazards Model for the Subdistribution of a Competing Risk. *J. Am. Stat. Assoc.* **1999**, *94*, 496–509. [CrossRef]
23. Riggs, B.L.; Melton, L.J.; Robb, R.A.; Camp, J.J.; Atkinson, E.J.; Oberg, A.L.; A Rouleau, P.; McCollough, C.H.; Khosla, S.; Bouxsein, M.L. Population-Based Analysis of the Relationship of Whole Bone Strength Indices and Fall-Related Loads to Age- and Sex-Specific Patterns of Hip and Wrist Fractures. *J. Bone Miner. Res.* **2005**, *21*, 315–323. [CrossRef] [PubMed]
24. Sigurdsson, G.; Aspelund, T.; Chang, M.; Jonsdottir, B.; Sigurdsson, S.; Eiriksdottir, G.; Gudmundsson, A.; Harris, T.B.; Gudnason, V.; Lang, T.F. Increasing sex difference in bone strength in old age: The Age, Gene/Environment Susceptibility-Reykjavik study (AGES-REYKJAVIK). *Bone* **2006**, *39*, 644–651. [CrossRef] [PubMed]

25. Lane, N.E. Epidemiology, etiology, and diagnosis of osteoporosis. *Am. J. Obstet. Gynecol.* **2006**, *194*, S3–S11. [CrossRef] [PubMed]
26. Kanis, J.A. Osteoporosis III: Diagnosis of osteoporosis and assessment of fracture risk. *Lancet* **2002**, *359*, 1929–1936. [CrossRef]
27. González López-Valcárcel, B.; Sosa Henríquez, M. Estimación del riesgo de fractura osteoporótica a los 10 años para la pobla-ción española. *Med. Clin.* **2013**, *140*, 104–109. [CrossRef]
28. Borgström, F.; for the International Osteoporosis Foundation; Karlsson, L.; Ortsäter, G.; Norton, N.; Halbout, P.; Cooper, C.; Lorentzon, M.; McCloskey, E.V.; Harvey, N.C.; et al. Fragility fractures in Europe: Burden, management and opportunities. *Arch. Osteoporos.* **2020**, *15*, 1–21. [CrossRef] [PubMed]
29. Tsuda, T. Epidemiology of fragility fractures and fall prevention in the elderly: A systematic review of the literature. *Curr. Orthop. Pr.* **2017**, *28*, 580–585. [CrossRef]
30. Azagra, R.; Roca, G.; Encabo, G.; Prieto, D.; Aguye, A.; Zwart, M.; Güell, S.; Puchol, N.; Gené, E.; Casado, E.; et al. Prediction of absolute risk of fragility fracture at 10 years in a Spanish population: Validation of the WHO FRAX ™ tool in Spain. *BMC Musculoskelet. Disord.* **2011**, *12*, 30. [CrossRef]
31. Bynum, J.P.W.; Bell, J.E.; Cantu, R.V.; Wang, Q.; McDonough, C.M.; Carmichael, D.; Tosteson, T.D.; Tosteson, A.N.A. Second fractures among older adults in the year following hip, shoulder, or wrist fracture. *Osteoporos. Int.* **2016**, *27*, 2207–2215. [CrossRef]
32. Schnell, S.; Friedman, S.M.; Mendelson, D.A.; Bingham, K.W.; Kates, S.L. The 1-Year Mortality of Patients Treated in a Hip Fracture Program for Elders. *Geriatr. Orthop. Surg. Rehabil.* **2010**, *1*, 6–14. [CrossRef] [PubMed]
33. Guzon-Illescas, O.; Fernandez, E.P.; Villarias, N.C.; Donate, F.J.Q.; Peña, M.; Alonso-Blas, C.; García-Vadillo, A.; Mazzucchelli, R. Mortality after osteoporotic hip fracture: Incidence, trends, and associated factors. *J. Orthop. Surg. Res.* **2019**, *14*, 1–9. [CrossRef] [PubMed]
34. Kanis, J.; Oden, A.; Johnell, O.; De Laet, C.; Jonsson, B.; Oglesby, A. The components of excess mortality after hip fracture. *Bone* **2003**, *32*, 468–473. [CrossRef]
35. Kanis, J.A.; Cooper, C.; Rizzoli, R.; Abrahamsen, B.; Al-Daghri, N.M.; Brandi, M.L.; Cannata-Andia, J.; Cortet, B.; Dimai, H.P.; Ferrari, S.; et al. Identification and management of patients at increased risk of osteoporotic fracture: Outcomes of an ESCEO expert consensus meeting. *Osteoporos. Int.* **2017**, *28*, 2023–2034. [CrossRef] [PubMed]
36. Naranjo, A.; Ojeda, S.; Giner, M.; Balcells-Oliver, M.; Canals, L.; Cancio, J.M.; Duaso, E.; Mora-Fernández, J.; Pablos, C.; González, A.; et al. Best Practice Framework of Fracture Liaison Services in Spain and their coordination with Primary Care. *Arch. Osteoporos.* **2020**, *15*, 1–7. [CrossRef]

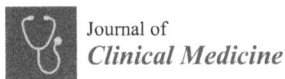

Article

Fractal-Based Analysis of Bone Microstructure in Crohn's Disease: A Pilot Study

Judith Haschka [1,2], Daniel Arian Kraus [1,2], Martina Behanova [2], Stephanie Huber [1,2], Johann Bartko [1,2], Jakob E. Schanda [3,4], Philip Meier [5], Arian Bahrami [6], Shahin Zandieh [6], Jochen Zwerina [1,2] and Roland Kocijan [1,2,7,*]

1. 1st Medical Department, Hanusch Hospital, 1140 Vienna, Austria; judith.haschka@osteologie.lbg.ac.at (J.H.); daniel.arian.kraus@gmail.com (D.A.K.); huberstephy@yahoo.com (S.H.); johann.bartko@oegk.at (J.B.); jochen.zwerina@osteologie.lbg.ac.at (J.Z.)
2. Ludwig Boltzmann Institute of Osteology, Hanusch Hospital of OEGK, AUVA Trauma Center Vienna-Meidling, 1140 Vienna, Austria; martina.behanova@osteologie.lbg.ac.at
3. Department of Trauma Surgery, AUVA Trauma Center Vienna-Meidling, 1120 Vienna, Austria; jakob.schanda@gmail.com
4. Ludwig Boltzmann Institute for Experimental and Clinical Traumatology, 1200 Vienna, Austria
5. ImageBiopsy Lab., 1140 Vienna, Austria; p.meier@imagebiopsy.com
6. Department of Radiology and Nucelar Medicine, Hanusch Hospital Vienna, 1140 Vienna, Austria; arian.bahrami@oegk.at (A.B.); shahin.zandieh@oegk.at (S.Z.)
7. Medical Faculty of Bone Diseases, Sigmund Freud University, 1020 Vienna, Austria
* Correspondence: roland.kocijan@osteologie.lbg.ac.at; Tel.: +43-191-021-57368

Received: 9 November 2020; Accepted: 13 December 2020; Published: 20 December 2020

Abstract: Crohn's disease (CD) is associated with bone loss and increased fracture risk. TX-Analyzer™ is a new fractal-based technique to evaluate bone microarchitecture based on conventional radiographs. The aim of the present study was to evaluate the TX-Analyzer™ of the thoracic and lumbar spine in CD patients and healthy controls (CO) and to correlate the parameters to standard imaging techniques. 39 CD patients and 39 age- and sex-matched CO were analyzed. Demographic parameters were comparable between CD and CO. Bone structure value (BSV), bone variance value (BVV) and bone entropy value (BEV) were measured at the vertebral bodies of T7 to L4 out of lateral radiographs. Bone mineral density (BMD) and trabecular bone score (TBS) by dual energy X-ray absorptiometry (DXA) were compared to TX parameters. BSV and BVV of the thoracic spine of CD were higher compared to controls, with no difference in BEV. Patients were further divided into subgroups according to the presence of a history of glucocorticoid treatment, disease duration > 15 years and bowel resection. BEV was significantly lower in CD patients with these prevalent risk factors, with no differences in BMD at all sites. Additionally, TBS was reduced in patients with a history of glucocorticoid treatment. Despite a not severely pronounced bone loss in this population, impaired bone quality in CD patients with well-known risk factors for systemic bone loss was assessed by TX-Analyzer™.

Keywords: Crohn's disease; bone microstructure; bone loss; fractal-based analysis; glucocorticoid treatment; risk factors; imaging methods

---

1. Introduction

Bone loss and increased fracture risk are well-known extraintestinal complications of Crohn's disease (CD) [1,2]. As has been recently shown by our study group, CD patients have an increased risk for hip fractures and an associated higher mortality risk after fracture compared to the general population [3]. However, overall data on osteoporosis and fracture risk are conflicting in literature and largely depend on the patient population, severity of disease, disease duration and different imaging techniques in assessing bone mineral density (BMD) [4]. Further, patients with CD have many risk factors contributing to bone loss and therefore need special attention to identify patients at risk and prevent fractures. Bone strength is not only determined by BMD, but also by bone microarchitecture. To date, the gold-standard for examination of BMD is dual X-ray absorptiometry (DXA), a two-dimensional imaging method. With respect to the methodology of this imaging technique, no information on bone microstructure is assessed. Furthermore, anterior–posterior DXA scanning may not accurately reflect true changes in BMD, e.g., due to calcification of the aorta or osteophytes within the region of interest (ROI) [5–7].

Trabecular bone score (TBS), a grey-level texture parameter, can be applied to lumbar spine DXA scans as an add-on tool and provides information on the trabecular network of vertebral bodies. Additionally, TBS does not seem to be affected by degenerative changes of lumbar spine in contrast to BMD [8].

To date there is only one study addressing TBS assessment in adult CD patients in the literature. Interestingly, no differences in BMD or TBS compared to controls in the total cohort of CD patients were detected, but TBS was decreased in patients with a severe course of disease while BMD showed no difference [9]. Another method for assessing bone microarchitecture in vivo even more precisely is high-resolution peripheral quantitative computed tomography (HR-pQCT) of the distal radius and tibia. Bone microarchitecture assessed by HR-pQCT in inflammatory bowel disease (IBD) patients showed that CD patients have a severe deterioration of cortical and trabecular bone despite a reduced volumetric BMD at the distal radius. In this study, female sex, the diagnosis of CD, lower body mass index (BMI) and a lack of disease remission were identified as independently associated factors with bone loss in IBD [10].

The implementation of novel imaging techniques for the assessment of bone microarchitecture into clinical practice is of major interest. Fractal analysis techniques are based on the fractal model by Mandelbrot [11] and can be used to measure and express complex structures in numeric dimensions and for distinguishing image textures. Extensions of this model led to different techniques examining bone structure from two-dimensional X-ray projections. Fractal analysis of calcaneus radiographs in patients with previous osteoporotic fractures allowed to distinguish patients with fractures from those without fractures, independently and more exactly than BMD [12,13]. In another study, Caligiuri P et al. identified patients with vertebral fractures more accurately using fractal analysis of radiographs of the spine compared to DXA [14].

These results support the hypothesis, that fractal analysis provides complementary information out of conventional radiographs and can improve fracture risk evaluation, independently of BMD and additional radiation exposure.

TX-Analyzer™ is a novel software for fractal-based analysis of radiographs and features three texture algorithms—bone structure value (BSV), bone variance value (BVV) and bone entropy value (BEV). To date, the primary use is for research purposes on different skeletal sites. Until now, only one study on lumbar spine using TX-Analyzer™ was performed. In this retrospective analysis of a large randomized trial in postmenopausal women treated with the monoclonal antibody denosumab over eight years, Dimai HP et al. reported an increase of BMD and BSV of lumbar spine [15].

The aim of the present pilot study was to evaluate bone microstructure assessed by TX-Analyzer™ of the thoracic and lumbar spine in CD patients and for the first time, in the general population to correlate and compare the parameters to standard imaging techniques such as DXA and TBS.

2. Patients and Methods

2.1. Patients and Study Design

A total number of 40 patients and 40 age and sex-matched controls were analyzed in this case-controlled study. All patients participated in the "Crohn-Bone-Study", a non-interventional, prospective, cross-sectional, single-center study with the aim to create a database of patients with

Crohn's disease and assess the effects on bone. The patients were recruited in the gastroenterology outpatient clinic of the 1st Medical Department of the Hanusch Hospital of the Austrian Health Insurance in Vienna. Inclusion criteria were a histologically verified diagnosis of CD and patients had to be at least 18 years of age. Out of 51 patients included in the Crohn-Bone-Study, 40 patients underwent DXA scans of the lumbar spine and the hip and radiographs of the thoracic and lumbar spine and were, therefore, selected for this pilot study. Demographic parameters, information on disease duration (DD), treatment including glucocorticoid (GC) therapy, conventional or biological immunosuppressive therapy and history of surgery were assessed. Laboratory results including serum C-reactive protein (CRP), and bone turnover markers including calcium, phosphate, alkaline phosphatase (AP), beta-crosslaps, osteocalcin, parathyroid hormone (PTH) and 25(OH)-vitamin D levels as well as levels of fecal calprotectin were analyzed. Laboratory assessment was performed using immunoturbidimetric assay for CRP, photometric color test for calcium, photometric UV test for phosphate, 2-site immunometric (sandwich) electrochemiluminescence detection assay for beta-crosslaps, chemiluminescence immunoassay for osteocalcin, PTH, 25(OH)-vitamin D and calprotectin. The lower limits of quantification were as follows: 0.2 mg/L for CRP, 0.01 mmol/L for calcium, 0.11 mmol/L for phosphate, 5 U/L for AP, 0.01 ng/mL for beta-crosslaps, 3 ng/mL for osteocalcin, 1 pg/mL for parathyroid hormone, 11 nmol/L for 25(OH)-vitamin D and <5 mg/kg for fecal calprotectin.

Selection of controls was randomly chosen with respect to available conventional radiographs of the thoracic and lumbar spine. In total, 81 subjects who underwent X-ray examinations of the spine at the Radiological Department of the Hanusch Hospital Vienna were screened. Healthy controls were than matched 1:1 to CD, based on age- and sex-distribution of CD. Exclusion criteria for controls were a documented medical history of osteoporosis, low traumatic fractures, diabetes mellitus type 1 or 2, renal insufficiency CKD III-V (chronic kidney disease), hepatic cirrhosis (CHILD B or C), chronic alcohol abuse, rheumatologic disease, malignancy within 5 years or any eating disorder.

Two patients were excluded from the analysis (1 CD and 1 control) due to degenerative changes on the lumbar spine resulting into inaccurate BMD and TX lumbar spine values. In addition, both patients had extremely outranged high BMI (>41 kg/m^2) and (i) no DXA software for obese patients was available, (ii) TBS cannot be interpreted appropriately in patients with BMI > 40 and (iii) the influence of severe obesity on TX values is unclear.

The final analytical sample therefore comprised 39 CD patients and 39 controls. The study flow-chart is shown in supplementary Figure 1.

The study was approved by the local ethical committee (EK-16-252-1216) and conducted in accordance with the Declaration of Helsinki. All patients agreed to participate to the study and signed an informed consent form.

2.1.1. TX-Analyzer™

The software TX-Analyzer™ (ImageBiopsy Lab., Vienna, Austria) determines structural three-dimensional information of bone architecture non-invasively using a fractal-based analysis out of two-dimensional plain radiographs [16,17]. The software features the three unitless texture algorithms BSV, BVV and BEV. To date, no normative values for these parameters are available.

In detail, BSV reflects the quantification of the fractal dimension of the bone texture via an implementation of a maximum-likelihood estimator of the Hurst coefficient. The Hurst coefficient represents a measure of long-range dependency of data and therefore a good descriptor of wide range of natural phenomena [12,18,19]. This Hurst coefficient was measured in vertical and horizontal directions, for further analysis mean BSV was used. BVV quantifies the Hurst coefficient via the variance of pixel-intensity differences in four directions (0, 45, 90 and 135 degrees) and therefore, the extracted values include the vertical, horizontal and diagonal as well as the mean value, which was further analyzed. BSV and BVV range between 0 and 1; the maximum value of 1 indicates the highest possible homogeneity. The BEV represents the Shannon entropy originating from the field information theory and quantifies the average information content and complexity of the ROI [20].

The analysis of all radiographs was performed by two trained investigators (SH, JES). All X-rays were obtained using Philips DigitalDiagnost.

DICOM files of lateral-view radiographs of the thoracic and lumbar spine were analyzed using a semi-automatic software application (IB Lab TX-Analyzer™, IBL, Vienna, Austria). The annotation of the radiographs was carried out and the region of interest was defined. For positioning and analysis of the ROI the preset biopsy mask was used, according to the manufacturers' recommendation. After marking the front and back corners of each vertebral body, the software places the ROI within the vertebral body. For each subject, all vertebral bodies from the seventh thoracic vertebral body to the fourth lumbar vertebral body were analyzed (Figure 1). Fractured vertebral bodies were excluded from analysis and the mean of the remaining parameters calculated. If only one vertebral body was eligible for analysis, the patient was excluded.

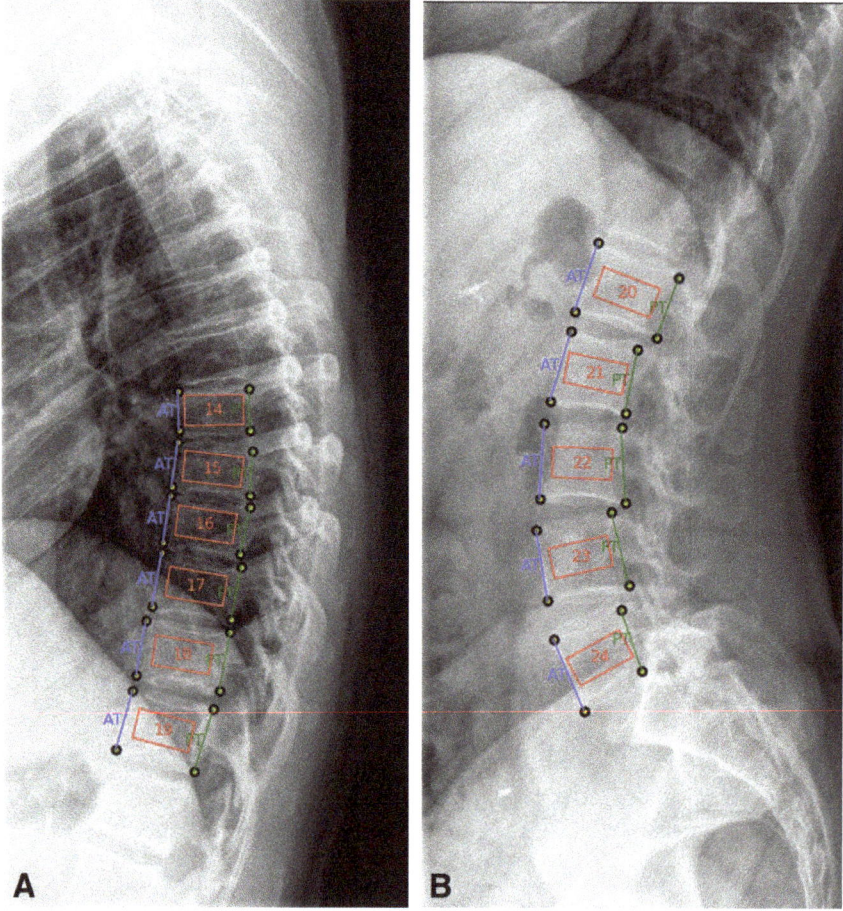

Figure 1. Application of TX-Analyzer™ software on lateral-view radiographs of the thoracic and lumbar spine of patients with Crohn's disease and controls. Definition of region of interest (ROI) using a preset biopsy mask, after definition of the upper and lower and the anterior and posterior corner of the vertebral bodies the ROI box is placed by the software. (**A**) thoracic spine and (**B**) lumbar spine.

2.1.2. Dual X-ray Absorptiometry (DXA) and Trabecular Bone Score (TBS)

DXA scanning and analysis was performed of the lumbar spine, the total femur and the femoral neck using GE Healthcare Lunar Prodigy (GE©, Boston, MA, USA). BMD and *T*-scores at all three sites were assessed. Analysis of DXA scans was performed according to international guidelines [21] and non-evaluable vertebral bodies excluded, accordingly. If only one vertebral body was evaluable, the measurement was excluded. TBS analysis was performed using TBS iNsight software version 3.

2.1.3. Statistics

Characteristics of CD patients and controls were described using frequencies and percentages for categorical variables and medians and interquartile ranges (IQR) for continuous variables if not stated otherwise. We assessed the distribution of each parameter via normality plots and Kolmogorov–Smirnov test. For group comparisons we used *T*-test or Mann–Whitney *U* test for continuous variables and Chi-square test for categorical variables, as appropriate. *p*-values were two sided, and the statistical significance level was set at 0.05. In case of multiple comparisons, we applied a Bonferroni correction.

For exploration of an association between two continuous variables we calculated either Pearson's correlation coefficient or Spearman's rank correlation coefficient, according to the normality of variable distribution. When both variables were normally distributed, we used Pearson's correlation coefficient, otherwise we used Spearman's correlation coefficient.

We stratified CD patients by glucocorticoid use ($\geq$5 mg prednisolone-equivalent daily > 3 months users vs. non-users), the disease duration (below or above 15 years), the history of bowel resection (yes vs. no) and compared these groups in demographic, DXA and TX parameters. Due to the study design the selection of healthy controls was solely based on the availability of X-rays, therefore no data of DXA parameters or TBS were available.

In order to test the robustness of our findings, we performed a sensitivity analysis by excluding patients with extreme values for TX parameters and repeated all the analysis. Extreme outliers were defined as values below and above the interquartile range multiplied by 3 (Q1 − 3 × IQR and Q3 + 3 × IQR).

All statistical analyses were conducted in IBM SPSS Statistics for Windows, Version 26 [22].

3. Results

3.1. Patient Population and Demographic Characteristics

Table 1 summarizes patient characteristics of CD patients and controls. There were no significant differences between CD patients and controls in age, sex or BMI. The disease duration was 8.0 (18) years and the median calprotectin level 88.9 (221.9) mg/kg.

Table 1. Demographics and disease specific characteristics of patients with Crohn's disease (CD) and controls.

	Crohn's Disease *n* = 39	Controls *n* = 39	*p*
Demographics and Disease Duration			
Sex [male/female]	13/26	14/25	0.812
Age [years]	53.9 (40.4–60.7)	44.8 (41.3–55.9)	0.439
Height [m]	1.68 (1.6–1.74)	1.67 (1.62–1.72)	0.859
Weight [kg]	75 (59–94)	78 (64.8–85.3)	0.895
BMI [kg/m^2]	27.4 (22.1–32.3)	27.1 (23.4–30.2)	0.924
Laboratory Results			
CRP [mg/L, 0.0–4.9]	2.80 (1.40–7.30)	-	-
Ca [mmol/L, 2.20–2.65]	2.37 (2.31–2.53)	-	-

Table 1. Cont.

	Crohn's Disease n = 39	Controls n = 39	p
Ph [mmol/L, 0.81–1.45]	1.14 (1.00–1.27)	-	-
AP [U/L, 30–120]	78 (65–95)	-	-
Beta-crosslaps [ng/mL, 0.03–0.37]	0.390 (0.28–0.58)	-	-
PTH [pg/mL, 12–88]	45.5 (31–73)	-	-
Osteocalcin [ng/mL, 4.6–65.4]	16.5 (14.1–21.9)	-	-
25(OH)-vitamin D [nmol/L, 75–250]	64 (52–76)	-	-
Calprotectin [mg/kg, 0.0–50.0]	88.9 (26.1–248)	-	-
Disease Characteristics			
Disease duration [years]	8 (2–20)	-	-
cDMARDs, n (%)	21 (55.3)	-	-
bDMARDs, n (%)	20 (52.6)	-	-
GC-Treatment > 3 mo, n (%)	23 (59)	-	-
History of bowel resection due to CD, n (%) *	14 (35.9) *	-	-
Ileocoecal Resection, n (%)	13 (34.2)	-	-
Small bowel resection, n (%)	4 (10.5)	-	-
Colonic resection, n (%)	5 (13.2)	-	-

Notes: BMI, body mass index; laboratory results [unit, reference range]; CRP, C-reactive protein; Ca, calcium; Ph, phosphate; AP, alkaline phosphatase; PTH, parathyroid hormone; cDMARDs, conventional disease modifying immunosuppressive drugs (including 6-mercaptopurine, azathioprine, budesonide or mesalazine); bDMARDs, biologic disease modifying immunosuppressive drugs (including adalimumab, infliximab, ustekinumab, vedolizumab); GC-treatment > 3 mo, glucocorticoid treatment over 3 months ≥ 5 mg; * some patients had joint procedures therefore the numbers do not sum up; and all parameters are reported as median (25th–75th percentile) or number (%), respectively, level of significance $p < 0.05$.

Fifty-nine percent of patients had a history of glucocorticoid treatment > 5 mg daily over more than 3 months. In total, 55.3% of CD patients were treated with conventional disease modifying immunosuppressive drugs (cDMARDs; 6-mercaptopurine, azathioprine, budesonide or mesalazine) and 52.6% with biological DMARDs therapy (bDMARDs; adalimumab, infliximab, ustekinumab, vedolizumab). Laboratory results showed no increase in CRP levels or alterations of bone turnover markers. The median level of 25(OH)-vitamin D in CD patients was 64 (24) nmol/L.

3.2. Bone Mineral Density and Bone Microarchitecture

Overall median T-score in lumbar spine of CD patients was −1.4 (2.2) and BMD 1.030 (0.2) g/cm^2. At the total hip and femoral neck, the BMD was 0.921 (0.13) g/cm^2 and 0.885 (0.15) g/cm^2, respectively, with a corresponding T-score of −0.9 (1.2) and −0.9 (1.3). TBS of CD patients was 1.307 (0.2).

At the lumbar spine the TX analysis revealed no differences of BSV, BVV or BEV between CD and controls. BSV and BVV of the thoracic spine were higher in CD patients compared to control patients ($p = 0.016$ and 0.012). All results are summarized in Table 2.

Table 2. Results of TX analysis, dual X-ray absorptiometry (DXA) and trabecular bone score (TBS) of patients with Crohn's disease and controls.

	Crohn's Disease n = 39	Controls n = 39	p
DXA and TBS			
Lumbar Spine (L1–L4)			
BMD [g/cm^2]	1.030 (0.955–1.183)	-	-
T-Score [SD]	−1.4 (−2.1–0.1)	-	-
TBS [units]	1.307 (1.218–1.402)	-	-
Total Hip			
BMD [g/cm^2]	0.921 (0.847–0.978)	-	-
T-Score [SD]	−0.9 (−1.4, −0.2)	-	-

Table 2. *Cont.*

	Crohn's Disease n = 39	Controls n = 39	p
	Femoral Neck		
BMD [g/cm^2]	0.885 (0.787–0.938)	-	-
T-Score [SD]	−0.9 (−1.8, −0.5)	-	-
	TX Analysis		
	Thoracic Spine (T7–T12)		
BSV	0.293 (0.268–0.309)	0.270 (0.225–0.302)	0.016
BVV	0.282 (0.260–0.302)	0.251 (0.214–0.288)	0.012
BEV	12.2 (12.1–12.3)	12.2 (12.1–12.3)	0.919
	Lumbar Spine (L1–L4)		
BSV	0.109 (0.093–0.128)	0.110 (0.104–0.125)	0.310
BVV	0.100 (0.092–0.118)	0.103 (0.010–0.119)	0.301
BEV	11.5 (11.4–11.6)	11.5 (11.4–11.6)	0.154

Notes: BMD, bone mineral density; SD, standard deviation; BSV, bone structure value; BVV, bone variance value; BEV, bone entropy value; BSV, BVV and BEV are unitless; and all parameters are reported as median (25th–75th percentile), level of significance $p < 0.05$.

3.3. Correlation of Imaging Parameters

All results of correlation analysis are reported in Table 3. BSV, BVV and BEV were correlated with each other within the region of investigation—in lumbar spine BSV and BVV we observed a strong positive correlation ($r = 0.800$, $R^2 = 0.88$, $p < 0.001$) and for BSV and BEV a moderate positive correlation ($r = 0.660$, $p < 0.001$). Comparable significant correlations were found for TX parameters at the thoracic spine. In contrast to the correlations within the two regions, no correlations of TX parameters between the thoracic and the lumbar spine were observed.

BSV, BVV and BEV of the thoracic spine showed no correlation to demographic parameters. At the lumbar spine, for BSV and BVV moderate negative correlations with weight ($r = -0.647$, $p < 0.001$ and $r = -0.605$, $p < 0.001$) and BMI ($r = -0.568$, $p < 0.001$ and $r = -0.403$, $p < 0.001$) were observed. No significant correlations were found between the TX parameters and TBS.

Further, correlations of TX parameters and BMD at all three measuring sites with laboratory results presented in Table 1 were performed. No correlation was found between TX parameters or BMD with the level of 25(OH)-vitamin D. BSV, BVV and BEV at the lumbar spine were moderately correlated with calprotectin levels ($r = 0.438$, $p = 0.009$; $r = 0.458$, $p = 0.006$; and $r = 0.518$, $p < 0.001$). A negative moderate correlation was observed for BSV and BVV with PTH ($r = -0.465$, $p = 0.004$ and $r = -0.524$, $p = 0.001$), but not for BEV. All results are presented in a Supplemental Table S1.

3.4. Glucocorticoid Use in Crohn's Disease Patients

Patients with a GC intake > 3 months had a significantly lower TBS of lumbar spine compared to patients without long-term GC treatment ($p = 0.014$). All further DXA parameters revealed no difference between these two groups.

TX analysis showed a significantly reduced BEV of the thoracic spine in GC treated patients, with no difference in BSV and BVV. At the lumbar spine no difference in BSV, BVV or BEV was found. All parameters are summarized in Table 4.

Table 3. Correlations of demographics and imaging parameters assessed by TX analysis, bone mineral density and trabecular bone score.

	Age	Weight	Height	BMI	BSV T7–T12	BSV L1–L4	BVV T7–T12	BVV L1–L4	BEV T7–T12	BEV L1–L4	BMD L1–L4	BMD Fem.Neck	BMD Total Fem
Weight	0.220												
Height	0.151	0.498 **											
BMI	0.159	0.876 **	0.025										
BSV T7–T12	0.029	−0.046	0.032	−0.078									
BSV L1–L4	−0.200	−0.647 *	−0.359 **	−0.568 **	0.109								
BVV T7–T12	0.054	−0.093	0.070	−0.151	0.966 **	0.134							
BVV L1–L4	−0.304 **	−0.605 **	−0.250 *	−0.594 **	0.152	0.800 *	0.196						
BEV T7–T12	−0.086	−0.082	−0.142	−0.019	0.476 **	0.041	0.349 **	−0.003					
BEV L1–L4	−0.154	−0.476 **	−0.259 **	−0.403 **	0.060	0.666 **	0.047	0.452 **	0.151				
BMD L1–L4	−0.095	0.407 *	0.204	0.360 *	0.014	−0.250	−0.121	−0.134	0.417 **	0.115			
BMD fem.neck	−0.273	0.454 **	0.337 *	0.353 **	0.010	−0.314	−0.097	−0.122	0.349 *	−0.029	0.785 **		
BMD total fem	−0.120	0.545 **	0.256	0.507 **	−0.064	−0.472 **	−0.177	−0.264	0.358 *	−0.238	0.771 **	0.881 **	
TBS	−0.525 **	0.154	−0.037	0.191	−0.102	−0.067	−0.165	0.067	0.217	0.116	0.417 *	0.466 **	0.451 **

Note: fem, femoral; and * level of significance $p < 0.05$; ** level of significance $p < 0.001$, (with adjustment for a Bonferroni correction). Values in bold are considered as statistically significant also after Bonferroni correction.

Table 4. Analysis of TX parameters, DXA and TBS in patients distributed according to disease duration, glucocorticoid (GC) use and history of bowel resection.

	History of GC Treatment			Disease Duration			History for Surgery for CD		
	<3 months N = 16	>3 months N = 23	p	≤15 years N = 25	>15 years N = 14	p	No N = 25	Yes N = 14	p
	Demographics and Disease Duration								
Sex [male/female]	5/11	8/15	0.818	6/19	7/7	0.098	4/21	9/5	0.002
Age [years]	44.4 (35.9–56.4)	54.8 (41.8–61.4)	0.228	54.3 (36.0–62.6)	52.7 (42.1–56.9)	0.883	53.9 (38.8–58.6)	50.8 (39.9–62.6)	0.972
Height [m]	1.65 (1.56–1.7)	1.69 (1.63–1.74)	0.579	1.66 (1.59–1.7)	1.70 (1.62–1.78)	0.268	1.67 (1.59–1.7)	1.74 (1.65–1.79)	0.016
Weight [kg]	70 (55–94.8)	80 (61–90)	0.346	75 (60.5–94.5)	73 (49.8–89.3)	0.519	73 (59–85)	88.5 (57.8–105.5)	0.111
BMI [kg/m²]	26.3 (21.7–32.9)	28.3 (22.7–31.6)	0.908	28.3 (23.1–32.6)	26.7 (18.2–30.3)	0.170	26.6 (22.3–32.0)	29.2 (21.5–32.4)	0.613
Dis. duration [years]	6.5 (2–13)	12 (5–25)	0.053	5 (1.5–8)	22 (17.8–30.5)	<0.001	5 (1.5–14)	17 (8–22.8)	0.013

Table 4. Cont.

	History of GC Treatment			Disease Duration			History for Surgery for CD		
	<3 months N = 16	>3 months N = 23	p	≤15 years N = 25	>15 years N = 14	p	No N = 25	Yes N = 14	p
	DXA and TBS								
	Lumbar Spine (L1-L4)								
BMD [g/cm²]	1.062 (0.994–1.282)	0.976 (0.912–1.183)	0.145	1.086 (0.972–1.223)	0.963 (0.874–1.047)	0.337	1.036 (0.952–1.223)	1.029 (0.919–1.076)	0.567
T-Score [SD]	−1.2 (−1.6–0.8)	−1.8 (−2.2–0.1)	0.146	−1.1 (−1.8–0.3)	−1.9 (−2.6–1.4)	0.412	−1.2 (−2.0–0.3)	−1.5 (−2.3–1.2)	0.357
TBS [units]	1.397 (1.299–1.459)	1.257 (1.186–1.356)	0.014	1.336 (1.222–1.403)	1.274 (1.210–1.390)	0.361	1.302 (1.202–1.399)	1.323 (1.240–1.407)	0.527
	Total Hip								
BMD [g/cm²]	0.921 (0.895–1.040)	0.922 (0.814–0.978)	0.251	0.943 (0.886–1.024)	0.855 (0.770–0.931)	0.598	0.921 (0.849–0.990)	0.926 (0.838–1.003)	0.942
T-Score [SD]	−0.8 (−1.5–0.3)	−1.1 (−1.7–0.2)	0.159	−0.6 (−1.1–0.2)	−1.4 (−2.3–0.6)	0.425	−0.8 (−1.3–0.1)	−1.2 (−1.6–0.3)	0.443
	Femoral Neck								
BMD [g/cm²]	0.900 (0.813–1.015)	0.857 (0.766–0.938)	0.224	0.900 (0.829–0.943)	0.813 (0.757–0.947)	0.724	0.885 (0.786–0.936)	0.901 (0.781–1.015)	0.536
T-Score [SD]	−0.8 (−1.5–0.3)	−1.0 (−1.8–0.6)	0.215	−0.8 (−1.3–0.5)	−1.4 (−2.3–0.6)	0.373	−0.8 (−1.7–0.5)	−1.1 (−2.1–0.3)	0.844
	TX Analysis								
	Thoracic Spine (T7-T12)								
BSV	0.295 (0.270–0.305)	0.290 (0.259–0.315)	0.932	0.298 (0.269–0.308)	0.284 (0.266–0.313)	0.761	0.293 (0.269–0.308)	0.284 (0.266–0.314)	0.919
BVV	0.275 (0.260–0.294)	0.286 (0.243–0.310)	0.475	0.282 (0.251–0.303)	0.278 (0.255–0.309)	0.806	0.276 (0.251–0.303)	0.286 (0.255–0.304)	0.828
BEV	12.3 (12.2–12.4)	12.2 (12.1–12.3)	0.015	12.3 (12.2–12.4)	12.1 (12.0–12.2)	0.001	12.2 (12.1–12.3)	12.2 (12.1–12.4)	0.784

Table 4. Cont.

	History of GC Treatment			Disease Duration			History for Surgery for CD		
	<3 months N = 16	>3 months N = 23	p	≤15 years N = 25	>15 years N = 14	p	No N = 25	Yes N = 14	p
	Lumbar Spine (L1–L4)								
BSV	0.115 (0.093–0.131)	0.103 (0.096–0.126)	0.797	0.109 (0.093–0.126)	0.106 (0.093–0.176)	0.478	0.115 (0.096–0.132)	0.100 (0.090–0.117)	0.228
BVV	0.107 (0.092–0.118)	0.099 (0.086–0.122)	0.549	0.099 (0.091–0.118)	0.105 (0.091–0.146)	0.515	0.099 (0.092–0.124)	0.101 (0.086–0.115)	0.675
BEV	11.6 (11.4–11.6)	11.5 (11.3–11.6)	0.138	11.5 (11.4–11.6)	11.5 (11.3–11.6)	0.303	11.6 (11.5–11.6)	11.4 (11.3–11.5)	0.011

Note: Dis.duration, disease duration; BSV, BVV and BEV are unitless; and all parameters are reported as median (25th–75th percentile), level of significance $p < 0.05$.

3.5. Disease Duration in Crohn's Disease Patients

Of the CD patients, 14 patients had a DD of >15 years and 25 patients a DD of ≤15 years. Patients with longer disease duration showed no difference in BMD of the lumbar spine or hip. Further, no difference in TBS was found compared to patients with a shorter disease duration. TX analysis revealed a significantly decreased BEV of the thoracic spine in patients with a DD of >15 years ($p = 0.001$). At the lumbar spine no difference of BEV between the two groups was observed. BSV and BVV showed no differences at the thoracic and the lumbar spine (Table 4).

3.6. History of Bowel Resection in Crohn's Disease Patients

Of the CD patients, 14 patients had a history of surgery, 34.2% of these patients with a resection of the terminal ileum, 10.5% had small bowel resection and 13.2% had a segmental colonic resection—some of the patients had joint procedures therefore the numbers do not sum up. The group of patients with a history of surgery included more male patients, patients were taller ($p = 0.016$) and had a longer disease duration ($p = 0.013$). BMD at the lumbar spine and hip showed no difference between the two groups of CD patients. Additionally, TBS was the same within these two groups. Regarding TX parameters, again BEV was significantly lower in patients with a history of bowel resection ($p = 0.011$), in this group at the lumbar spine. No further differences in TX parameters have been found (Table 4).

3.7. Sensitivity Analysis

For sensitivity analyses six patients were excluded with extreme values for TX parameters. A total of 34 CD patients and 38 controls were analyzed. The results with regard to differences between CD and controls in TX parameters remained practically unchanged (Supplemental Table S2). Concerning the analysis of CD patients there were no differences in DXA measures between patients with disease duration below or above 15 years, neither in patients with or without bowel resection. A more pronounced deterioration of bone microarchitecture in GC treated patients represented by lower levels of BSV and BVV at the lumbar spine was observed.

4. Discussion

In this pilot study spinal bone microstructure of Crohn's disease patients and controls of the general population was assessed for the first time using TX-Analyzer™, a novel fractal-based analysis. BSV and BVV of the thoracic spine were higher in CD patients compared to controls, with no difference in BEV. However, a significant impact of risk factors, like disease duration, glucocorticoid treatment and a history of bowel resection, on TX parameters was found in CD patients.

Patients with CD have multiple risk factors for bone loss like malnutrition, inflammatory state, malabsorption associated with vitamin D deficiency and glucocorticoid treatment. In literature, data on osteoporosis and fracture risk in CD patients are incongruent depending on patient population, disease duration and differences in imaging techniques [4]. The BMD measurement of CD patients in the present cohort using DXA technique, the gold standard in clinical practice, revealed overall no severe bone loss. Additional, trabecular bone assessed by TBS showed overall, that only a partially degraded microstructure at the lumbar spine of CD patients. The fact that BSV and BVV showed higher levels of CD patients compared to healthy controls is conflicting, but this should be considered as a result of an overall group, not severely affected bone of the present CD cohort. A recent large retrospective analysis of 393 CD patients revealed that only 19.8% of patients were diagnosed with osteoporosis, whereas the rest had normal BMD (39.9%) or the diagnosis of osteopenia (40.2%). Reduced BMD was associated with risk factors like male sex, low BMI and a history of bowel resection and longitudinal evaluation showed a further reduction of BMD in GC treated patients [23]. These findings indicate that by a modern management of CD using anti-inflammatory medications bone loss overall is not severe, but patients with one or even multiple risk factors and especially those treated with GC treatment should be identified and evaluated.

Further, in the present study, a fractal-based analysis of the spine using TX-Analyzer™ in the general population was performed for the first time. To date no reference values on TX parameters of the spine are available. Due to the study design, no information on BMD or TBS of the control group was available and therefore a deterioration of bone assessed by standardized measurements cannot be ruled out. However, a previous study of Dimai HP et al. focused on a prospective analysis of BSV at the lumbar spine in postmenopausal women on antiresorptive treatment with denosumab and an additional increase of BSV to a gain of BMD was observed [15]. Comparing the presented absolute levels of BSV in this population of women with postmenopausal osteoporosis to those in the present study, levels of BSV and BMD of patients with postmenopausal osteoporosis were much lower compared to CD patients and controls in the present cohort. This supports further the hypothesis of an overall not severely pronounced bone loss in the presented cohort.

It is important to note, that after dividing the population according to three above-mentioned risk factors, significant changes of bone microstructure assessed by TX parameters have been observed. Patients with GC treatment in the medical history, with long standing disease duration and with a history of bowel resection showed a reduction of BEV compared to controls despite no differences in BMD. This highlights that despite an overall not severely pronounced bone loss, deterioration of bone microstructure is assessable at an early time point using BEV.

Additionally, in patients with GC use, this finding is further supported by a reduction of TBS. Interestingly, no differences in BMD were observed. To date, there is only one study assessing TBS in adult CD patients in the literature. Krajcovicova A et al. showed that CD patients with severe disease course showed a reduction of TBS while BMD remained the same as controls [9]. These findings are in accordance with the present findings, since patients treated repeatedly with GC over time can be assumed to have a more severe course of disease.

However, long-term GC treatment itself is a well-known risk factor for bone loss due to inhibition of calcium absorption and promotion of renal calcium loss [24,25] and a promotion of osteoblast apoptosis and decreasing levels of osteoprotegerin [26,27]. Further, significant alterations of bone microarchitecture in patients treated with GC have been previously described in literature [28,29]. In a study of Leib ES et al. TBS was significantly lower in patients treated with GC due to different diseases compared to patients without GC treatment, while areal BMD at the lumbar spine showed no difference. Therefore, the authors stated, that GC use is associated with an impairment of microarchitectural texture of the central skeleton measured by TBS, preceding changes of BMD [30].

Deteriorations of bone microstructure in CD patients have been described previously in the literature. HR-pQCT scans of CD patients in a tertiary care center showed a severe deterioration of cortical and trabecular bone despite a reduced volumetric BMD of the ultradistal radius [10]. Nevertheless, those patients overall had a more severe course of disease compared to the present cohort and for the clinical setting this method has a limitation due to its rare availability. The most accurate information on bone microstructure is gained by performing a transiliac bone biopsy with histomorphometry. In a study by Oostlander AE et al. transiliac bone biopsies of 23 CD patients in remission were analyzed and histomorphometric analysis showed a reduction in bone mass characterized by trabecular thinning, caused by reduced bone formation [31]. All these studies provide important information on the risk of trabecular bone loss in patients with CD. Due to the limitations of availability and invasiveness, new imaging tools such as TX-Analyzer™ are of major interest for the clinical setting since pre-existing radiographs can be analyzed without additional radiation exposure.

TBS is the only available texture parameter in clinical practice to gain additional information on bone microstructure out of DXA scans. Spinal osteoarthrosis has no significant effect on TBS, while BMD increases in contrast [8]. Therefore, imaging techniques assessing bone microstructure within the vertebral body are of major interest. Since lower TBS as well as BEV values in the patient population with prior GC treatment despite normal BMD levels were found, one can suggest, that a fractal-based analysis using TX-Analyzer™ may as well elucidate early degradation of bone microstructure, prior to a loss of BMD and irrespectively of degenerative spinal changes. The acquisition of conventional radiographs due to different reasons is much more widespread compared to the performance of DXA scans, especially in younger patients. Therefore, TX-Analyzer™ may identify patients at risk at an early time point and before fractures even occur.

This pilot study is not without limitations. The main limitation is, that the size of the cohort was overall relatively small and therefore not suitable for building a regression model to address the question if two or further risk factors contribute to trabecular bone loss. Further studies with bigger study populations are required to confirm our preliminary results.

Additional, correlation analysis showed a positive correlation of lumbar and thoracic TX parameters, but no correlation between the different areas. Further, since there is a negative correlation observed of BSV, BVV and BEV of the lumbar spine with demographic parameters like height, weight and BMI, while there were no correlations with thoracic spine parameters, an influence of visceral fat on results of the lumbar spine may be a potential explanation. Furthermore, these results have to be further investigated and validated in a bigger cohort, since the present patient population and controls was overall well balanced and did not meet the recommendations of the World Health Organization for nutrition state with a median BMI of 27 kg/m^2. Nevertheless, taking this limitation into account, BEV reduction at the thoracic spine was present in two subgroups, despite an overall not reduced BMD. Further, validated imaging methods like TBS were lower in GC treated patients in addition to low BEV at the thoracic spine, supporting the findings. To date only limited information and experience with the TX-Analyzer™ at the spine is available and no reference values of the general population have been assessed previously. Therefore, we were able to demonstrate data on TX parameters of the thoracic and lumbar spine in healthy subjects for the first time.

5. Conclusions

In conclusion, the software TX-Analyzer™ is a non-invasive tool for indirect assessment of bone microstructure based on existing conventional radiographs. In the present study, CD patients were not severely affected by systemic bone loss and therefore, no typical microstructure pattern by this method was assessable compared to controls. However, well-known risk factors for systemic bone loss like glucocorticoid treatment, disease duration and history of bowel resection resulted in impaired bone quality assessed by TX-Analyzer™. Especially patients with GC treatment showed pronounced changes in BEV in accordance with a reduction of TBS despite normal BMD assessed by DXA.

Supplementary Materials: The following are available online at http://www.mdpi.com/2077-0383/9/12/4116/s1, Figure S1: Study flow-chart, Table S1: Correlations of imaging parameters assessed by TX analysis, Bone Mineral Density and Trabecular Bone Score and laboratory results, Table S2: Analysis of TX parameters, DXA and TBS in patients distributed according to disease duration, GC use and history of bowel resection after exclusion of extreme outliers.

Author Contributions: J.B., D.A.K. and J.H. collected the data. P.M. provided software. A.B. and S.Z. provided radiographs and D.A.K. scans. S.H. and J.E.S. performed TX-Analyzer™ measurements. J.Z. and R.K. contributed to the study design. M.B. performed the statistical analysis. J.H., M.B. and R.K. interpreted the data. J.H. drafted the manuscript. D.A.K., M.B. and R.K. were involved in drafting the manuscript. All authors read and approved the final manuscript.

Funding: This research received no external funding.

Conflicts of Interest: Judith Haschka, Daniel Arian Kraus, Martina Behanova, Stephanie Huber, Johann Bartko, Jakob E Schanda, Arian Bahrami, Shahin Zandieh, Jochen Zwerina and Roland Kocijan declare no conflict of interest. Philip Meier is shareholder and employee of ImageBiopsy Lab.

References

1. Targownik, L.E.; Bernstein, C.N.; Nugent, Z.; Johansson, H.; Oden, A.; McCloskey, E.; Kanis, J.A.; Leslie, W.D. Inflammatory bowel disease and the risk of fracture after controlling for FRAX. *J. Bone Miner. Res.* **2013**, *28*, 1007–1013. [CrossRef] [PubMed]
2. van Staa, T.P.; Cooper, C.; Brusse, L.S.; Leufkens, H.; Javaid, M.K.; Arden, N.K. Inflammatory bowel disease and the risk of fracture. *Gastroenterology* **2003**, *125*, 1591–1597. [CrossRef] [PubMed]

3. Bartko, J.; Reichardt, B.; Kocijan, R.; Klaushofer, K.; Zwerina, J.; Behanova, M. Inflammatory Bowel Disease: A Nationwide Study of Hip Fracture and Mortality Risk After Hip Fracture. *J. Crohn's Colitis* **2020**, *14*, 1256–1263. [CrossRef] [PubMed]
4. Targownik, L.E.; Bernstein, C.N.; Nugent, Z.; Leslie, W.D. Inflammatory bowel disease has a small effect on bone mineral density and risk for osteoporosis. *Clin. Gastroenterol. Hepatol.* **2013**, *11*, 278–285. [CrossRef] [PubMed]
5. Drinka, P.J.; DeSmet, A.A.; Bauwens, S.F.; Rogot, A. The effect of overlying calcification on lumbar bone densitometry. *Calcif. Tissue Int.* **1992**, *50*, 507–510. [CrossRef] [PubMed]
6. Orwoll, E.S.; Oviatt, S.K.; Mann, T. The Impact of Osteophytic and Vascular Calcifications on Vertebral Mineral Density Measurements in Men*. *J. Clin. Endocrinol. Metab.* **1990**, *70*, 1202–1207. [CrossRef]
7. Greenspan, S.L.; Maitland-Ramsey, L.; Myers, E. Classification of osteoporosis in the elderly is dependent on site-specific analysis. *Calcif. Tissue Int.* **1996**, *58*, 409–414. [CrossRef]
8. Dufour, R.; Winzenrieth, R.; Heraud, A.; Hans, D.; Mehsen, N. Generation and validation of a normative, age-specific reference curve for lumbar spine trabecular bone score (TBS) in French women. *Osteoporos. Int. J. Establ. Result Coop. Eur. Found. Osteoporos. Natl. Osteoporos. Found. USA* **2013**, *24*, 2837–2846. [CrossRef]
9. Krajcovicova, A.; Kuzma, M.; Hlavaty, T.; Hans, D.; Koller, T.; Jackuliak, P.; Leskova, Z.; Sturdik, I.; Killinger, Z.; Payer, J. Decrease of trabecular bone score reflects severity of Crohn's disease: Results of a case-control study. *Eur. J. Gastroenterol. Hepatol.* **2018**, *30*, 101–106. [CrossRef]
10. Haschka, J.; Hirschmann, S.; Kleyer, A.; Englbrecht, M.; Faustini, F.; Simon, D.; Figueiredo, C.P.; Schuster, L.; Muschitz, C.; Kocijan, R.; et al. High-resolution Quantitative Computed Tomography Demonstrates Structural Defects in Cortical and Trabecular Bone in IBD Patients. *J. Crohn's Colitis* **2016**, *10*, 532–540. [CrossRef]
11. Mandelbrot, B.B.; Freeman, W.H. *The Fractal Geometry of Nature*; Henry Holt and Company: New York, NY, USA, 1983.
12. Benhamou, C.L.; Poupon, S.; Lespessailles, E.; Loiseau, S.; Jennane, R.; Siroux, V.; Ohley, W.; Pothuaud, L. Fractal analysis of radiographic trabecular bone texture and bone mineral density: Two complementary parameters related to osteoporotic fractures. *J. Bone Miner. Res.* **2001**, *16*, 697–704. [CrossRef] [PubMed]
13. Pothuaud, L.; Lespessailles, E.; Harba, R.; Jennane, R.; Royant, V.; Eynard, E.; Benhamou, C.L. Fractal analysis of trabecular bone texture on radiographs: Discriminant value in postmenopausal osteoporosis. *Osteoporos. Int.* **1998**, *8*, 618–625. [CrossRef] [PubMed]
14. Caligiuri, P.; Giger, M.L.; Favus, M. Multifractal radiographic analysis of osteoporosis. *Med. Phys.* **1994**, *21*, 503–508. [CrossRef] [PubMed]
15. Dimai, H.P.; Ljuhar, R.; Ljuhar, D.; Norman, B.; Nehrer, S.; Kurth, A.; Fahrleitner-Pammer, A. Assessing the effects of long-term osteoporosis treatment by using conventional spine radiographs: Results from a pilot study in a sub-cohort of a large randomized controlled trial. *Skeletal. Radiol.* **2019**, *48*, 1023–1032. [CrossRef] [PubMed]
16. Pentland, A.P. Fractal-based description of natural scenes. *IEEE Trans. Pattern Anal. Mach. Intell.* **1984**, *6*, 661–674. [CrossRef]
17. Nehrer, S.; Ljuhar, R.; Steindl, P.; Simon, R.; Maurer, D.; Ljuhar, D.; Bertalan, Z.; Dimai, H.P.; Goetz, C.; Paixao, T. Automated Knee Osteoarthritis Assessment Increases Physicians' Agreement Rate and Accuracy: Data from the Osteoarthritis Initiative. *Cartilage* **2019**. [CrossRef]
18. Prouteau, S.; Ducher, G.; Nanyan, P.; Lemineur, G.; Benhamou, L.; Courteix, D. Fractal analysis of bone texture: A screening tool for stress fracture risk? *Eur. J. Clin. Investig.* **2004**, *34*, 137–142. [CrossRef]
19. Lundahl, T.; Ohley, W.J.; Kay, S.M.; Siffert, R. Fractional brownian motion: A maximum likelihood estimator and its application to image texture. *IEEE Trans. Med. Imaging* **1986**, *5*, 152–161. [CrossRef]
20. Shannon, C.E. The mathematical theory of communication. 1963. *MD Comput.* **1997**, *14*, 306–317.
21. 2019 ISCD Official Positions—Adult. Available online: https://www.iscd.org/official-positions/2019-iscd-official-positions-adult/ (accessed on 19 December 2020).
22. IBM Corp. *Released 2019. IBM SPSS Statistics for Windows, Version 26.0*; IBM Corp.: Armonk, NY, USA, 2019.
23. Hoffmann, P.; Krisam, J.; Kasperk, C.; Gauss, A. Prevalence, Risk Factors and Course of Osteoporosis in Patients with Crohn's Disease at a Tertiary Referral Center. *J. Clin. Med.* **2019**, *8*, 2178. [CrossRef]
24. Suzuki, Y.; Ichikawa, Y.; Saito, E.; Homma, M. Importance of increased urinary calcium excretion in the development of secondary hyperparathyroidism of patients under glucocorticoid therapy. *Metab. Clin. Exp.* **1983**, *32*, 151–156. [CrossRef]

25. Hahn, T.J.; Halstead, L.R.; Baran, D.T. Effects off short term glucocorticoid administration on intestinal calcium absorption and circulating vitamin D metabolite concentrations in man. *J. Clin. Endocrinol. Metab.* **1981**, *52*, 111–115. [CrossRef] [PubMed]
26. Kondo, T.; Kitazawa, R.; Yamaguchi, A.; Kitazawa, S. Dexamethasone promotes osteoclastogenesis by inhibiting osteoprotegerin through multiple levels. *J. Cell. Biochem.* **2008**, *103*, 335–345. [CrossRef] [PubMed]
27. Adami, G.; Saag, K.G. Glucocorticoid-induced osteoporosis: 2019 concise clinical review. *Osteoporos. Int.* **2019**, *30*, 1145–1156. [CrossRef]
28. Dalle Carbonare, L.; Arlot, M.E.; Chavassieux, P.M.; Roux, J.P.; Portero, N.R.; Meunier, P.J. Comparison of trabecular bone microarchitecture and remodeling in glucocorticoid-induced and postmenopausal osteoporosis. *J. Bone Miner. Res. Off. J. Am. Soc. Bone Miner. Res.* **2001**, *16*, 97–103. [CrossRef]
29. Dempster, D.W. Bone histomorphometry in glucocorticoid-induced osteoporosis. *J. Bone Miner. Res. Off. J. Am. Soc. Bone Miner. Res.* **1989**, *4*, 137–141. [CrossRef]
30. Leib, E.S.; Winzenrieth, R. Bone status in glucocorticoid-treated men and women. *Osteoporos. Int. J. Establ. Result Coop. Eur. Found. Osteoporos. Natl. Osteoporos. Found. USA* **2016**, *27*, 39–48. [CrossRef]
31. Oostlander, A.E.; Bravenboer, N.; Sohl, E.; Holzmann, P.J.; van der Woude, C.J.; Dijkstra, G.; Stokkers, P.C.; Oldenburg, B.; Netelenbos, J.C.; Hommes, D.W.; et al. Histomorphometric analysis reveals reduced bone mass and bone formation in patients with quiescent Crohn's disease. *Gastroenterology* **2011**, *140*, 116–123. [CrossRef]

Publisher's Note: MDPI stays neutral with regard to jurisdictional claims in published maps and institutional affiliations.

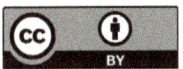

© 2020 by the authors. Licensee MDPI, Basel, Switzerland. This article is an open access article distributed under the terms and conditions of the Creative Commons Attribution (CC BY) license (http://creativecommons.org/licenses/by/4.0/).

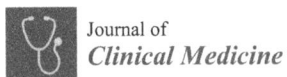

Article

Impact of Hormonal Replacement Therapy on Bone Mineral Density in Premature Ovarian Insufficiency Patients

Agnieszka Podfigurna [1,†], Marzena Maciejewska-Jeske [1,†], Malgorzata Nadolna [2,†], Paula Mikolajska-Ptas [2,†], Anna Szeliga [1], Przemyslaw Bilinski [3,4], Paulina Napierala [1] and Blazej Meczekalski [1,*]

[1] Department of Gynecological Endocrinology, Poznan University of Medical Sciences, 33 Polna Street, 60-535 Poznan, Poland; agnieszkapodfigurna@gmail.com (A.P.); marzena@jeske.pl (M.M.-J.); anna.mariaszeliga@gmail.com (A.S.); napierala.anna92@gmail.com (P.N.)
[2] Students Scientific Society of the Department of Gynecological Endocrinology, Poznan University of Medical Sciences, 33 Polna Street, 60-535 Poznan, Poland; mnadolna@hotmail.com (M.N.); pola.wiktoria@wp.pl (P.M.-P.)
[3] The President Stanislaw Wojciechowski State University of Applied Sciences in Kalisz, 62-800 Kalisz, Poland; bildom@gmail.com
[4] Copernicus Memorial Multidisciplinary Comprehensive Cancer and Traumatology Center, 93-513 Lodz, Poland
* Correspondence: blazejmeczekalski@yahoo.com
† The authors contributed to the paper equally.

Received: 25 October 2020; Accepted: 2 December 2020; Published: 7 December 2020

Abstract: Abstract: Introduction Premature ovarian insufficiency (POI) is a type of hypergonadotropic hypogonadism caused by impaired ovarian function before the age of 40. Due to the hypoestrogenism, women with POI experience a variety of health complications, including an increased risk of bone mineral density loss and developing osteopenia and osteoporosis, which poses an important problem for public health. **Purpose:** The aim of this study was to evaluate and compare the values of bone mineral density (BMD), T-score and Z-score within the lumbar spine (L1-L4) using the dual energy X-ray absorptiometry method. The dual-energy X-ray absorptiometry (DXA) scans described in this original prospective article were performed at the time of POI diagnosis and after treatment with sequential hormone replacement therapy (HRT). **Materials and methods:** This study included 132 patients with a mean age of 31.86 ± 7.75 years who had been diagnosed with idiopathic POI. The control group consisted of 17 healthy women with regular menstrual cycles, with a mean age of 23.21 ± 5.86 years. Serum follicle-stimulating hormone (FSH), luteinizing hormone (LH), 17-estradiol (E2), prolactin (PRL), testosterone (T), dehydroepiandrosterone sulfate (DHEA-S), thyroid-stimulating hormone (TSH), free thyroxine (fT4), insulin, and fasting serum glucose were measured. Lumbar spine (L1-L4) BMD was assessed by means of dual-energy X-ray absorptiometry. DXA scans were performed at the time of diagnosis and following treatment with sequential hormone replacement therapy (HRT) comprised of daily oral 2 mg 17-β-estradiol and 10 mg dydrogesterone. The mean time of observation was 3 ± 2 years. **Results:** Patients in the POI group presented with characteristic hypergonadotropic hypogonadism. They had a significantly decreased mean lumbar spine BMD when compared to healthy controls (1.088 ± 0.14 g/cm^2 vs. 1.150 ± 0.30 g/cm^2) ($p = 0.04$) as well as a decreased T-score (0.75 ± 1.167 vs. -0.144 ± 0.82) ($p = 003$). There was a significant increase in BMD (1.088 ± 0.14 vs. 1.109 ± 0.14; $p < 0.001$), T-score (-0.75 ± 1.17 vs. -0.59 ± 1.22; $p < 0.001$), and Z-score (-0.75 ± 1.12 vs. -0.49 ± 1.11; $p < 0.001$) after the implementation of HRT when compared to pre-treatment results. **Conclusions:** In conclusion, this study has demonstrated that patients with POI often have decreased bone mineral density and that the implementation of HRT has a significant and positive influence on bone mass. The implementation of full-dose HRT and monitoring of bone status is particularly important in these patients.

Keywords: premature ovarian insufficiency; DXA; osteoporosis; menopause; bone mineral density

1. Introduction

Premature ovarian insufficiency (POI) is a type of hypergonadotropic hypogonadism caused by impaired ovarian function before the age of 40 [1,2]. It affects 1:100 women before the age of 40 and 1:10,000 before the age of 20 [2]. Due to the hypoestrogenism, women with POI experience a variety of health complications. The natural progression of POI includes a short period of oligomenorrhea with subsequent secondary amenorrhea. If POI occurs before the age of 16 years, patients often present with primary amenorrhea. Vasomotor symptoms (hot flashes, night sweats), genitourinary symptoms (vaginal dryness, dyspareunia), neurological impairment, increased cardiovascular risk, and bone health deterioration are all part of the natural sequalae of POI [1].

The impact of estrogen deficiency on bone mass in postmenopausal patients is well described in the literature. Bone mass reduction progresses as a result of increased osteoclast action [3] causing cancellous bone perforation. Similarly, POI has adverse long-term effects on bone health. Various studies have demonstrated that patients with POI concomitantly develop decreased bone mineral density (BMD) [4]. Thus, according to recent discussions in the literature [5,6], it is reasonable to expect that these patients are likely to experience an increased risk of developing osteopenia and osteoporosis, and potential fractures in later life.

Fracture prevention is a worldwide public health priority; osteoporosis is a major healthcare problem leading to a high incidence of various fractures causing morbidity and mortality in the ageing population. Therefore, care should be taken to provide patients with effective treatment to prevent long-term health complications. The efficacy of hormone replacement therapy (HRT) as a protection against adverse outcomes in POI, however, has been poorly evaluated. The potential benefits these patients can gain form HRT may not fully correspond with the body of trials carried out on populations of postmenopausal women [6].

HRT has a favorable effect on BMD in postmenopausal women and decreases their overall risk of bone fractures [7–9]. The evidence suggests that supplementing estrogen levels in POI and restoring it to normal levels through the use of HRT replaces ovarian function and may also have a positive impact on bone mass. Implementation of HRT raises the level of serum estradiol, which is a stimulus for bone formation and slows bone resorption [10].

Taking into consideration the limited data regarding BMD in POI and the influence of different HRT regimens on BMD in this group of patients, the aim of this study was to compare the BMD of POI patients with that of healthy controls and to evaluate the effect of sequential hormonal replacement therapy on BMD in this group of patients. The medical problem presented in this study represents the importance to public health of understanding the risks of osteopenia, osteoporosis in populations of young women with premature ovarian insufficiency (POI).

2. Materials and Methods

2.1. Materials

This study included 132 patients with a mean age of 31.86 ± 7.75 years. They had been diagnosed with spontaneous POI and treated by the Department of Gynecological Endocrinology, Poznan University of Medical Sciences, Poznan, Poland during the period from 2013 to 2016. BMD was assessed in each individual before and after the use of estro-progestin hormone therapy.

Qualifying participants had an established diagnosis of POI based on the following the criteria [11]

(1) Onset before 40 years of age
(2) Secondary amenorrhea for a duration of at least 4 months
(3) FSH level above 25 IU/L measured on two separate occasions at least 4 months apart

(4) Estrogen level below 50 pg/mL

To maintain homogeneity in the study population, only patients with an idiopathic etiology of POI were included. Subjects with karyotype abnormalities and genetic defects, and those with an autoimmune, infectious or iatrogenic etiology of POI were disqualified.

The control group consisted of 17 healthy women with a mean age of 23.21 ± 5.86 years and regular menstrual cycles.

Exclusion criteria for the control group were:

(1) Any preexisting endocrine disorders—based on laboratory parameters and anamnesis
(2) Chronic diseases, particularly diseases affecting the musculoskeletal system
(3) Any hormonal treatment taken in the 3 months preceding the examination.

2.2. Methods

Each qualifying study participant had a thorough medical history taken, and a physical and gynecological examination and a transvaginal ultrasound were performed. Weight (kg) and height (m) were measured and BMI was calculated (kg/m^2).

Venous blood samples were collected between 7:00 am and 9:00 am in a fasting state. Blood samples in the control group were drawn in the late follicular phase; between the 10th and 12th day of the menstrual cycle.

Serum follicle-stimulating hormone (FSH), luteinizing hormone (LH), 17-estradiol (E2), prolactin (PRL), testosterone (T), dehydroepiandrosterone sulfate (DHEA-S), thyroid-stimulating hormone (TSH), free thyroxine (fT4), insulin, and fasting serum glucose were measured in all participants. Serum concentration was determined using electrochemiluminescence immunoassay (ECLIA) on a Cobas E601 analyzer (Roche Diagnostics, Indianapolis, IN, USA).

BMD measurement of the lumbar spine (L1-L4) was performed using dual-energy X-ray absorptiometry (DXA, Lunar Prodigy Primo, General Electric, USA). The results were expressed as g/cm^2, Z-score, and T-score. The T-score was calculated from mean peak BMD and SD obtained from database analysis of normative data for the lumbar spine of young healthy adults. T-score values of between −1 and −2.5 were used as thresholds for diagnosing osteopenia, and values lower than −2.5 were characterized as osteoporosis.

DXA was performed at the time of diagnosis and following treatment with sequential hormone replacement therapy (HRT). Treatment consisted of daily oral 2 mg 17-β-estradiol and 10 mg dydrogesterone. The mean time of observation was 3 ± 2 years.

This study may be limited by the inconsistent durations of hormone replacement therapy, as in some patients it was shorter, and in some it was longer; however, it lasted at least 12 months in all cases.

2.3. Statistical Analysis

Statistical analysis was performed using StatSoft 2012 STATISTICA Version 12. The normality of data distribution was assessed using the Shapiro–Wilk test. The Pearson's linear correlation coefficient and Spearman's rank correlation coefficient were used for correlation assessment. For comparison, Student's t-test or the Mann–Whitney test were used where appropriate. Comparison between more than 2 groups was performed using analysis of variance (ANOVA test). A p-value of 0.05 was considered statistically significant.

All participants provided written informed consent before enrolling in the study. The study protocol was approved by the Ethics Committee of Poznan University of Medical Sciences in Poznan, Poland.

3. Results

Patients in the POI group presented with characteristic hypergonadotropic hypogonadism (significantly elevated serum concentrations of FSH and LH with concomitantly low serum level of estradiol). They were also found to have a significantly higher fasting glucose level when compared to healthy controls (Table 1).

Table 1. Characterization of POI group and control group.

	POI Group			Control Group	
	Before Treatment	After Treatment	p1		p2
BMI [kg/m^2]	23.68 ± 4.42	23.81 ± 4.67	0.25	20.71 ± 5.15	0.06
FSH [mIU/ml]	100.14 ± 36.93	82.56 ± 48.72	<0.001	9.83 ± 2.44	<0.001
LH [mIU/ml]	49.64 ± 18.02	50.67 ± 30.77	0.76	10.47 ± 2.62	<0.001
E2 [pg/mL]	13.43 ± 18.91	56.1 ± 68.83	<0.001	94.12 ± 24.86	<0.001
T [ng/mL]	0.28 ± 0.19	0.44 ± 1.09	0.02	0.32 ± 0.18	0.31
DHEA-S [μmol/L]	5.94 ± 2.89	5.98 ± 2.89	0.51	7.38 ± 4.79	0.46
fT4 [ng/dL]	1.29 ± 0.18	1.45 ± 1.19	0.24	1.23 ± 0.3	0.98
TSH [μIU/mL]	2.58 ± 1.94	2.1 ± 1.72	0.01	2.76 ± 1.69	0.53
Glucose [mg/dl]	90.45 ± 9.97	87.75 ± 14.43	0.35	71.32 ± 17.72	<0.001
Insulin [mU/mL]	8.9 ± 4.64	9.58 ± 6.9	0.28	7.43 ± 3.6	0.31
PRL [ng/mL]	12.35 ± 10.19	11.64 ± 6.07	0.82	8.42 ± 3.66	0.16

Data presented as mean ± SD; p1-comparison of data before and after treatment (comparisons made using the Wilcoxon signed-rank test); p2-comparison between TS before treatment and control group (comparisons made using t-student test (data consistent with normal distribution) or Mann-Whitney U test (data inconsistent with normal distribution)); $p < 0.05$ considered significant.

Women in the POI group had a significantly decreased lumbar spine mean BMD (1088 ± 0.14 g/cm^2 vs. 1150 ± 0.30 g/cm^2) (p = 0.04), (median 1099 g/cm^2 vs. 1169 g/cm^2) (Figure 1) and T-score (0.75 ± 1167 vs. −0.144 ± 0.82) (p = 0.03) when compared to healthy controls (Figure 2).

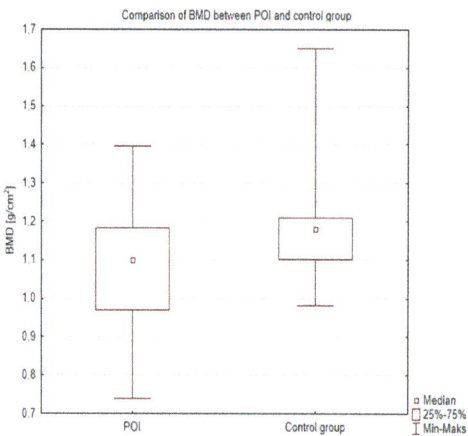

Figure 1. Comparison of BMD between POI and control group.

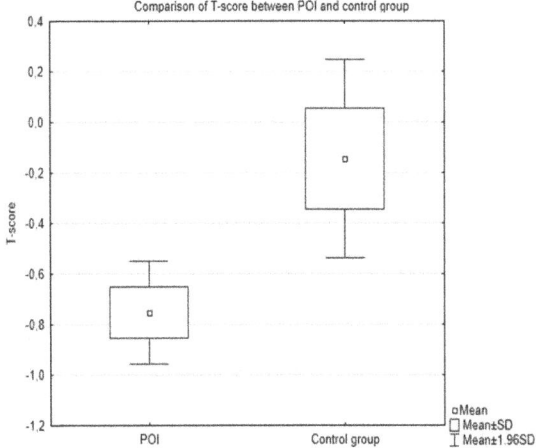

Figure 2. Comparison of T-score between POI and control group.

Comparative analysis of BMD, T-scores, and Z-scores was performed in the study group. Values at baseline were compared with post-treatment scores and a significant increase in BMD, T-score, and Z-score was observed following implementation of HRT in these patients (Table 2).

Table 2. BMD in POI group before and after treatment.

	POI Group		
	Before Treatment	After Treatment	p
BMD [g/cm2]	1.088 ± 0.14	1,109 ± 0.14	<0.001
T-score	−0.75 ± 1.17	−0.59 ± 1.22	<0.001
Z-score	−0.75 ± 1.12	−0.49 ± 1.11	<0.001

Data presented as mean ± SD; comparisons made using the Wilcoxon signed-rank test; $p < 0.05$ considered significant.

Before commencing HRT, 8.94% of 132 patients in the POI group fulfilled the T-score criteria for osteoporosis and 30.08% were found to suffer from osteopenia. After HRT only 1.69% of the patients were found to meet diagnostic criteria for osteoporosis, whereas 42.37% were found to be osteopenic.

The group of patients with POI was additionally divided into two groups based on baseline T-score values. The first subgroup included patients with a baseline T-score within the normal reference range. The second subgroup comprised POI patients with an abnormal baseline T-score defined as osteoporosis or osteopenia. It was noted, that the second subgroup (with abnormal baseline T-score) had a significantly higher serum LH concentration when compared to the group with normal baseline T-score. No additional differences were observed in other serum parameters. Moreover, analysis of variance found no significant difference between any measured parameter in the POI group when comparing normal BMD, osteopenia, and osteoporosis.

4. Discussion

POI is most often associated with impaired ovarian function and results in ovarian hormone deficiency. This lack of estrogens exerts an influence on osteoclasts, and leads to exacerbated bone reduction exceeding the rate of bone formation. As a consequence, estrogen deprivation in patients with POI has a negative impact on bone health, which may lead to decreased bone mineral density and an increased risk of osteoporosis and fractures in later life.

This study was conducted to investigate the bone mineral density in a significant sample of patients with POI and compare it to age and weight-matched premenopausal controls. It then evaluated and quantified the influence of estroprogestative replacement therapy (using 17β-estradiol and dydrogesterone) on lumbar spine bone mass in this patient group.

Following this study, we report that women with POI have lower baseline lumbar spine BMD when compared to age and weight matched controls. The implementation of HRT increased BMD in these patients compared to their values at the baseline.

Soong et al. [12] was one of the first studies to evaluate BMD in premenopausal amenorrhoeic patients. They studied a group of 21 patients with premature ovarian insufficiency. The mean BMD for all participant groups in this study (including one group of patients with POI) was reduced when compared to the control group [12].

In another study, Popat et al. [13] compared a cohort of patients with spontaneous POI to age-matched women with regular menstrual cycles. They discovered that the POI population had a significantly lower (2–3%) BMD in the lumbar spine, femoral neck, and total hip. In total, 15% of women in the POI group were found to have a Z-score below −2.0, a result which was below the expected value for age. In total, 8% of women with POI were shown to have a T-score below −2.5, a result characteristic of osteoporosis [13].

A number of later studies went on to confirm the association between low BMD and POI patients: idiopathic POI [13], Turner syndrome [14], chemotherapy [15], ovariectomy [16], gonadal dysgenesis [17], and mixed etiology POI [18]. The results demonstrated in our study are reflective of the findings mentioned above and support the thesis that women with POI have a significantly decreased BMD and, in some cases, even T-score values in the osteopenic and osteoporotic range at the moment of diagnosis. These profound early changes may be explained by the fact that impairment of ovarian function and subsequent estrogen deficiency can proceed insidiously prior to the diagnosis of POI. Alzubaidi et al. [19] reports that diagnosis is delayed in up to half of cases, and in 25% of cases this delay can be more than 5 years.

Popat et al. [13] have reported on certain modifiable factors correlating with significant low-for-age Z-score. These included vitamin D levels below 32 ng/mL, body weight below 55 kg, lack of regular exercise, calcium intake below 1000 mg/d, and no HRT implementation.

In order to protect bone health and decrease fracture risk, non-pharmacological strategies which are shown to be beneficial for postmenopausal women [20] are also advised for patients with POI. These recommendations include maintaining appropriate body weight, consuming a balanced diet, practicing weight-bearing exercises, moderating alcohol consumption, and smoking cessation [20]. According to WHO guidelines, maintaining a minimum recommended calcium intake of 1000 mg/day and a vitamin D intake of 800IU/day is essential to maintaining bone health and reducing the risk of fractures [21,22].

The results of BMD measurements should be taken into consideration at the time of management initiation for all patients, and particularly in those who present following a long period of estrogen deficiency and additional risk factors for decreased bone mass [23]. DXA is regarded as the gold standard in BMD assessment and is a first-line method for monitoring BMD in POI patients. It is important to note that the estimated yearly increase in BMD following the initiation of treatment is only 2%, which does not exceed the reported error margin of a DXA absorptiometer (1–2%). It is therefore recommended to perform a BMD assessment by DXA scan at 5 year intervals to ensure adequate monitoring [23,24]. The ideal measurement site for determining BMD has not yet been specified. It is known, however, that estrogens exert stronger antiresorptive action on trabecular bone, a structure making up a larger volume in the spine than in the total hip [25].

5. Estrogen Formulation

The use of estrogen therapy is an accepted method of improving POI-related health sequelae. This is in spite of the fact that trials comparing the efficacy of treatment regimens and their safety profiles with regard to symptom mitigation and the prevention of disease progression are deficient. Evidence has accumulated, however, showing that the use of HRT can restore bone mass in POI patients [26]. The available estrogen formulations commonly used to treat POI include 17β-estradiol (E2), ethinylestradiol (EE), and conjugated equine estrogens (CEE). A growing body of literature has supported the use of estradiol as the preferred form of estrogen replacement [11].

In 2014, Popat et al. [26] evaluated the influence of HRT on BMD in POI. In their study, preparations of 100 µg transdermal E2 and 10mg oral medroxyprogesterone were administered for a 3-year period. These were noted to significantly improve BMD measured at both the lumbar spine and femoral neck when compared to their baseline BMD values. The addition of testosterone did not have any beneficial effect on BMD levels in these patients. At the end of the study period, patients with POI exhibited no significant difference in BMD compared to the control group.

Similar results were observed by Cartwright et al. [27] who determined the superiority of HRT (2 mg oral E2 and 0.075 mg levonorgestrel daily) over a combined oral contraceptive pill (30 µg EE and 0.150 mg levonorgestrel daily for 21 days followed by a 7 day break) in improving the BMD of the lumbar spine in POI patients following 12 and 24 months of treatment. In POI patients receiving E2, significant gains in BMD were observed at all timepoints compared to EE. BMD in total hip and femoral neck did not differ significantly between the E2 and EE groups. The E2 group appeared to have a slightly greater influence on bone turnover markers (procollagen type I N-terminal propeptide (P1NP) and C-terminal telopeptide of type 1 collagen (CTX)) but statistical significance was not achieved. A possible explanation of these findings is the fact that EE leads to a considerable increase in the level of sex hormone binding globulin (SHBG) which decreases bioavailable estrogens and results in a reduced action on bone and BMD gain.

Nevertheless, oral estrogen administration is subject to hepatic first-pass metabolism and has an inhibitory impact on insulin-like growth factor-1 (IGF-1) production, which is known to be an important factor in bone formation. Therefore, this has been proposed as the main reason oral use of estrogen in menopause suppresses IGF-1 levels, while estrogen taken through the transdermal route does not cause this downregulation. So far, it is still unclear whether this effect of the route-dependent metabolic action of estrogens can be extrapolated to patients with POI. Mauras et al. [28] analyzed metabolic rates and parameters in patients with Turner Syndrome who were undergoing growth-hormone treatment. They found no statistical difference in the level of the IGF-1 between patients receiving estrogen via oral and transdermal routes, despite higher serum estrogen levels after oral administration [28]. In a similar study, Nabhan et al. [29] noted no statistical difference in IGF-1 levels between patients with Turner Syndrome receiving estrogen by either route. Nevertheless, patients receiving estrogen transdermally were found to have significantly higher spine BMD compared to the group receiving estrogen via oral administration [29].

Estrogen Dose

Current standards of practice dictate that the dose of exogenous estradiol should achieve replacement levels comparable to natural serum estrogen. Currently recommended formulations for patients with POI include daily doses of: 1–2 mg micronized oral E2; 100 µg transdermal E2; or 0.625–1.25 mg oral conjugated EE [1,30].

However, dose–response trials that include patients with POI are sparse and there is evidence supporting the observation that standard postmenopausal dosages are inadequate for patients with POI. In a study examining the etiology of idiopathic POI, Giraldo et al. [31] observed that standard HRT estrogen dosing (1 mg 17β-estradiol or 0.625 mg conjugated estrogen) was insufficient to sustain adequate BMD in POI patients. Moreover, the loss in BMD in these patients was similar or even more pronounced than that seen in women who did not receive estrogen therapy at all.

Nevertheless, further studies are required to confirm this finding and extend its scope to patients with various other etiologies of POI. The results obtained in our study pertain to patients with idiopathic POI and provide support to observations that a 2 mg dose of 17β-estradiol is sufficient to restore bone mass in these patients.

6. Conclusions

In conclusion, this study demonstrates that patients with POI have decreased bone mineral density, and treatment with HT has the potential to greatly influence and improve bone mass. Further investigation, however, is needed to determine appropriate effective dosages.

Author Contributions: Conceptualization, A.P. and B.M.; methodology, A.S.; software, A.P.; validation, A.S., M.N. and P.M.-P.; formal analysis, M.M.-J.; investigation, A.P., A.S.; resources, A.P., A.S., B.M.; data curation, M.N., P.M.-P.; writing, M.N., P.M.-P.; writing—review and editing, A.S., A.P., P.N., B.M.; visualization, A.S., M.N., P.M.-P.; supervision, A.P., B.M., P.B., M.M.-J.; project administration, A.P., B.M.; funding acquisition. All authors have read and agreed to the published version of the manuscript.

Funding: The authors received no financial support for the research, authorship, and/or publication of this article.

Acknowledgments: The authors wish to thank to Grzegorz Bala M.D. for help in English language editing.

Conflicts of Interest: The authors declare that they have no conflict of interest.

References

1. Nelson, L.M. Primary Ovarian Insufficiency. *N. Engl. J. Med.* **2009**, *360*, 606–614. [CrossRef]
2. Podfigurna-Stopa, A.; Czyzyk, A.; Grymowicz, M.; Smolarczyk, R.; Katulski, K.; Czajkowski, K.; Meczekalski, B. Premature Ovarian Insufficiency: The context of long-term effects. *J. Endocrinol. Investig.* **2016**, *39*, 983–990. [CrossRef]
3. Steiniche, T.; Hasling, C.; Charles, P.; Eriksen, E.F.; Mosekilde, L.; Melsen, F. A randomized study on the effects of estrogen/gestagen or high dose oral calcium on trabecular bone remodeling in postmenopausal osteoporosis. *Bone* **1989**, *10*, 313–320. [CrossRef]
4. Amarante, F.; Vilodre, L.C.; Maturana, M.A.; Spritzer, P.M. Women with primary ovarian insufficiency have lower bone mineral density. *Braz. J. Med. Biol. Res.* **2011**, *44*, 78–83. [CrossRef]
5. van der Voort, D.J.M.; van der Weijer, P.H.M.; Barentsen, R. Early menopause: Increased fracture risk at older age. *Osteoporos Int.* **2003**, *14*, 525–530. [CrossRef]
6. Svejme, O.; Ahlborg, H.; Nilsson, J.-Å.; Karlsson, M. Early menopause and risk of osteoporosis, fracture and mortality: A 34-year prospective observational study in 390 women. *BJOG Int. J. Obstet. Gynaecol.* **2012**, *119*, 810–816. [CrossRef]
7. Papadakis, G.; Gonzalez Rodriguez, E.; Marques-Vidal, P.; Hans, D.; Vollenweider, P.; Waeber, G.; Lamy, O. Menopausal hormone therapy. Effects on bone and body composition. *Rev. Med. Suisse* **2019**, *15*, 836–839. [CrossRef]
8. Wells, G.; Tugwell, P.; Shea, B.; Guyatt, G.; Peterson, J.; Zytaruk, N.; Robinson, V.; Henry, D.; O'Connell, D.; Cranney, A. Osteoporosis Methodology Group and The Osteoporosis Research Advisory Group. Meta-analyses of therapies for postmenopausal osteoporosis. V. Meta-analysis of the efficacy of hormone replacement therapy in treating and preventing osteoporosis in postmenopausal women. *Endocr. Rev.* **2002**, *23*, 529–539. [PubMed]
9. Cauley, J.A.; Robbins, J.; Chen, Z.; Cummings, S.R.; Jackson, R.D.; LaCroix, Z.; LeBoff, M.; Lewis, C.E.; McGowan, J.; Neuner, J.; et al. Women's Health Initiative Investigators. Effects of estrogen plus progestin on risk of fracture and bone mineral density: The Women's Health Initiative randomized trial. *JAMA* **2003**, *290*, 1729–1738. [CrossRef] [PubMed]
10. Khastgir, G.; Studd, J.W.; Fox, S.W.; Jones, J.; Alaghband-Zadeh, J.; Chow, J.W. A Longitudinal Study of the Effect of Subcutaneous Estrogen Replacement on Bone in Young Women with Turner's Syndrome. *J. Bone Miner. Res.* **2003**, *18*, 925–932. [CrossRef] [PubMed]
11. European Society for Human Reproduction and Embryology (ESHRE) Guideline Group on POI; Webber, L.; Davies, M.; Anderson, R.; Bartlett, J.; Braat, D.; Cartwright, B.; Cifkova, R.; de Muinck Keizer-Schrama, S.; Hogervorst, E.; et al. ESHRE Guideline: Management of women with premature ovarian insufficiency. *Hum. Reprod.* **2016**, *31*, 926–937.
12. Soong, Y.K.; Hsu, J.J.; Tzen, K.Y. Measurement of bone mineral density in amenorrheic women with dual photon absorptiometry. *Taiwan Yi Xue Hui Za Zhi* **1989**, *88*, 1097–1103. [PubMed]

13. Popat, V.B.; Calis, K.A.; Vanderhoof, V.H.; Cizza, G.; Reynolds, J.C.; Sebring, N.; Troendle, J.F.; Nelson, L.M. Bone Mineral Density in Estrogen-Deficient Young Women. *J. Clin. Endocrinol. Metab.* **2009**, *94*, 2277–2283. [CrossRef] [PubMed]
14. Freriks, K.; Timmermans, J.; Beerendonk, C.C.; Verhaak, C.M.; Netea-Maier, R.T.; Otten, B.J.; Braat, D.D.; Smeets, F.; Kunst, D.H.; Hermus, A.R.; et al. Standardized Multidisciplinary Evaluation Yields Significant Previously Undiagnosed Morbidity in Adult Women with Turner Syndrome. *J. Clin. Endocrinol. Metab.* **2011**, *96*, E1517–E1526. [CrossRef] [PubMed]
15. Ratcliffe, M.A.; Lanham, S.A.; Reid, D.M.; Dawson, A.A. Bone mineral density (BMD) in patients with lymphoma: The effects of chemotherapy, intermittent corticosteroids and premature menopause. *Hematol. Oncol.* **1992**, *10*, 181–187. [CrossRef] [PubMed]
16. Lindsay, R.; Hart, D.M.; Forrest, C.; Baird, C. Prevention of spinal osteoporosis in oophorectomised women. *Lancet* **1980**, *2*, 1151–1154. [CrossRef]
17. Han, T.S.; Goswami, D.; Trikudanathan, S.; Creighton, S.M.; Conway, G.S. Comparison of bone mineral density and body proportions between women with complete androgen insensitivity syndrome and women with gonadal dysgenesis. *Eur. J. Endocrinol.* **2008**, *159*, 179–185. [CrossRef]
18. Bidet, M.; Bachelot, A.; Bissauge, E.; Golmard, J.L.; Gricourt, S.; Dulon, J.; Coussieu, C.; Badachi, Y.; Touraine, P. Resumption of Ovarian Function and Pregnancies in 358 Patients with Premature Ovarian Failure. *J. Clin. Endocrinol. Metab.* **2011**, *96*, 3864–3872. [CrossRef]
19. Alzubaidi, N.H.; Chapin, H.L.; Vanderhoof, V.H.; Calis, K.A.; Nelson, L.M. Meeting the needs of young women with secondary amenorrhea and spontaneous premature ovarian failure. *Obstet. Gynecol.* **2002**, *99*, 720–725.
20. Christianson, M.S.; Shen, W. Osteoporosis Prevention and Management. *Clin. Obstet. Gynecol.* **2013**, *56*, 703–710. [CrossRef]
21. Boyle, P.; Wojtyla, A. Health, wellbeing and family. *J. Health Inequal.* **2019**, *5*, 20. [CrossRef]
22. Food and Agricultural Organization of the United Nations. *World Health Organization Human Vitamin and Mineral Requirements: Report of a Joint FAO/WHO Expert Consultation*; Food and Agricultural Organization of the United Nations: Bangkok, Thailand, 2001.
23. Kanis, J.A.; Cooper, C.; Rizzoli, R.; Reginster, J.-Y. Scientific Advisory Board of the European Society for Clinical and Economic Aspects of Osteoporosis (ESCEO) and the Committees of Scientific Advisors and National Societies of the International Osteoporosis Foundation (IOF): European guidance for the diagnosis and management of osteoporosis in postmenopausal women. *Osteoporos. Int.* **2019**, *30*, 3–44. [PubMed]
24. Baim, S.; Wilson, C.R.; Lewiecki, E.M.; Luckey, M.M.; Downs, R.W.; Lentle, B.C. Precision assessment and radiation safety for dual-energy X-ray absorptiometry: Position paper of the International Society for Clinical Densitometry. *J. Clin. Densitom.* **2005**, *8*, 371–378. [CrossRef]
25. Genant, H.K.; Cann, C.E.; Ettinger, B.; Gordan, G.S. Quantitative Computed Tomography of Vertebral Spongiosa: A Sensitive Method for Detecting Early Bone Loss After Oophorectomy. *Ann. Intern. Med.* **1982**, *97*, 699–705. [CrossRef] [PubMed]
26. Popat, V.B.; Calis, K.A.; Kalantaridou, S.N.; Vanderhoof, V.H.; Koziol, D.; Troendle, J.F.; Reynolds, J.C.; Nelson, L.M. Bone Mineral Density in Young Women with Primary Ovarian Insufficiency: Results of a Three-Year Randomized Controlled Trial of Physiological Transdermal Estradiol and Testosterone Replacement. *J. Clin. Endocrinol. Metab.* **2014**, *99*, 3418–3426. [CrossRef] [PubMed]
27. Cartwright, B.; Robinson, J.; Seed, P.T.; Fogelman, I.; Rymer, J. Hormone Replacement Therapy Versus the Combined Oral Contraceptive Pill in Premature Ovarian Failure: A Randomized Controlled Trial of the Effects on Bone Mineral Density. *J. Clin. Endocrinol. Metab.* **2016**, *101*, 3497–3505. [CrossRef]
28. Mauras, N.; Shulman, D.; Hsiang, H.Y.; Balagopal, P.; Welch, S. Metabolic Effects of Oral Versus Transdermal Estrogen in Growth Hormone-Treated Girls with Turner Syndrome. *J. Clin. Endocrinol. Metab.* **2007**, *92*, 4154–4160. [CrossRef]
29. Nabhan, Z.M.; DiMeglio, L.A.; Qi, R.; Perkins, S.M.; Eugster, E.A. Conjugated Oral versus Transdermal Estrogen Replacement in Girls with Turner Syndrome: A Pilot Comparative Study. *J. Clin. Endocrinol. Metab.* **2009**, *94*, 2009–2014. [CrossRef] [PubMed]
30. Committee on Gynecologic Practice. Committee Opinion No. 698. *Obstet. Gynecol.* **2017**, *129*, e134–e141. [CrossRef]

31. Giraldo, H.; Benetti-Pinto, C.; Ferreira, V.; Garmes, H.; Yela, D.; Giraldo, P. Standard hormone therapy is inadequate for bone density in premature ovarian insufficiency. *Gynecol. Endocrinol.* **2017**, *33*, 283–286. [CrossRef]

Publisher's Note: MDPI stays neutral with regard to jurisdictional claims in published maps and institutional affiliations.

© 2020 by the authors. Licensee MDPI, Basel, Switzerland. This article is an open access article distributed under the terms and conditions of the Creative Commons Attribution (CC BY) license (http://creativecommons.org/licenses/by/4.0/).

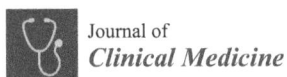

Article

Metformin Attenuates Osteoporosis in Diabetic Patients with Carcinoma in Situ: A Nationwide, Retrospective, Matched-Cohort Study in Taiwan

Chieh-Hua Lu [1,2], Chi-Hsiang Chung [3,4], Feng-Chih Kuo [1], Kuan-Chan Chen [1], Chia-Hao Chang [1], Chih-Chun Kuo [1], Chien-Hsing Lee [1], Sheng-Chiang Su [1], Jhih-Syuan Liu [1], Fu-Huang Lin [3], Chang-Huei Tsao [5,6], Po-Shiuan Hsieh [2,7,8], Yi-Jen Hung [1], Chang-Hsun Hsieh [1,*] and Wu-Chien Chien [2,3,*]

1. Department of Internal Medicine, Division of Endocrinology and Metabolism, Tri-Service General Hospital, School of Medicine, National Defense Medical Center, Taipei 11490, Taiwan; undeca2001@gmail.com (C.-H.L.); shoummie@hotmail.com (F.-C.K.); kuanchanndmc@gmail.com (K.-C.C.); kittyrvyi@gmail.com (C.-H.C.); lg1001010@gmail.com (C.-C.K.); doc10383@gmail.com (C.-H.L.); shiyuan71@yahoo.com.tw (S.-C.S.); ajleonn21@hotmail.com.tw (J.-S.L.); metahung@yahoo.com (Y.-J.H.)
2. Department of Medical Research, National Defense Medical Center, Taipei 11490, Taiwan; pshsieh@hotmail.com
3. School of Public Health, National Defense Medical Center, Taipei 11490, Taiwan; g694810042@gmail.com (C.-H.C.); noldling@ms10.hinet.net (F.-H.L.)
4. Taiwanese Injury Prevention and Safety Promotion Association, Taipei 10048, Taiwan
5. Department of Medical Research, Tri-Service General Hospital, National Defense Medical Center, Taipei 11490, Taiwan; changhuei@mail.ndmctsgh.edu.tw
6. Department of Microbiology & Immunology, National Defense Medical Center, Taipei 11490, Taiwan
7. Department of Physiology and Biophysics, National Defense Medical Center, Taipei 11490, Taiwan
8. Institute of Preventive Medicine, National Defense Medical Center, Taipei 11490, Taiwan
* Correspondence: 10324@yahoo.com.tw (C.-H.H.); chienwu@mail.ndmctsgh.edu.tw (W.-C.C.); Tel.: +886-2-8792-7182 (C.-H.H.); +886-2-8792-3311 (W.-C.C.); Fax: +886-2-8792-7235 (C.-H.H.); +886-2-8792-7183 (W.-C.C.)

Received: 30 July 2020; Accepted: 30 August 2020; Published: 2 September 2020

Abstract: Patients with diabetes are at increased risk of cancer development and osteoporosis. Metformin is an effective agent for diabetes management. Epidemiological studies have identified an association between metformin use and cancer prevention. This article outlines the potential for metformin to attenuate the rate of osteoporosis in diabetic patients with carcinoma in situ (CIS). From the National Health Insurance Research Database of Taiwan, 7827 patients with diabetes with CIS who were receiving metformin therapy were selected, along with 23,481 patients as 1:3 sex-, age- and index year-matched controls, who were not receiving metformin therapy. A Cox proportional hazard analysis was used to compare the rate of osteoporosis during an average of 15-year follow-up. Of the subjects who were enrolled, 801 (2.56%) had osteoporosis, including 168 from the metformin group (2.15%) and 633 from the without metformin group (2.70%). The metformin group presented a lower rate of osteoporosis at the end of follow-up ($p = 0.009$). The Cox proportional hazard regression analysis revealed a lower rate of osteoporosis for the metformin group (adjusted hazard ratio of 0.820; 95% confidence interval = 0.691–0.972, $p = 0.022$). Diabetic patients with CIS under metformin therapy presented lower osteoporosis rate than those who were not receiving metformin therapy.

Keywords: osteoporosis; diabetes; metformin; carcinoma in situ; National Health Insurance Research Database

1. Introduction

Patients with diabetes are at increased risk of cancer development [1] and associated with an increased risk of fragility fractures compared to the general population [2]. Type 2 diabetes mellitus (T2DM) and cancer share many risk factors, such as age, obesity, diet and physical inactivity [3]. The possible mechanisms for a direct link between T2DM and cancer include hyperinsulinemia [4], hyperglycemia [5] and inflammation [6,7].

Diabetes and cancer are clinical risk factors used for fragility fracture probability assessments across the general population [8,9]. Osteoporosis is a skeletal disorder that is characterized by low bone mass and compromised bone strength [10]. T2DM may affect bone metabolism and leads to osteoporosis [11] and cancer may affect both, through the direct effects of cancer cells on the skeleton and the deleterious effects of cancer-specific therapies on bone cells [9].

Metformin is an effective agent for T2DM management [12]. Furthermore, epidemiological studies have identified an association between metformin use and cancer prevention [13]. Fractures are a clinically important consequence of osteoporosis and result not only in disabilities, but also in excess mortality; however, the pathogenic mechanisms that underlie the relationship between osteoporosis, diabetes and cancer remain incompletely understood. The aim of this study was to determine the potential for metformin to attenuate the rate of osteoporosis in diabetic patients with carcinoma in situ using data from the Taiwan National Health Insurance Research Database (NHIRD), which is a nationwide health insurance database.

2. Materials and Methods

2.1. Data Sources

Our study used data from the NHIRD to investigate whether metformin therapy in diabetic patients with carcinoma in situ could lower osteoporosis rates, compared to a group of individuals who were not receiving metformin, over a 15-year period, from the outpatient Longitudinal Health Insurance Database (LHID) in Taiwan (2000–2015). The National Health Insurance (NHI) Program was launched in Taiwan in 1995, and as of June 2009, it included contracts with 97% of the medical providers in Taiwan, with approximately 23 million beneficiaries or more than 99% of the entire Taiwan population [14]. The NHIRD uses International Classification of Diseases, 9th Revision, Clinical Modification (ICD-9-CM) codes to record diagnoses [15]. All diagnoses of T2DM, carcinoma in situ, and osteoporosis were made by a board-certified medical specialist. The Bureau of NHI randomly reviews the records of 1 in 100 ambulatory care visits and 1 in 20 in-patient claims, to verify the accuracy of the diagnoses [16]. Several studies have demonstrated the accuracy and validity of the diagnoses in the NHIRD [17,18].

2.2. Study Design and Sampled Participants

Our study was a retrospective matched-cohort design. Patients with diagnosed T2DM, carcinoma in situ, and osteoporosis were selected from 1 January 2000 to 31 December 2015, according to ICD-9-CM 230.XX-234.XX (carcinoma in situ), ICD-9-CM 733.XX (osteoporosis) and ICD-9-CM 250.XX (T2DM). Furthermore, each enrolled patient was required to have made at least three outpatient visits within the study period, according to these ICD-9-CM codes whether or not they were receiving metformin therapy. Patients with osteoporosis diagnoses before 2000 and those less than 18 years of age were excluded. Furthermore, patients with diabetes who received thiazolidinedione or canagliflozin therapy were also excluded.

The covariates included Charlson comorbidity index (CCI), T2DM, sex, age, geographical area of residence (north, center, south and east of Taiwan) and urbanization level of residence (level 1 to 4). The urbanization level of residence was defined according to the population and various indicators of the level of development. Level 1 was defined as a population >1,250,000 and a specific economic, cultural, metropolitan and political development designation. Level 2 was defined as a population between 500,000 and 1,249,999 that played an important role in the political system, culture and economy. Urbanization levels 3 and 4 were defined as either populations between 149,999 and 499,999 or <149,999, respectively [19].

2.3. Outcome Measures

All of the study participants were followed from the index date until the onset of osteoporosis, from the NHI program, before the end of 2015.

2.4. Statistical Analysis

All statistical analyses were performed using SPSS software version 22 for Windows (SPSS, Inc., Chicago, IL, USA). chi-squared and *t*-tests were used to evaluate the distributions of categorical and continuous variables, respectively. A regression analysis of multivariate Cox proportional hazards was used to determine the risk of osteoporosis under metformin therapy in patients with diabetes and carcinoma in situ. The statistical analyses were presented as hazard ratio (HR) with ninety-five percent confidence interval (CI). The difference in the risk of osteoporosis for patients with diabetes and carcinoma in situ, with or without metformin therapy, was estimated using the log rank test—Kaplan-Meier method. A two-tailed test *p*-value less than 0.05 was considered to indicate statistical significance.

2.5. Ethics

Our study was conducted in accordance with the Code of Ethics of the World Medical Association (Declaration of Helsinki). The Institutional Review Board of Tri-Service General Hospital (TSGH) approved our study and waived the need for individual written informed consent (TSGH IRB No.2-105-05-082).

3. Results

Of the 61,307 enrolled patients, 11,151 were excluded and 50,156 patients with cancer and T2DM were included. Furthermore, 9030 of the included patients were receiving metformin therapy, of which 1203 patients had used metformin for less than 90 days and were excluded and 7827 were enrolled (case group). For the control group, we enrolled 41,126 individuals who were not receiving metformin therapy to represent the 1:3 sex-, age- and index year-matched control group and excluded 17,645 patients used metformin less than 90 days, for a final count of 23,481 subjects (control group) (Figure 1). Overall, the diabetic patients with carcinoma in situ under metformin therapy presented a lower rate of osteoporosis than those who were not receiving metformin (adjusted HR 0.820 (95% CI = 0.691–0.972, $p = 0.022$). Figure 2 shows the Kaplan-Meier analysis for the cumulative risk of osteoporosis in patient and control groups and the difference is statistically significant (log rank, $p = 0.017$).

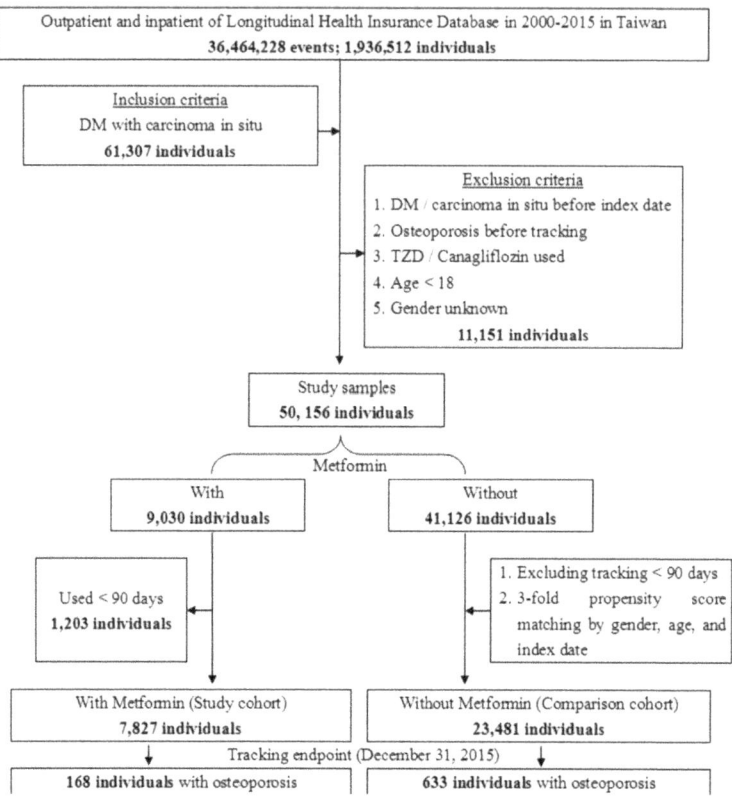

Figure 1. Flowchart of study patient selection from the National Health Insurance Research Database in Taiwan. DM—Diabetes mellitus: ICD-9-CM 250; Carcinoma in situ: ICD-9-CM 230–234; Osteoporosis: ICD-9-CM 733.0; Metformin: ≥90 days.

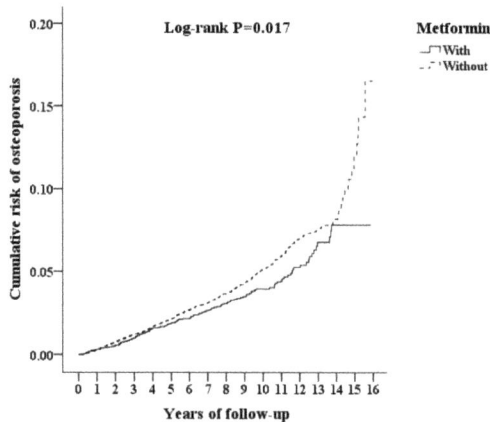

Figure 2. Kaplan-Meier analysis of cumulative risk of osteoporosis among patients with diabetes mellitus with carcinoma in situ aged 18 and over, stratified by metformin use and analyzed using a log-rank test.

The baseline sex, age, comorbidities, location, urbanization, level of care and income of the study subjects and controls is presented in Table 1. Of the 31,308 adult diabetic patients with carcinoma in situ, 13,284 (42.43%) were male, 12,928 (41.29%) were ≥60 year of age and the mean age was 55.95 ± 14.28 years (Table 1). There were no significant differences between the metformin and control groups in age distribution, sex, comorbidities and covariates, after propensity-score matching.

Table 1. Characteristics of study in the baseline.

Metformin	Total		With		Without		p
Variables	n	%	n	%	n	%	
Total	31,308	-	7827	25.00	23,481	75.00	-
Gender	-	-	-	-	-	-	0.999
Male	13,284	42.43	3321	42.43	9963	42.43	-
Female	18,024	57.57	4506	57.57	13,518	57.57	-
Age (years)	55.95 ± 14.28		55.91 ± 14.36		55.96 ± 14.25		0.759
Age groups (years)	-	-	-	-	-	-	0.999
18–49	11,960	38.20	2990	38.20	8970	38.20	-
50–59	6420	20.51	1605	20.51	4815	20.51	-
≥60	12,928	41.29	3232	41.29	9696	41.29	-
Low-income	-	-	-	-	-	-	0.952
Without	30,998	99.01	7749	99.00	23,249	99.01	-
With	310	0.99	78	1.00	232	0.99	-
Catastrophic Illness	-	-	-	-	-	-	0.206
Without	25,374	81.05	6382	81.54	18,992	80.88	-
With	5934	18.95	1445	18.46	4489	19.12	-
Marital status	-	-	-	-	-	-	0.073
Without	12,841	41.02	3278	41.88	9563	40.73	-
With	18,467	58.98	4549	58.12	13,918	59.27	-
Education (years)	-	-	-	-	-	-	0.683
<12	13,692	43.73	3407	43.53	10,285	43.80	-
≥12	17,616	56.27	4420	56.47	13,196	56.20	-
CCI_R	0.61 ± 1.75		0.60 ± 1.70		0.61 ± 1.77		0.641
Season	-	-	-	-	-	-	0.866
Spring (Mar–May)	8070	25.78	2037	26.03	6033	25.69	-
Summer (Jun–Aug)	8425	26.91	2101	26.84	6324	26.93	-
Autumn (Sep–Nov)	7896	25.22	1982	25.32	5914	25.19	-
Winter (Dec–Feb)	6917	22.09	1707	21.81	5210	22.19	-
Location	-	-	-	-	-	-	0.659
Northern Taiwan	13,289	42.45	3335	42.61	9954	42.39	-
Middle Taiwan	8492	27.12	2150	27.47	6342	27.01	-
Southern Taiwan	8227	26.28	2017	25.77	6210	26.45	-
Eastern Taiwan	1253	4.00	315	4.02	938	3.99	-
Outlets islands	47	0.15	10	0.13	37	0.16	-
Urbanization level	-	-	-	-	-	-	0.877
1 (Highest)	12,423	39.68	3115	39.80	9308	39.64	-
2	14,419	46.06	3603	46.03	10,816	46.06	-
3	1346	4.30	324	4.14	1022	4.35	-
4 (Lowest)	3120	9.97	785	10.03	2335	9.94	-
Level of care	-	-	-	-	-	-	0.083
Hospital center	16,949	54.14	4319	55.18	12,630	53.79	-
Regional hospital	10,975	35.05	2668	34.09	8307	35.38	-
Local hospital	3384	10.81	840	10.73	2544	10.83	-

P—chi-squared/Fisher's exact test on category variables and t-test on continue variables.

At the end of the follow-up period, 801 enrolled subjects (2.56%) had osteoporosis, including 168 from the metformin group (2.15%) and 633 from the without metformin group (2.70%), as shown in Table 2. The metformin group was associated with a lower rate of osteoporosis at the end of the follow-up ($p = 0.009$). There were no significant differences between the metformin and control groups in age distribution, sex, comorbidities and covariates at the end of the follow-up period.

Table 2. Characteristics of study in the endpoint.

Metformin	Total		With		Without		p
Variables	n	%	n	%	n	%	
Total	31,308	-	7827	25.00	23,481	75.00	-
Osteoporosis	-	-	-	-	-	-	0.009
Without	30,507	97.44	7659	97.85	22,848	97.30	-
With	801	2.56	168	2.15	633	2.70	-
Gender	-	-	-	-	-	-	0.999
Male	13,284	42.43	3321	42.43	9963	42.43	-
Female	18,024	57.57	4506	57.57	13,518	57.57	-
Age (yrs)	61.37 ± 15.55		61.32 ± 15.60		61.39 ± 15.54		0.707
Age groups (yrs)	-	-	-	-	-	-	0.393
18–49	8106	25.89	2061	26.33	6045	25.74	-
50–59	6647	21.23	1625	20.76	5022	21.39	-
≥60	16,555	52.88	4141	52.91	12,414	52.87	-
Low-income	-	-	-	-	-	-	0.336
Without	30,936	98.81	7726	98.71	23,210	98.85	-
With	372	1.19	101	1.29	271	1.15	-
Catastrophic Illness	-	-	-	-	-	-	0.652
Without	22,517	71.92	5647	72.15	16,870	71.85	-
With	8791	28.08	2180	27.85	6611	28.15	-
Marital status	-	-	-	-	-	-	0.058
Without	12,846	41.03	3283	41.94	9563	40.73	-
With	18,462	58.97	4544	58.06	13,918	59.27	-
Education (years)	-	-	-	-	-	-	0.659
<12	13,687	43.72	3405	43.50	10,282	43.79	-
≥12	17,621	56.28	4422	56.50	13,199	56.21	-
CCI_R	1.96 ± 3.70		1.99 ± 3.76		1.95 ± 3.68		0.320
Season	-	-	-	-	-	-	0.486
Spring	7236	23.11	1782	22.77	5454	23.23	-
Summer	7995	25.54	2017	25.77	5978	25.46	-
Autumn	8780	28.04	2232	28.52	6548	27.89	-
Winter	7297	23.31	1796	22.95	5501	23.43	-
Location	-	-	-	-	-	-	0.499
Northern Taiwan	12,321	39.35	3067	39.18	9254	39.41	-
Middle Taiwan	9222	29.46	2340	29.90	6882	29.31	-
Southern Taiwan	8108	25.90	1993	25.46	6115	26.04	-
Eastern Taiwan	1548	4.94	399	5.10	1149	4.89	-
Outer islands	109	0.35	28	0.36	81	0.34	-
Urbanization level	-	-	-	-	-	-	0.727
1 (Highest)	10,135	32.37	2522	32.22	7613	32.42	-
2	14,118	45.09	3502	44.74	10,616	45.21	-
3	2131	6.81	537	6.86	1594	6.79	-
4 (Lowest)	4924	15.73	1266	16.17	3658	15.58	-
Level of care	-	-	-	-	-	-	0.590
Hospital center	12,771	40.79	3156	40.32	9615	40.95	-
Regional hospital	13,322	42.55	3340	42.67	9982	42.51	-
Local hospital	5215	16.66	1331	17.01	3884	16.54	-

P—chi-squared/Fisher's exact test on category variables and t-test on continue variables.

The results of the Cox regression analysis of the factors associated with osteoporosis are shown in Table 3. The Cox proportional hazard regression analysis showed a lower rate of osteoporosis for patients receiving metformin therapy (adjusted hazard ratio of 0.820; 95% confidence interval = 0.691–0.972, $p = 0.022$).

Table 3. Factors of osteoporosis by using Cox regression.

Variables	Crude HR	95% CI	95% CI	p	Adjusted HR	95% CI	95% CI	p
Metformin	-	-	-	-	-	-	-	-
Without	1	-	-	-	1	-	-	-
With	0.813	0.686	0.964	0.017	0.820	0.691	0.972	0.022
Gender	-	-	-	-	-	-	-	-
Male	0.662	0.497	0.883	0.005	0.576	0.431	0.770	<0.001
Female	1	-	-	-	1	-	-	-
Age groups (yrs)	-	-	-	-	-	-	-	-
18–49	1	-	-	-	1	-	-	-
50–59	2.827	1.648	4.851	<0.001	3.113	1.813	5.345	<0.001
≥60	13.133	8.114	21.257	<0.001	15.456	9.533	25.059	<0.001
Low-income	-	-	-	-	-	-	-	-
Without	1	-	-	-	1	-	-	-
With	1.083	0.490	1.973	0.961	1.505	0.747	3.030	0.253
Catastrophic Illness	-	-	-	-	-	-	-	-
Without	1	-	-	-	1	-	-	-
With	0.521	0.426	0.638	<0.001	1.030	0.883	1.214	0.166
Marital status	-	-	-	-	-	-	-	-
Without	1	-	-	-	1	-	-	-
With	1.234	0.724	2.013	0.306	1.305	0.896	2.284	0.299
Education (years)	-	-	-	-	-	-	-	-
<12	1	-	-	-	1	-	-	-
≥12	0.903	0.512	1.894	0.376	0.865	0.483	1.881	0.425
CCI_R	0.892	0.860	0.925	<0.001	0.880	0.840	0.921	<0.001
Season	-	-	-	-	-	-	-	-
Spring	1	-	-	-	1	-	-	-
Summer	0.946	0.778	1.150	0.576	0.993	0.817	1.208	0.946
Autumn	0.785	0.644	0.957	0.017	0.769	0.653	0.971	0.024
Winter	1.008	0.827	1.229	0.938	1.013	0.831	1.235	0.898
Location	-	-	-	-				
Northern Taiwan	1	-	-	-				
Middle Taiwan	1.318	1.111	1.563	0.002				
Southern Taiwan	1.151	0.958	1.383	0.113	Multicollinearity with urbanization level			
Eastern Taiwan	1.675	1.274	2.204	<0.001				
Islands outer of Taiwan	1.584	0.590	4.253	0.362				
Urbanization level	-	-	-	-	-	-	-	-
1 (Highest)	0.525	0.374	0.736	<0.001	0.560	0.420	0.827	0.002
2	0.707	0.591	0.846	<0.001	0.856	0.706	1.038	0.113
3	0.725	0.598	0.878	0.001	0.912	0.733	1.135	0.410
4 (Lowest)	1	-	-	-	1	-	-	-
Level of care	-	-	-	-	-	-	-	-
Hospital center	0.646	0.536	0.778	<0.001	0.712	0.594	0.853	<0.001
Regional hospital	0.670	0.560	0.800	<0.001	0.761	0.615	0.942	0.012
Local hospital	1	-	-	-	1	-	-	-

HR—hazard ratio; CI—confidence interval; Adjusted HR—adjusted variables listed in table.

For the subgroups in which osteoporosis factors were stratified by the variables listed in Table 4, the Cox regression analysis showed that the male, age < 60 years, better income, without catastrophic illness, unmarried, longer education, live in the higher urbanization level and care in hospital center were associated with a much lower osteoporosis rate.

Table 4. Factors of osteoporosis stratified by variables listed in table by using Cox regression.

Metformin		With				Without			Ratio	With vs. Without (Reference)			
Stratified	Events	PYs	Rate (per 10^5 PYs)		Events	PYs	Rate (per 10^5 PYs)			Adjusted HR	95% CI	95% CI	p
Total	168	83,045.71	202.30		633	254,028.18	249.18		0.812	0.820	0.691	0.972	0.022
Gender	-	-	-		-	-	-		-	-	-	-	-
Male	8	24,313.43	32.90		42	72,902.21	57.61		0.571	0.572	0.483	0.689	0.007
Female	160	58,732.28	272.42		591	181,125.97	326.29		0.835	0.843	0.710	1.006	0.054
Age groups (yrs)	-	-	-		-	-	-		-	-	-	-	-
18–49	1	16,823.43	5.94		16	48,608.18	32.92		0.181	0.180	0.150	0.218	<0.001
50–59	7	18,252.93	38.35		52	56,989.26	91.25		0.420	0.422	0.352	0.513	<0.001
≥60	160	47,969.35	333.55		565	148,430.74	380.65		0.876	0.886	0.746	1.072	0.241
Low-income	-	-	-		-	-	-		-	-	-	-	-
Without	166	82,125.32	202.13		626	251,334.43	249.07		0.812	0.818	0.682	0.954	0.019
With	2	920.40	217.30		7	2693.75	259.86		0.836	0.845	0.703	0.998	0.047
Catastrophic Illness	-	-	-		-	-	-		-	-	-	-	-
Without	148	63,571.83	232.81		562	192,669.45	291.69		0.798	0.806	0.672	0.958	0.020
With	20	19,473.89	102.70		71	61,358.72	115.71		0.888	0.899	0.758	1.094	0.182
Marital status	-	-	-		-	-	-		-	-	-	-	-
Without	70	38,033.11	184.05		295	120,005.45	245.82		0.749	0.754	0.632	0.891	<0.001
With	98	45,012.60	217.72		338	134,022.73	252.20		0.863	0.870	0.731	0.984	0.022
Education (years)	-	-	-		-	-	-		-	-	-	-	-
<12	88	38,948.45	225.94		320	122,940.53	260.29		0.868	0.867	0.721	0.979	0.023
≥12	80	44,097.26	181.42		313	131,087.65	238.77		0.760	0.765	0.634	0.910	<0.001
Season	-	-	-		-	-	-		-	-	-	-	-
Spring	38	18,725.29	202.93		155	57,375.11	270.15		0.751	0.759	0.632	0.902	0.001
Summer	39	20,940.50	186.24		165	65,150.71	253.26		0.735	0.743	0.621	0.880	<0.001
Autumn	40	25,007.28	159.95		162	72,600.25	223.14		0.717	0.724	0.608	0.863	<0.001
Winter	51	18,372.65	277.59		151	58,902.11	256.36		1.083	1.094	0.924	1.286	0.388

Table 4. Cont.

Metformin	With			Without				With vs. Without (Reference)			
Stratified	Events	PYs	Rate (per 10⁵ PYs)	Events	PYs	Rate (per 10⁵ PYs)	Ratio	Adjusted HR	95% CI	95% CI	p
Urbanization level											
1 (Highest)	42	24,936.20	168.43	182	79,857.63	227.91	0.739	0.742	0.611	0.897	<0.001
2	66	37,254.28	177.16	269	112,534.77	239.04	0.741	0.749	0.620	0.903	0.002
3	11	5966.48	184.36	36	18,479.15	194.81	0.946	0.953	0.798	1.138	0.265
4 (Lowest)	49	14,888.76	329.11	146	43,156.63	338.30	0.973	0.981	0.824	1.206	0.402
Level of care											
Hospital center	54	31,037.93	173.98	214	97,437.34	219.63	0.792	0.799	0.635	0.950	0.009
Regional hospital	71	37,481.36	189.43	270	114,617.84	235.57	0.804	0.812	0.682	0.964	0.018
Local hospital	43	14,526.42	296.01	149	41,973.00	354.99	0.834	0.843	0.710	0.997	0.047

PYs—person-years; Adjusted HR—adjusted hazard ratio, adjusted for the variables listed in Table 3; CI—confidence interval.

4. Discussion

We found that diabetic patients with carcinoma in situ under metformin therapy presented lower osteoporosis rates than those who were not receiving metformin. The overall adjusted HR was 0.820 ($p = 0.022$), even after adjusting for comorbidities and other covariates. The Kaplan-Meier analysis revealed that the study subjects had a significantly lower 15-year risk of osteoporosis than the controls. This study is the first to indicate that diabetic patients with carcinoma in situ under metformin therapy have a lower osteoporosis risk in a nationwide, population-based study.

Prior research that has found that patients with diabetes have a relatively high risk of fracture [20], and one systematic review that showed that patients with diabetes have up to a three-fold greater fracture risk than the average person, with hip fracture being the largest [21]. Cancer is a major risk factor for osteoporosis, which is a common bone disease characterized by reduced bone mass and increased risk of fracture. Furthermore, these factors are associated both with the direct effects of cancer cells on the skeleton and the deleterious effects of cancer-specific therapies on bone cells [9]. One review article showed that certain key factors, osteoprotegerin (OPG)/ receptor activator of NF-κB ligand (RANKL)/receptor activator of NF-κB (RANK), underlie the molecular mechanism of osteoclastogenesis [22], and the anti-human RANKL monoclonal antibody has been successfully applied to the treatment of osteoporosis and cancer-related bone disorders [23,24].

Metformin is the preferred initial pharmacologic medicine for T2DM treatment, unless there are contraindications [25]. First-line metformin therapy has beneficial effects on HbA1C and weight [26] and may reduce the risk of cardiovascular events and death [27]. Patients with diabetes who received thiazolidinedione or canagliflozin therapy were excluded, due to the potential risk of osteoporosis [28]. Some studies have reported that older age, diabetes, and cancer under chemotherapy were associated with increased fracture risk, which was associated with elevated bone resorption [29,30].

Will metformin treatment reduce the incidence of osteoporosis in diabetic patients with carcinoma in situ? No study has investigated this in the past, and therefore, we used a cohort investigation to evaluate this issue. We found that the diabetic patients with carcinoma in situ under metformin therapy presented lower osteoporosis rates than those who were not receiving metformin. Evans and other scholars first proposed that metformin could reduce the cancer risk of patients with diabetes through epidemiological studies [31], in accordance with our results.

The impact of metformin on osteoporosis has been studied in the past. In vitro data on metformin suggest a protective effect on bones [32] and that metformin improves bone quality and decreases the risk of fractures in patients with diabetes, in addition to improving glycemic control and insulin sensitivity [33]. Recent studies have shown that metformin can be osteogenic in vitro through the activation of AMP-activated protein kinase (AMPK), which results in osteoblastic cells differentiation, bone matrix synthesis and osteoblasts proliferation [34,35]. An in vivo study in mice showed that metformin enhances osteoblast proliferation and inhibits osteoclast differentiation to attenuate cancellous bone loss [36]. Furthermore, molecular research has found that metformin reduces RANKL and stimulates OPG expression in osteoblasts, which further inhibits osteoclast differentiation and prevents bone loss in ovariectomized rats [37]. Furthermore, metformin has been found to promote the proliferation of murine preosteoblasts by regulating the AMPK-mechanistic target of rapamycin 2 (mTOR2) and the AKT-mTORC1 signaling axis [38]. Additionally, metformin promotes the proliferation and differentiation of murine preosteoblasts by regulating the expression of sirtuin 6 (sirt6) and oct4 [39].

We therefore hypothesized that diabetic patients with carcinoma in situ who are on metformin therapy may present attenuated cancellous bone loss through metformin regulation of AMPK signaling in preosteoblasts, which reduces RANKL and stimulates OPG expression. Hence, metformin could be associated with reduced osteoporosis. Our findings are similar to many studies that have shown that females and older patients have a greater risk of osteoporosis. Clinical factors could be associated with those projected by demographic changes, with regards to age- and sex-specific risks [40]. Otherwise, the reasons why the subgroups that lived in higher urbanized areas and received therapy in hospital centers showed lower rates of osteoporosis are unknown and warrant further studies.

The present study has a few limitations. First, our study lacks analyses of disease duration, disease severity and patient parameters, such as body weight, BMI and waistline. Hip fracture risk is increased in patients with diabetes, whereas BMD is increased in patients with T2DM [41]. While the pathophysiological mechanism is only partially understood, a common complication may explain the increased fracture risk, whereas BMI may ameliorate the increased fracture risk in patients with T2DM [42]. Finally, a longer follow-up period may be necessary to clarify the osteoporosis risk for diabetic patients with carcinoma in situ.

In conclusion, diabetic patients with carcinoma in situ under metformin therapy presented a lower osteoporosis rate than those who were not receiving metformin therapy, and this effect may be attributed to the decreased levels of proinflammatory factors and the potential for metformin to modulate molecular pathways involved in cancer cell signaling and metabolism.

Author Contributions: C.-H.L. (Chieh-Hua Lu), F.-C.K., K.-C.C., C.-H.C. (Chia-Hao Chang), C.-C.K., C.-H.L. (Chien-Hsing Lee), S.-C.S., J.-S.L., F.-H.L., C.-H.T., P.-S.H. and Y.-J.H. participated in the conceptualization of the manuscript. C.-H.C. (Chi-Hsiang Chung) participated in data curation and the formal analysis of this study. C.-H.L. (Chieh-Hua Lu) wrote the original draft of the manuscript. C.-H.H. and W.-C.C. participated in manuscript review and editing. All authors have read and approved the final version of the manuscript.

Funding: This study was funded by the Tri-Service General Hospital Research Foundation (TSGH-C108-003, TSGH-C108-142, TSGH-C108-143, TSGH-C108-144) and the National Defense Medical Center, Ministry of National Defense-Medical Affairs Bureau (MAB-109–062) and the Teh-Tzer Study Group for Human Medical Research Foundation.

Conflicts of Interest: The authors declare no conflict of interest.

References

1. Giovannucci, E.; Harlan, D.M.; Archer, M.C.; Bergenstal, R.M.; Gapstur, S.M.; Habel, L.A.; Pollak, M.; Regensteiner, J.G.; Yee, D. Diabetes and cancer. *Diabetes Care* **2010**, *33*, 1674–1685. [CrossRef] [PubMed]
2. Sozen, T.; Ozisik, L.; Başaran, N.Ç.; Özışık, L. An overview and management of osteoporosis. *Eur. J. Rheumatol.* **2017**, *4*, 46–56. [CrossRef]
3. Calle, E.E.; Rodriguez, C.; Walker-Thurmond, K.; Thun, M.J. Overweight, obesity, and mortality from cancer in a prospectively studied cohort of U.S. adults. *N. Engl. J. Med.* **2003**, *348*, 1625–1638. [CrossRef] [PubMed]
4. Pollak, M. Insulin and insulin like growth factor signalling in neoplasia. *Nat. Rev. Cancer* **2008**, *8*, 915–928. [CrossRef] [PubMed]
5. Yun, J.; Rago, C.; Cheong, I.; Pagliarini, R.; Angenendt, P.; Rajagopalan, H.; Schmidt, K.; Willson, J.K.V.; Markowitz, S.; Zhou, S.; et al. Glucose deprivation contributes to the development of KRAS Pathway Mutations in Tumor Cells. *Science* **2009**, *325*, 1555–1559. [CrossRef] [PubMed]
6. Kalaany, N.Y.; Sabatini, D.M. Tumours with PI3K activation are resistant to dietary restriction. *Nature* **2009**, *458*, 725–731. [CrossRef]
7. Yu, H.; Pardoll, E.; Jove, R. STATs in cancer inflammation and immunity: A leading role for STAT3. *Nat. Rev. Cancer* **2009**, *9*, 798–809. [CrossRef]
8. Poiana, C.; Capatina, C. Osteoporosis and fracture risk in patients with type 2 diabetes mellitus. *Acta Endocrinol. (Bucharest)* **2019**, *15*, 231–236. [CrossRef]
9. Drake, M.T. Osteoporosis and cancer. *Curr. Osteoporos. Rep.* **2013**, *11*, 163–170. [CrossRef]
10. Hodgson, S.F.; Watts, N.B.; Bilezikian, J.; Clarke, B.L.; Gray, T.K.; Harris, D.W.; Johnston, C.C.; Kleerekoper, M.; Lindsay, R.; Luckey, M.M.; et al. American association of clinical endocrinologists medical guidelines for clinical practice for the prevention and treatment of postmenopausal osteoporosis: 2001 edition, with selected updates for 2003. *Endocr. Pract.* **2003**, *9*, 544–564. [CrossRef]
11. Jackuliak, P.; Payer, J. Osteoporosis, fractures, and diabetes. *Int. J. Endocrinol.* **2014**, *2014*, 1–10. [CrossRef] [PubMed]
12. Rojas, L.B.A.; Gomes, M.B. Metformin: An old but still the best treatment for type 2 diabetes. *Diabetol. Metab. Syndr.* **2013**, *5*, 6. [CrossRef]
13. Kasznicki, J.; Sliwinska, A.; Drzewoski, J. Metformin in cancer prevention and therapy. *Ann. Transl. Med.* **2014**, *2*, 57.

14. Chamberlain, J.J.; Herman, W.H.; Leal, S.; Rhinehart, A.S.; Shubrook, J.H.; Skolnik, N.; Kalyani, R.R. Pharmacologic therapy for type 2 diabetes: Synopsis of the 2017 American diabetes association standards of medical care in diabetes. *Ann. Intern. Med.* **2017**, *166*, 572. [CrossRef] [PubMed]
15. Chinese Hospital Association. *ICD-9-CM English-Chinese Dictionary*; Chinese Hospital Association Press: Taipei, Taiwan, 2000.
16. Guilherme, A.; Virbasius, J.V.; Puri, V.; Czech, M.P. Adipocyte dysfunctions linking obesity to insulin resistance and type 2 diabetes. *Nat. Rev. Mol. Cell Biol.* **2008**, *9*, 367–377. [CrossRef] [PubMed]
17. Chang, C.-H.; Toh, S.; Lin, J.-W.; Chen, S.-T.; Kuo, C.-W.; Chuang, L.-M.; Lai, M.-S. Cancer risk associated with insulin glargine among adult type 2 diabetes patients—A nationwide cohort study. *PLoS ONE* **2011**, *6*, e21368. [CrossRef]
18. Rau, H.-H.; Hsu, M.-H.; Lin, Y.-A.; Atique, S.; Fuad, A.; Wei, L.-M.; Hsu, M.-H. Development of a web-based liver cancer prediction model for type II diabetes patients by using an artificial neural network. *Comput. Methods Programs Biomed.* **2016**, *125*, 58–65. [CrossRef]
19. Chang, C.-Y.; Chen, W.-L.; Liou, Y.-F.; Ke, C.-C.; Lee, H.-C.; Huang, H.-L.; Ciou, L.-P.; Chou, C.-C.; Yang, M.-C.; Ho, S.-Y.; et al. Increased Risk of major depression in the three years following a femoral neck fracture A National population-based follow-up study. *PLoS ONE* **2014**, *9*, e89867. [CrossRef]
20. Leslie, W.D.; Lix, L.M.; Prior, H.J.; Derksen, S.; Metge, C.; O'Neil, J. Biphasic fracture risk in diabetes: A population-based study. *Bone* **2007**, *40*, 1595–1601. [CrossRef]
21. Janghorbani, M.; Van Dam, R.M.; Willett, W.C.; Hu, F.B. Systematic Review of Type 1 and Type 2 Diabetes mellitus and risk of fracture. *Am. J. Epidemiol.* **2007**, *166*, 495–505. [CrossRef]
22. Yasuda, H. RANKL, a necessary chance for clinical application to osteoporosis and cancer-related bone diseases. *World J. Orthop.* **2013**, *4*, 207–217. [CrossRef]
23. Cummings, S.R.; Martín, J.S.; McClung, M.; Siris, E.S.; Eastell, R.; Reid, I.R.; Delmas, P.; Zoog, H.B.; Austin, M.; Wang, A.; et al. Denosumab for prevention of fractures in postmenopausal women with osteoporosis. *N. Engl. J. Med.* **2009**, *361*, 756–765. [CrossRef] [PubMed]
24. Smith, M.R.; Egerdie, B.; Toriz, N.H.; Feldman, R.; Tammela, T.L.; Saad, F.; Heracek, J.; Szwedowski, M.; Ke, C.; Kupic, A.; et al. Denosumab in Men receiving androgen-deprivation therapy for prostate cancer. *N. Engl. J. Med.* **2009**, *361*, 745–755. [CrossRef] [PubMed]
25. American Diabetes Association. 9. Pharmacologic Approaches to glycemic treatment: Standards of medical care in diabetes—2019. *Diabetes Care* **2018**, *42*, S90–S102. [CrossRef]
26. Maruthur, N.; Tseng, E.; Hutfless, S.; Wilson, L.M.; Suarez-Cuervo, C.; Berger, Z.; Chu, Y.; Iyoha, E.; Segal, J.B.; Bolen, S. Diabetes medications as monotherapy or metformin-based combination therapy for type 2 diabetes. *Ann. Intern. Med.* **2016**, *164*, 740. [CrossRef] [PubMed]
27. Holman, R.R.; Paul, S.; Bethel, M.A.; Matthews, D.R.; Neil, H.A.W. 10-Year Follow-up of Intensive Glucose Control in Type 2 Diabetes. *N. Engl. J. Med.* **2008**, *359*, 1577–1589. [CrossRef]
28. Paschou, S.A.; DeDe, A.D.; Anagnostis, P.G.; Vryonidou, A.; Morganstein, D.; Goulis, D.G. Type 2 Diabetes and osteoporosis: A guide to optimal management. *J. Clin. Endocrinol. Metab.* **2017**, *102*, 3621–3634. [CrossRef]
29. Iki, M.; Fujita, Y.; Kouda, K.; Yura, A.; Tachiki, T.; Tamaki, J.; Sato, Y.; Moon, J.-S.; Hamada, M.; Kajita, E.; et al. Increased risk of osteoporotic fracture in community-dwelling elderly men 20 or more years after gastrectomy: The Fujiwara-kyo Osteoporosis Risk in Men (FORMEN) Cohort Study. *Bone* **2019**, *127*, 250–259. [CrossRef]
30. Seo, G.H.; Kang, H.Y.; Choe, E.K. Osteoporosis and fracture after gastrectomy for stomach cancer. *Medicine* **2018**, *97*, e0532. [CrossRef]
31. Evans, J.M.M.; Donnelly, L.A.; Emslie-Smith, A.M.; Alessi, D.R.; Morris, A.D. Metformin and reduced risk of cancer in diabetic patients. *BMJ* **2005**, *330*, 1304–1305. [CrossRef]
32. Vestergaard, P.; Rejnmark, L.; Mosekilde, L. Relative fracture risk in patients with diabetes mellitus, and the impact of insulin and oral antidiabetic medication on relative fracture risk. *Diabetologia* **2005**, *48*, 1292–1299. [CrossRef] [PubMed]
33. Bahrambeigi, S.; Yousefi, B.; Rahimi, M.; Shafiei-Irannejad, V. Metformin; an old antidiabetic drug with new potentials in bone disorders. *Biomed. Pharmacother.* **2019**, *109*, 1593–1601. [CrossRef] [PubMed]
34. Shah, M.; Kola, B.; Bataveljic, A.; Arnett, T.; Viollet, B.; Saxon, L.; Korbonits, M.; Chenu, C. AMP-activated protein kinase (AMPK) activation regulates in vitro bone formation and bone mass. *Bone* **2010**, *47*, 309–319. [CrossRef] [PubMed]

35. Sofer, E.; Shargorodsky, M. Effect of metformin treatment on circulating osteoprotegerin in patients with nonalcoholic fatty liver disease. *Hepatol. Int.* **2015**, *10*, 169–174. [CrossRef] [PubMed]
36. Liu, Q.; Xu, X.; Yang, Z.; Liu, Y.; Wu, X.; Huang, Z.; Liu, J.; Huang, Z.; Kong, G.; Ding, J.; et al. Metformin alleviates the bone loss induced by ketogenic diet: An in vivo study in mice. *Calcif. Tissue Int.* **2018**, *104*, 59–69. [CrossRef]
37. Mai, Q.-G.; Zhang, Z.-M.; Xu, S.; Lu, M.; Zhou, R.-P.; Zhao, L.; Jia, C.; Wen, Z.-H.; Jin, D.; Bai, X.-C. Metformin stimulates osteoprotegerin and reduces RANKL expression in osteoblasts and ovariectomized rats. *J. Cell. Biochem.* **2011**, *112*, 2902–2909. [CrossRef]
38. Hay, N.; Sonenberg, N. Upstream and downstream of mTOR. *Genes Dev.* **2004**, *18*, 1926–1945. [CrossRef]
39. Mu, W.; Wang, Z.; Ma, C.; Jiang, Y.; Zhang, N.; Hu, K.; Li, L.; Wang, Z. Metformin promotes the proliferation and differentiation of murine preosteoblast by regulating the expression of sirt6 and oct4. *Pharmacol. Res.* **2018**, *129*, 462–474. [CrossRef]
40. Hernlund, E.; Svedbom, A.; Ivergard, M.; Compston, J.; Cooper, C.; Stenmark, J.; McCloskey, E.V.; Jonsson, B.; Kanis, J.A. Osteoporosis in the European Union: Medical management, epidemiology and economic Burden: A report prepared in collaboration with the International Osteoporosis Foundation (IOF) and the European Federation of Pharmaceutical Industry Associations (EFPIA). *Arch. Osteoporos.* **2013**, *8*, 136. [CrossRef]
41. Vestergaard, P. Discrepancies in bone mineral density and fracture risk in patients with type 1 and type 2 diabetes—A meta-analysis. *Osteoporos. Int.* **2006**, *18*, 427–444. [CrossRef]
42. De Laet, C.; Kanis, J.; Odén, A.; Johanson, H.; Johnell, O.; Delmas, P.; Eisman, J.A.; Kröger, H.; Fujiwara, S.; Garnero, P.; et al. Body mass index as a predictor of fracture risk: A meta-analysis. *Osteoporos. Int.* **2005**, *16*, 1330–1338. [CrossRef] [PubMed]

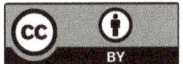

© 2020 by the authors. Licensee MDPI, Basel, Switzerland. This article is an open access article distributed under the terms and conditions of the Creative Commons Attribution (CC BY) license (http://creativecommons.org/licenses/by/4.0/).

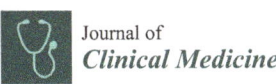

Review

Testosterone and Bone Health in Men: A Narrative Review

Kazuyoshi Shigehara *, Kouji Izumi, Yoshifumi Kadono and Atsushi Mizokami

Department of Integrative Cancer Therapy and Urology, Kanazawa University Graduate School of Medical Science, 13-1, Kanazawa, Ishikawa 920-8641, Japan; azuizu2003@yahoo.co.jp (K.I.); yskadono@yahoo.co.jp (Y.K.); mizokami@staff.kanazawa-u.ac.jp (A.M.)
* Correspondence: kshigehara0415@yahoo.co.jp; Tel.: +81-76-265-2393

Abstract: Bone fracture due to osteoporosis is an important issue in decreasing the quality of life for elderly men in the current aging society. Thus, osteoporosis and bone fracture prevention is a clinical concern for many clinicians. Moreover, testosterone has an important role in maintaining bone mineral density (BMD) among men. Some testosterone molecular mechanisms on bone metabolism have been currently established by many experimental data. Concurrent with a decrease in testosterone with age, various clinical symptoms and signs associated with testosterone decline, including decreased BMD, are known to occur in elderly men. However, the relationship between testosterone levels and osteoporosis development has been conflicting in human epidemiological studies. Thus, testosterone replacement therapy (TRT) is a useful tool for managing clinical symptoms caused by hypogonadism. Many recent studies support the benefit of TRT on BMD, especially in hypogonadal men with osteopenia and osteoporosis, although a few studies failed to demonstrate its effects. However, no evidence supporting the hypothesis that TRT can prevent the incidence of bone fracture exists. Currently, TRT should be considered as one of the treatment options to improve hypogonadal symptoms and BMD simultaneously in symptomatic hypogonadal men with osteopenia.

Keywords: testosterone; men; osteoporosis; bone mineral density

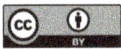

1. Introduction

Serum testosterone levels decrease by 1% annually with age in elderly men [1], which may induce various clinical symptoms of late-onset hypogonadism (LOH) syndrome [2]. LOH syndrome is involved in a cluster of clinical symptoms, including depression, irritability, sexual dysfunction, decreased muscle mass and strength, and decreased bone mineral density (BMD), visceral obesity, and metabolic syndrome, which have been thought to be associated with aging [3,4]. These symptoms and signs often impair the quality of life (QOL) in elderly men and are considered a serious public health concern in the current aging society. Thus, testosterone replacement therapy (TRT) is expected to be one of the tools for improving these clinical conditions and QOL in men with LOH syndrome. Consequently, its clinical use has substantially increased over the past years [5].

In particular, osteoporosis often causes compression spine fractures and femoral neck fractures in elderly men, resulting in a decrease of activities of daily living (ADL) and QOL. Estrogen, which is important for maintaining BMD, decreases immediately in women during menopause. However, testosterone, which decreases slowly with age, plays an important role in maintaining BMD in men. Therefore, osteoporosis occurs more commonly in elderly women than in men [6,7]. The prevalence of osteoporosis increases with age at <10%, 13%, 18%, and 21% for 40, 70–75, 75–80, and >80 years old men in Japan, respectively [8]. Moreover, about 12 million people are estimated to suffer from osteoporosis [6,7]. The incidence frequency of femoral neck fracture is fourfold more in men than in women with osteoporosis [9]. Thus, osteoporosis prevention is an important issue in maintaining ADL and QOL in elderly men.

BMD has a close correlation with serum testosterone levels in men. Moreover, testosterone levels immediately decrease because of androgen deprivation therapy (ADT) for prostate cancer, resulting in a decrease of BMD and osteoporosis. In addition, estradiol (E2) converted from testosterone by aromatase is deeply related to BMD maintenance. A relative decrease in estrogen level due to ADT also poses a risk for BMD loss [10,11]. In general, BMD decreases by about 2%–8% in 1 year after the commencement of ADT [12]. Furthermore, ADT increases the risk of decreased BMD at five- to tenfold compared to prostate cancer patients with normal testosterone levels. A meta-analysis demonstrated that 9%–53% of osteoporosis incidence was caused by ADT [13]. Consequently, patients with ADT have a definite higher risk of sustaining a fracture. Furthermore, ADT can increase the risk of proximal femur fractures by 1.5- to 1.8-fold [14,15]. The BMD decrease in these patients is caused by a decline in serum testosterone and estrogen levels by ADT.

As aforementioned, the association between testosterone deficiency and BMD loss has been currently clarified. It is believed that TRT can contribute to maintaining and increasing BMD among hypogonadal men. However, the efficacy of TRT for bone health in hypogonadal men has been currently less in consensus and more conflicting [16–21]. Therefore, this article reviewed the relationship between testosterone and BMD in men and mentioned the benefits of TRT on BMD among hypogonadal men.

2. Materials and Methods

A review of PubMed, MEDLINE, and EMBASE databases was conducted to search for original articles, systematic review, and meta-analysis under key words as following; "testosterone" or "hypogonadism", "bone mineral density" or "osteoporosis" or "bone fracture", and "men". There was no limitation on language, publication status, and study design. Papers published from January 1990 through to October 2020 were collected. We also checked the references of systematic reviews and meta-analyses carefully to identify additional original articles for inclusion. Two reviewers screened the search results, and the data were collected on 4 November 2020.

All papers suitable for three topics including "The Relationship between Hypogonadism and BMD in human", "The Relationship between Testosterone and Bone Fracture", and "The Effects of TRT on Bone Health among Hypogonadal Men" from the journal databases were adopted for the present analysis.

3. Molecular Roles of Sex Hormones on Bone Metabolism

Testosterone is converted to highly active dihydrotestosterone (DHT) by 5α-reductase in the cytoplasm of target cells [22,23]. Consequently, DHT can induce androgenic activity by binding to the androgen receptor (AR). Moreover, testosterone is converted to E2 by aromatase. E2 binds to the estrogen receptor (ER) and exerts estrogenic action. ERα and ERβ are the two ER subtypes. ERα is mainly associated with bone metabolism [10,24].

AR is present in chondrocytes and osteoblasts, although its expression level widely varies by age and bone sites. Testosterone acts directly on osteoblasts by AR and can consequently promote bone formation [17]. In addition, testosterone has some indirect effects on bone metabolism through various cytokines and growth factors [17,25–28] (Figure 1). Furthermore, testosterone can increase AR expression level in osteoblasts, resulting in differentiation promotion and osteoblast and chondrocyte apoptosis proliferation [17,29]. Consequently, less evidence supporting the hypothesis that testosterone has any direct effects on osteoclasts has been shown [30].

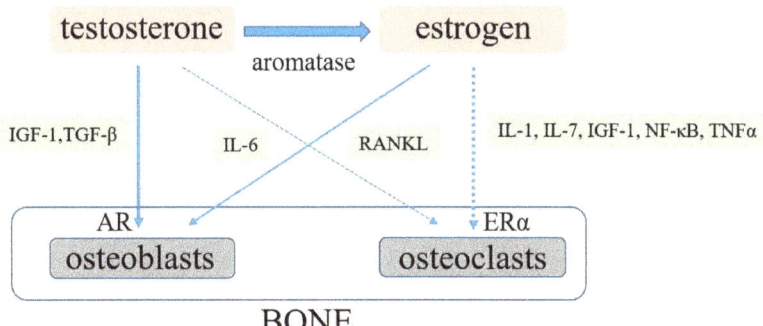

Figure 1. Molecular rules of testosterone and estrogen in bone metabolism. AR, androgen receptor; ERα, estrogen receptor α; IGF-1, insulin growth factor-1; TGFβ, transforming growth factor-β; IL, interleukins; RANKL, receptor activator of NF-κB ligand; NF-κB, nuclear factor-κB; TNFα, tumor necrotic factor-α.

In addition, testosterone deficiency promotes the activation of nuclear factor kappa-B ligand (RANKL) production from osteoblasts, which contributes to the promotion of the differentiations and functions in osteoclasts. Increased RANKL level progresses bone resorption and decreases BMD [25,26]. Thus, testosterone positively regulates the expression of insulin-like growth factor-1 (IGF-1) and IGF-binding protein (IGF-BP) in osteoblasts. The differentiation and proliferation of chondrocytes and osteoblasts are induced by IGF and IGF-BP, and the suppression of apoptosis of chondrocytes promotes bone formation. Moreover, testosterone activates the expression of transforming growth factor-β (TGF-β) in osteoblasts and promotes the differentiation of osteoblasts [27]. Testosterone suppresses the activity of interleukins (IL)-6, which activates osteoclasts and promotes bone resorption. However, testosterone deficiency decreases in BMD through increased IL-6 activation [28].

E2 and ERα also play important roles in maintaining BMD in men and women. Estrogen has a greater effect than androgen in inhibiting bone resorption in men. Consequently, men with loss of ERα function exhibit extremely low BMD [31]. Male patients with aromatase deficiency have a marked decrease in BMD in trabecular and cortical bone. Thus, estrogen replacement therapy in these patients can improve BMD [32,33]. E2 generally regulates apoptosis and function of osteoclast, which contributes to BMD maintenance. Moreover, E2 deficiency may accelerate osteoclast apoptosis by increased tumor growth factor-β production [34,35]. IL-1, IL-6, IL-7, IGF-1, nuclear factor-κB (NF-κB), RANKL, and tumor necrotic factor-α (TNFα) are the E2 target genes [36–39]. However, E2 deficiency increases IL-6, which reduces osteoblast proliferation and activity while increasing osteoclastic activity and increasing the expression of RANKL-mediated osteoclastogenesis [36,37]. Some experimental data showed that estrogen decrease also induces inflammatory cytokine, IL-1, and TNFα, resulting in BMD loss. However, this phenomenon does not occur in IL-1 receptor- or TNFα-deficient mice [38,39].

4. The Relationship between Hypogonadism and BMD in Humans

The apparent relationship between testosterone deficiency and low BMD has been currently established [5]. In particular, this relationship is much stronger in young adult men with moderate to severe hypogonadism [40,41]. However, epidemiological information on male osteoporosis attributed to hypogonadism, especially in elderly men, has been less available. Therefore, the prevalence of hypogonadism among men with osteoporosis or bone fracture has not been clarified.

Some previous studies demonstrated that hypogonadism was the cause of male osteoporosis (6.9%–58%) [42–47] (Table 1). However, these studies are limited by their small sizes and various potential biases. In addition, case–control studies comparing the prevalence of hypogonadism between subjects with osteoporosis and controls have been limited.

Table 1. Prevalence of hypogonadism in men with osteopenia or bone fracture.

Author	Year	Subjects	Prevalence of HG	Reference
Stanley	1991	17 with MTHF	58%	[42]
		61 controls	18%	
Baillie	1992	70 with vertebral fracture	16%	[43]
Kelepouris	1995	47 with atraumatic fracture	15%	[44]
Fink HA	2006	2447 community-dwelling men including 130 with osteoporosis	7%	[45]
Ryan	2011	234 with osteoporosis	24%	[46]
Kotwal N	2018	200 male attendants of patients attending endocrine outpatient department	35%	[47]

HG, hypogonadism; MTHF, minimal trauma hip fracture.

A case–control study found that the prevalence rates of hypogonadism in men with osteoporotic fracture and control were 58% and 18%, respectively [42]. A cross-sectional and longitudinal study involving 2447 community-dwelling elderly men stated that the prevalence rates of hypogonadism among men with osteoporosis and normal BMD were 6.9% and 3.2%. Conversely, the prevalence of osteoporosis in men with hypogonadism was significantly higher in those with eugonadism (12.3% and 6.0%, respectively) [45]. Furthermore, a recent meta-analysis involving 300 patients from five case–control studies revealed that no significant difference was observed in testosterone level in both cases and controls [48]. Fewer exercise habits, cigarette smoking, various medications, and underlying diseases (e.g., metabolic syndrome, especially in elderly men) may modify the exact relationship between testosterone and osteoporosis, resulting in conflicting data. Further case–control studies involving a large number of subjects are likely required to better clarify whether prevalence of osteoporosis is higher in hypogonadal compared with eugonadal men.

In addition, whether low testosterone is a potential risk factor for developing male osteoporosis in men is still unclear. Several large-population observational trials have been performed to investigate the effects of testosterone deficiency on osteoporosis risk factors in men [45,49–58] (Table 2). Some previous studies supported the potential relationship between testosterone decline and low BMD [45,49,51,54], and other studies denied this association [50,52,53,55–58]. Conversely, some previous studies found that E2 was significantly correlated with BMD loss in elderly men [45,49,50,54–57], supporting the hypothesis that E2 is also significantly correlated with BMD in men. In men, 85% of serum E2 derives from testosterone conversion by aromatase [59]. Therefore, low testosterone leads to low E2 production via aromatase, which could provoke deleterious effects on BMD, but also on bone quality as assessed in vivo by some different diagnostic tools [60,61]. A previous study demonstrated that 12-month administration of aromatase inhibitor in elderly men with hypogonadism resulted in a further decrease in BMD [62].

The conflicting results on the role of testosterone in BMD may also be because serum testosterone levels do not always reflect local testosterone levels within bone tissues and localized testosterone metabolism. A sub-analysis of the prospective MrOS study in Sweden involving 631 elderly men showed that glucuronidated androgen metabolites, but not serum TT, had a significant correlation with BMD in elderly men, suggesting that localized testosterone levels may have an important role in maintaining BMD [63].

Table 2. The relationship between testosterone and BMD in men.

Author	Year	Country	Study Subjects	Hormones	Results	Ref
Greendale (Rancho Bernardo Study)	1997	USA	457 women and 534 men (50–89 years)	TT, DHT, E2, E1, BioT	Higher bioavailable (but not total) testosterone levels were associated with higher BMD.	[49]
Amin (Framingham Study)	2000	USA	448 men (68–96 years)	TT, E2, LH	Hypogonadism related to aging has little influence on BMD.	[50]
Fink	2006	USA	2447 community-dwelling men (>65 years)	TT, E2	The incidence rates of hip bone loss in men with deficient and normal total testosterone were 22.5% and 8.6%.	[45]
Mellström (MrOS Sweden)	2006	Sweden	2908 men (69–80 years)	TT, E2, FT, FE2, SHBG	FT levels were positively correlated with BMD in the hip, femur, and arm but not in the lumbar spine.	[51]
Bjørnerem (Tromsø Study)	2007	Norway	927 women (37–80 years), 894 men (25–80 years)	TT, E2, cFT SHBG	The relationship between all gender steroids and bone loss was weak.	[52]
Kuchuk NO (Longitudinal Ageing Study Amsterdam)	2007	Netherlands	623 men and 634 women (65–88 years)	TT, E2 SHBG	TT had no correlations with BMD	[53]
LeBlanc (MrOS Research)	2009	USA	5995 community-dwelling men (>65 years)	BioT, BioE2 SHBG	The combination of low BioE2, low BaT, and high SHBG was associated with significantly faster rates of BMD loss.	[54]
Vanderschueren (EMAS study)	2010	Belgium	3140 men (40–79 years)	TT, FT, E2 SHBG	TT and FT had no correlations with BMD.	[55]
Cauley (MrOS Research)	2010	USA	1238 men (cross-sectional) 969 men (longitudinal) >65 years	BioT, BioE2 SHBG	No association existed between BioT and hip BMD loss.	[56]
Woo	2012	Hong Kong	1448 men (>65 years)	TT, FT, E2, BioE2, SHBG	TT and FT were not correlated with bone loss.	[57]
Hsu (CHAMP Cohort)	2016	Australia	1705, 1367, and 958 men (>70 men)	TT, DHT, E2 E1, SHBG, LH FSH, cFT	Both TT and cFT had no correlations with bone loss.	[58]

BMD, bone mineral density; TT, total testosterone; DHT, dihydrotestosterone; E2, estradiol; E1, estriol; Bio, bioavailability; LH, luteinizing hormone; FT, free testosterone; FE2, free estradiol; SHBG, sex hormone-binding globulin; cFT, calculated free testosterone; FSH, follicle-stimulating hormone.

5. The Relationship between Testosterone and Bone Fracture

Falling and fractures in elderly men have a great impact on ADL and life prognosis. Moreover, preventing them has become an important issue worldwide. The occurrence of fractures associated with aging is largely due to the decrease in physical function (e.g., muscle mass loss and muscle weakness, frailty, and sarcopenia) in addition to the decrease in BMD [64,65]. Consequently, various clinical conditions caused by testosterone deficiency with age can also affect falls and fractures [2–5]. Additionally, osteoporosis is a bone condition in which bone mass and strength decrease with aging [8]. Thus, falls are an important factor in the onset of fractures.

Many previous studies investigated the relationship between testosterone and bone fracture risk [45,51,57,58,66–74] (Table 3). In addition, several studies have found that elderly men with osteoporotic fractures had statistically significant lower testosterone levels compared with age-matched controls [45,51,66–68,70,72,74], and other studies failed to show any associations between testosterone levels and fracture risk [57,58,69,71]. A meta-analysis including 55 studies demonstrated that a significant association was observed in hypogonadism, independent of age, low body mass index, cigarette smoking, excessive alcohol drinking, steroid use, history of diabetes, and so on [62]. Many studies were likely to support the negative effect of testosterone deficiency on the incidences of fall and fracture [45,51,66–68,70,72,74], although a smaller number of studies denied this relationship [57,58,69,71]. The more predominant roles for testosterone bone fracture in comparison with BMD may be due to the other role of testosterone in muscle strength and physical performance in men, which leads to sarcopenia and falls risks.

Table 3. The relationship between testosterone and bone fractures risk.

Author	Year	Country	Study Subjects	Hormones	Results	Ref
Szulc (MINOS study)	2003	France	1040 elderly men (19–85 years)	TT, FT	Hypogonadal men had increased rates of falls and markers of bone resorption.	[66]
Kenny	2005	USA	83 community-dwelling white men (>65 years)	BioT	Fifty-two percent of men with low BioT levels had lower BMD and were likely at an increased risk of fracture.	[67]
Fink	2006	USA	2447 community-dwelling men (>65 years)	TT, E2	Prevalence rates of osteoporosis in men with deficient and normal total testosterone were 12.3% and 6.0%.	[45]
Mellström (MrOS Sweden)	2006	Sweden	2908 men (69–80 years)	TT, E2, FT, FE2, SHBG	FT levels below the median were independent predictors of prevalent osteoporosis-related fractures and X-ray-verified vertebral fractures.	[51]
Tuck	2008	UK	57 men with symptomatic vertebral fractures 57 age-matched controls	FT, BioT, SHBG	Calculated FT was lower in the fracture group than the controls.	[68]
Mellstrom (MrOS Sweden)	2008	Sweden	2639 men (69–80 years)	TT, E2, FT, FE2, SHBG	TT and FT were not significantly associated with fracture risk.	[69]
Meier (The Dubbo Study)	2008	Switzerland	609 men (>60 years)	TT, E2, SHBG	Lower testosterone increased the risk of osteoporotic fracture, particularly with hip and nonvertebral fractures.	[70]
Roddam (EPIC-Oxford Study)	2009	UK	155 men and 281 women	TT, E2, SHBG	There were no associations between fracture risk and testosterone levels.	[71]
Risto	2012	Sweden	39 treated for fracture 45 controls	TT, BioT, BioE2	BioT was a possible marker for increased fracture risk.	[72]
Woo	2012	Hong Kong	1448 men (>65 years)	TT, FT, E2, BioE2, SHBG	TT and FT had no correlations with an increased bone fracture.	[57]
Torremadé-Barreda	2013	Spain	54 men with hip fracture 54 age-matched controls	TT, FT, BioT	Men with hip fractures had significantly lower calculated FT and BiaT levels.	[73]
Hsu (CHAMP Cohort)	2016	Australia	1705, 1367, and 958 men over 70 men	TT, DHT, E2, E1, SHBG, LH FSH, cFT	Both TT and cFT had no correlations with incident fractures.	[58]
Tran	2017	Australia	602 men with incident fractures	TT	TT was significantly correlated with the incidence of fracture risk.	[74]

TT, total testosterone; FT, free testosterone; BioT, bioavailable testosterone; E2, estradiol; FE2, free estradiol; SHBG, sex hormone-binding globulin; BioE2, bioavailable estradiol; DHT, dihydrotestosterone; E1, estriol; LH, luteinizing hormone; FSH, follicle-stimulating hormone; cFT, calculated free testosterone.

Furthermore, one previous review stated that E2 levels predict the risk of bone fracture, independent of not only serum testosterone and androgens but also estrogens, which are important regulators of bone health in men [75].

6. The Effects of TRT on Bone Health among Hypogonadal Men

TRT for hypogonadal men can improve various symptoms (e.g., metabolic syndrome) and has been used worldwide for managing these symptoms and maintaining QOL [2,5]. Moreover, testosterone plays some potential roles in maintaining BMD among men, and TRT is expected to be useful for preventing and managing osteoporosis and improving BMD among hypogonadal men.

Many recent previous studies suggested the ameliorative effect of TRT on osteoporosis/osteopenia [76–84] (Table 4). A meta-analysis involving 1083 subjects from 29 randomized controlled studies (RCTs) demonstrated that TRT could improve BMD at the lumbar spine by +3.7% (confidence interval, 1.0%–6.4%) compared with placebo [20]. In particular, many of the previous reports published since 2010 suggest some benefits of TRT on BMD. By contrast, a smaller number of studies failed to find the positive effect of BMD [85–87]. However, the subjects of this study were limited to men with hypogonadism, but not always with a lower BMD at baseline. Three studies targeting hypogonadal men with osteopenia or osteoporosis demonstrated that TRT could significantly increase their BMD [76,78,83]. Currently, extremely limited studies, including long-term TRT over 3 years, are available.

Further larger and longer RCTs are likely to be required to reach a conclusive result regarding the effects of TRT on bone health and to investigate the benefit of the severity of hypogonadism, degree of baseline BMD loss, and dose of testosterone supplement.

Table 4. The effects of TRT on BMD in hypogonadal men (from papers published since 2010).

Author	Country	Design	Study Subjects	TRT	Periods	Results	Ref
Kenny (2010)	USA	RCT	131 men with hypogonadism, bone fracture, low BMD, frailty	Transdermal testosterone (5 mg/day)	12–24 months	TRT could increase axial BMD.	[76]
Permpongkosol (2010)	Thailand	Single arm	161 hypogonadal men	1000 mg TU (Nebido)	54–150 weeks	No change in BMD was observed in TRT.	[85]
Aversa (2012)	Italy	Case–control	40 hypogonadal men 20 aged-match control	Intramuscular TU (4 times/year)	36 months	TRT increased vertebral and femoral BMD.	[77]
Wang (2013)	China	RCT	186 men with osteoporosis and hypogonadism	TU (20 or 40 mg/day)	24 months	TRT improved the lumbar spine and femoral neck BMD.	[78]
Bouloux (2013)	UK	RCT	322 men with LOH syndrome	Oral TU (80, 160, 240 mg/day)	1 year	Treatment with oral TU led to BMD improvement.	[79]
Rodriguez-Tolrà (2013)	Spain	Single arm	50 men with LOH syndrome	TG (50 mg/day for 12 months) 1000 mg TU (every 2–3 months from 12–24 months)	2 years	TRT improved lumbar spine and hip BMD.	[80]
Permpongkosol (2016)	Thailand	Single arm	120 hypogonadal men	1000 mg TU (Nebido)	5–8 years	A statistically significant increase was found in vertebral and femoral BMD.	[81]
Rogol (2016)	USA	RCT	306 hypogonadal men	TG (22 or 33 mg)	90–360 days	BMD improved from baseline by TRT.	[82]
Konaka (2016)	Japan	RCT	334 hypogonadal men	TE (250 mg/4 W)	12 months	12-month TRT could not improve BMD.	[86]
Shigehara (2017)	Japan	RCT	74 hypogonadal men with osteopenia	TE (250 mg/4 W)	12 months	TRT for 12 months could improve BMD.	[83]
Snyder (2017)	USA	RCT	211 hypogonadal men	TG (5 mg/day initially)	1 year	TRT increased BMD and bone strength, more in trabecula.	[84]
Ng Tang Fui (2018)	Australia	RCT	100 obese men with hypogonadism	TU (1000 mg/0, 6, 26, 36, and 46 weeks)	56 weeks	No significant changes in the lumbar spine and femoral BMD were observed.	[87]

TRT, testosterone replacement therapy; BMD, bone mineral density; RCT, randomized controlled study; TU, testosterone undecanoate; TG, testosterone gel; TE, testosterone enanthate; LOH, late-onset hypogonadism.

Currently, some guidelines have recommended TRT for symptomatic hypogonadal men with osteoporosis to prevent bone loss and help in acquiring peak bone mass [41,88–91]. However, the effects of TRT for decreasing the risk of fracture in hypogonadal men with osteopenia and osteoporosis remain unclear. Testosterone therapies have various inverse effects, including erythrocytosis, worsening of prostate hypertrophy and lower urinary tract symptoms, worsening of sleep apnea syndrome, and cardiovascular effects, which are likely to outweigh the beneficial effect for BMD improvement [2,3,5]. Therefore, TRT is not recommended as a tool solely to enhance and maintain BMD for hypogonadal men. At present, vitamin D formulation and antiresorptive drugs are understandably recommended to treat hypogonadism-related osteoporosis in elderly men [92–95]. On the other hand, TRT should be considered for the patients with any hypogonadal symptoms, and TRT may be an alternative tool for improving hypogonadal symptoms and BMD simultaneously in such cases.

7. Conclusions

Testosterone plays an important role in maintaining BMD and bone health among men. In addition, many molecular mechanisms of testosterone on bone metabolism have been currently established by many experimental data. Several recent studies demonstrated the benefit of TRT on BMD, especially in hypogonadal men with osteopenia and osteoporosis. However, a few studies failed to demonstrate its effects, and no evidence supporting the hypothesis that TRT can prevent bone fracture incidence exists. Further studies involving a large number of subjects and longer treatment duration are required to reach a more conclusive result regarding the effects of TRT on bone health.

Current evidence suggests that TRT is not recommended as a tool solely to enhance and maintain BMD for hypogonadal men. TRT should be considered as one of the treatment options to improve hypogonadal symptoms and BMD simultaneously in symptomatic hypogonadal men with osteopenia.

Author Contributions: Data collection, K.S., K.I., Y.K.; writing—original draft preparation, K.S.; writing—review and editing, K.S., K.I.; supervision, A.M. All authors have read and agreed to the published version of the manuscript.

Funding: This research received no external funding.

Institutional Review Board Statement: Not applicable.

Informed Consent Statement: Not applicable.

Data Availability Statement: Data sharing not applicable.

Conflicts of Interest: The authors declare no conflict of interest.

References

1. Feldman, H.A.; Longcope, C.; Derby, C.A.; Johannes, C.B.; Araujo, A.B.; Coviello, A.D.; Bremner, W.J.; McKinlay, J.B. Age trends in the level of serum testosterone and other hormones in middle-aged men: Longitudinal results from the Massachusetts male aging study. *J. Clin. Endocrinol. Metab.* **2002**, *87*, 589–598. [CrossRef] [PubMed]
2. Lunenfeld, B.; Mskhalaya, G.; Zitzmann, M.; Arver, S.; Kalinchenko, S.; Tishova, Y.; Morgentaler, A. Recommendations on the diagnosis, treatment and monitoring of hypogonadism in men. *Aging Male* **2015**, *18*, 5–15. [CrossRef] [PubMed]
3. Lunenfeld, B.; Arver, S.; Moncada, I.; Rees, D.A.; Schulte, H.M. How to help the aging male? Current approaches to hypogonadism in primary care. *Aging Male* **2012**, *15*, 187–197. [CrossRef] [PubMed]
4. McBride, J.A.; Carson, C.C.; Coward, R.M. Diagnosis and management of testosterone deficiency. *Asian. J. Androl.* **2015**, *17*, 177–186.
5. Bassil, N.; Alkaade, S.; Morley, J.E. The benefits and risks of testosterone replacement therapy: A review. *Ther. Clin. Risk Manag.* **2009**, *5*, 427–448.
6. Yoshimura, N.; Muraki, S.; Oka, H.; Kawaguchi, H.; Nakamura, K.; Akune, T. Cohort profile: Research on osteoarthritis/osteoporosis disability study. *Int. J. Epidemiol.* **2010**, *39*, 988–995. [CrossRef]
7. Melton, L.J.; Atkinson, E.J.; O'Connor, M.K.; O'Fallon, W.M.; Riggs, B.L. Bone density and fracture risk in men. *J. Bone Miner. Res.* **1998**, *13*, 1915–1923. [CrossRef]
8. Yamamoto, L. Guideline for treatment of osteoporosis. *Nippon Rinsho.* **2002**, *60*, 280–287.
9. van Staa, T.P.; Dennison, E.M.; Leufkens, H.G.; Cooper, C. Epidemiology of fractures in England and Wales. *Bone* **2001**, *29*, 517–522. [CrossRef]
10. Almeida, M.; Laurent, M.R.; Dubois, V.; Claessens, F.; O'Brien, C.A.; Bouillon, R.; Vanderschueren, D.; Manolagas, S.C. Estrogens and Androgens in Skeletal Physiology and Pathophysiology. *Physiol. Rev.* **2017**, *97*, 135–187. [CrossRef]
11. El Badri, S.A.; Salawu, A.; Brown, J.E. Bone Health in Men with Prostate Cancer: Review Article. *Curr. Osteoporos. Rep.* **2019**, *17*, 527–537. [CrossRef] [PubMed]
12. Mitsuzuka, K.; Arai, Y. Metabolic changes in patients with prostate cancer during androgen deprivation therapy. *Int. J. Urol.* **2018**, *25*, 45–53. [CrossRef] [PubMed]
13. Lassemillante, A.C.; Doi, S.A.; Hooper, J.D.; Prins, J.B.; Wright, O.R. Prevalence of osteoporosis in prostate cancer survivors: A meta-analysis. *Endocrine* **2014**, *45*, 370–381. [CrossRef] [PubMed]
14. Shahinian, V.B.; Kuo, Y.F.; Freeman, J.L.; Goodwin, J.S. Risk of fracture after androgen deprivation for prostate cancer. *N. Engl. J. Med.* **2005**, *352*, 154–164. [CrossRef] [PubMed]
15. Brahamsen, B.; Nielsen, M.F.; Esklldsen, P.; Andersen, J.T.; Walter, S.; Brixen, K. Fracture risk in Danish men with prostate cancer: A nationwide register study. *BJU Int.* **2007**, *100*, 749–754. [CrossRef]

16. Junjie, W.; Dongsheng, H.; Lei, S.; Hongzhuo, L.; Changying, S. Testosterone Replacement Therapy Has Limited Effect on Increasing Bone Mass Density in Older Men: A Meta-analysis. *Curr. Pharm. Des.* **2019**, *25*, 73–84. [CrossRef]
17. Mohamad, N.V.; Soelaiman, I.N.; Chin, K.Y. A concise review of testosterone and bone health. *Clin. Interv. Aging* **2016**, *11*, 1317–1324. [CrossRef]
18. Zhang, Z.; Kang, D.; Li, H. The effects of testosterone on bone health in males with testosterone deficiency: A systematic review and meta-analysis. *BMC Endocr. Disord.* **2020**, *20*, 33. [CrossRef]
19. Drake, M.T.; Murad, M.H.; Mauck, K.F.; Lane, M.A.; Undavalli, C.; Elraiyah, T.; Stuart, L.M.; Prasad, C.; Shahrour, A.; Mullan, R.J.; et al. Clinical review. Risk factors for low bone mass-related fractures in men: A systematic review and meta-analysis. *J. Clin. Endocrinol. Metab.* **2012**, *97*, 1861–1870. [CrossRef]
20. Isidori, A.M.; Giannetta, E.; Greco, E.A.; Gianfrilli, D.; Bonifacio, V.; Isidori, A.; Lenzi, A.; Fabbri, A. Effects of testosterone on body composition, bone metabolism and serum lipid profile in middle-aged men: A meta-analysis. *Clin. Endocrinol.* **2005**, *63*, 280–293. [CrossRef]
21. Tracz, M.J.; Sideras, K.; Boloña, E.R.; Haddad, R.M.; Kennedy, C.C.; Uraga, M.V.; Caples, S.M.; Erwin, P.J.; Montori, V.M. Testosterone use in men and its effects on bone health. A systematic review and meta-analysis of randomized placebo-controlled trials. *J. Clin. Endocrinol. Metab.* **2006**, *91*, 2011–2016. [CrossRef] [PubMed]
22. Kaufman, J.M.; Vermeulen, A. The decline of androgen levels in elderly men and its clinical and therapeutic implications. *Endocr. Rev.* **2005**, *26*, 833–876. [CrossRef] [PubMed]
23. Labrie, F.; Cusan, L.; Gomez, J.L.; Martel, C.; Bérubé, R.; Bélanger, P.; Bélanger, A.; Vandenput, L.; Mellström, D.; Ohlsson, C. Comparable amounts of sex steroids are made outside the gonads in men and women: Strong lesson for hormone therapy of prostate and breast cancer. *J. Steroid Biochem. Mol. Biol.* **2009**, *113*, 52–56. [CrossRef] [PubMed]
24. Imai, Y.; Kondoh, S.; Kouzmenko, A.; Kato, S. Minireview: Osteoprotective action of estrogens is mediated by osteoclastic estrogen receptor-alpha. *Mol. Endocrinol.* **2010**, *24*, 877–885. [CrossRef] [PubMed]
25. Chin, K.Y.; Ima-Nirwana, S. The effects of orchidectomy and supraphysiological testosterone administration on trabecular bone structure and gene expression in rats. *Aging Male* **2015**, *18*, 60–66. [CrossRef]
26. Li, X.; Ominsky, M.S.; Stolina, M.; Warmington, K.S.; Geng, Z.; Niu, Q.T.; Asuncion, F.J.; Tan, H.L.; Grisanti, M.; Dwyer, D.; et al. Increased RANK ligand in bone marrow of orchiectomized rats and prevention of their bone loss by the RANK ligand inhibitor osteoprotegerin. *Bone* **2009**, *45*, 669–676. [CrossRef]
27. Gill, R.K.; Turner, R.T.; Wronski, T.J.; Bell, N.H. Orchiectomy markedly reduces the concentration of the three isoforms of transforming growth factor beta in rat bone, and reduction is prevented by testosterone. *Endocrinology* **1998**, *139*, 546–550. [CrossRef]
28. Bellido, T.; Jilka, R.L.; Boyce, B.F.; Girasole, G.; Broxmeyer, H.; Dalrymple, S.A.; Murray, R.; Manolagas, S.C. Regulation of interleukin-6, osteoclastogenesis, and bone mass by androgens. The role of the androgen receptor. *J. Clin. Investig.* **1995**, *95*, 2886–2895. [CrossRef]
29. Chen, Q.; Kaji, H.; Kanatani, M.; Sugimoto, T.; Chihara, K. Testosterone increases osteoprotegerin mRNA expression in mouse osteoblast cells. *Horm. Metab. Res.* **2004**, *36*, 674–678. [CrossRef]
30. Kawano, H.; Sato, T.; Yamada, T.; Matsumoto, T.; Sekine, K.; Watanabe, T.; Nakamura, T.; Fukuda, T.; Yoshimura, K.; Yoshizawa, T.; et al. Suppressive function of androgen receptor in bone resorption. *Proc. Natl. Acad. Sci. USA* **2003**, *100*, 9416–9421. [CrossRef]
31. Smith, E.P.; Boyd, J.; Frank, G.R.; Takahashi, H.; Cohen, R.M.; Specker, B.; Williams, T.C.; Lubahn, D.B.; Korach, K.S. Estrogen resistance caused by a mutation in the estrogen-receptor gene in a man. *N. Engl. J. Med.* **1994**, *331*, 1056–1061. [CrossRef] [PubMed]
32. Morishima, A.; Grumbach, M.M.; Simpson, E.R.; Fisher, C.; Qin, K. Aromatase deficiency in male and female siblings caused by a novel mutation and the physiological role of estrogens. *J. Clin. Endocrinol. Metab.* **1995**, *80*, 3689–3698. [PubMed]
33. Bilezikian, J.P.; Morishima, A.; Bell, J.; Grumbach, M.M. Increased bone mass as a result of estrogen therapy in a man with aromatase deficiency. *N. Engl. J. Med.* **1998**, *339*, 599–603. [CrossRef] [PubMed]
34. Hughes, D.E.; Dai, A.; Tiffee, J.C.; Li, H.H.; Mundy, G.R.; Boyce, B.F. Estrogen promotes apoptosis of murine osteoclasts mediated by TGF-beta. *Nat. Med.* **1996**, *2*, 1132–1136. [CrossRef]
35. Raisz, L.G. Pathogenesis of osteoporosis: Concepts, conflicts, and prospects. *J. Clin. Investig.* **2005**, *115*, 3318–3325. [CrossRef]
36. Ding, K.H.; Wang, Z.Z.; Hamrick, W.M.; Deng, Z.B.; Zhou, L.; Kang, B.; Yan, S.L.; She, J.X.; Stern, D.M.; Isales, C.M.; et al. Disordered osteoclast formation in RAGE-deficient mouse establishes an essential role for RAGE in diabetes related bone loss. *Biochem. Biophys. Res. Commun.* **2006**, *340*, 1091–1097. [CrossRef]
37. Xie, J.; Méndez, J.D.; Méndez-Valenzuela, V.; Aguilar-Hernández, M.M. Cellular signaling of the receptor for advanced glycation end products (RAGE). *Cell Signal* **2013**, *25*, 2185–2197. [CrossRef]
38. Kimble, R.B.; Matayoshi, A.B.; Vannice, J.L.; Kung, V.T.; Williams, C.; Pacifici, R. Simultaneous block of interleukin-1 and tumor necrosis factor is required to completely prevent bone loss in the early postovariectomy period. *Endocrinology* **1995**, *136*, 3054–3061. [CrossRef]
39. Lorenzo, J.A.; Naprta, A.; Rao, Y.; Alander, C.; Glaccum, M.; Widmer, M.; Gronowicz, G.; Kalinowski, J.; Pilbeam, C.C. Mice lacking the type I interleukin-1 receptor do not lose bone mass after ovariectomy. *Endocrinology* **1998**, *139*, 3022–3025. [CrossRef]
40. Antonio, L.; Caerels, S.; Jardi, F.; Delaunay, E.; Vanderschueren, D. Testosterone replacement in congenital hypogonadotropic hypogonadism maintains bone density but has only limited osteoanabolic effects. *Andrology* **2019**, *7*, 302–306. [CrossRef]

41. Rochira, V.; Antonio, L.; Vanderschueren, D. EAA clinical guideline on management of bone health in the andrological outpatient clinic. *Andrology* **2018**, *6*, 272–285. [CrossRef] [PubMed]
42. Stanley, H.L.; Schmitt, B.P.; Poses, R.M.; Deiss, W.P. Does hypogonadism contribute to the occurrence of a minimal trauma hip fracture in elderly men? *J. Am. Geriatr. Soc.* **1991**, *39*, 766–771. [CrossRef] [PubMed]
43. Baillie, S.P.; Davison, C.E.; Johnson, F.J.; Francis, R.M. Pathogenesis of vertebral crush fractures in men. *Age Ageing* **1992**, *21*, 139–141. [CrossRef]
44. Kelepouris, N.; Harper, K.D.; Gannon, F.; Kaplan, F.S.; Haddad, J.G. Severe osteoporosis in men. *Ann. Intern. Med.* **1995**, *123*, 452–460. [CrossRef] [PubMed]
45. Fink, H.A.; Ewing, S.K.; Ensrud, K.E.; Barrett-Connor, E.; Taylor, B.C.; Cauley, J.A.; Orwoll, E.S. Association of testosterone and estradiol deficiency with osteoporosis and rapid bone loss in older men. *J. Clin. Endocrinol. Metab.* **2006**, *91*, 3908–3915. [CrossRef]
46. Ryan, C.S.; Petkov, V.I.; Adler, R.A. Osteoporosis in men: The value of laboratory testing. *Osteoporos. Int.* **2011**, *22*, 1845–1853. [CrossRef]
47. Kotwal, N.; Upreti, V.; Nachankar, A.; Hari Kumar, K.V.S. A prospective, observational study of osteoporosis in men. *Indian J. Endocrinol. Metab.* **2018**, *22*, 62–66.
48. Liu, Z.Y.; Yang, Y.; Wen, C.Y.; Rong, L.M. Serum Osteocalcin and Testosterone Concentrations in Adult Males with or without Primary Osteoporosis: A Meta-Analysis. *Biomed Res. Int.* **2017**, *2017*, 9892048. [CrossRef]
49. Greendale, G.A.; Edelstein, S.; Barrett-Connor, E. Endogenous sex steroids and bone mineral density in older women and men: The Rancho Bernardo Study. *J. Bone Miner. Res.* **1997**, *12*, 1833–1843. [CrossRef]
50. Amin, S.; Zhang, Y.; Sawin, C.T.; Evans, S.R.; Hannan, M.T.; Kiel, D.P.; Wilson, P.W.; Felson, D.T. Association of hypogonadism and estradiol levels with bone mineral density in elderly men from the Framingham study. *Ann. Intern. Med.* **2000**, *133*, 951–963. [CrossRef]
51. Mellström, D.; Johnell, O.; Ljunggren, O.; Eriksson, A.L.; Lorentzon, M.; Mallmin, H.; Holmberg, A.; Redlund-Johnell, I.; Orwoll, E.; Ohlsson, C. Free Testosterone is an Independent Predictor of BMD and Prevalent Fractures in Elderly Men: MrOS Sweden. *J. Bone Miner. Res.* **2006**, *21*, 529–535. [CrossRef] [PubMed]
52. Bjørnerem, A.; Emaus, N.; Berntsen, G.K.; Joakimsen, R.M.; Fønnebø, V.; Wilsgaard, T.; Oian, P.; Seeman, E.; Straume, B. Circulating sex steroids, sex hormone-binding globulin, and longitudinal changes in forearm bone mineral density in postmenopausal women and men: The Tromsø study. *Calcif. Tissue Int.* **2007**, *81*, 65–72. [CrossRef] [PubMed]
53. Kuchuk, N.O.; van Schoor, N.M.; Pluijm, S.M.; Smit, J.H.; de Ronde, W.; Lips, P. The association of sex hormone levels with quantitative ultrasound, bone mineral density, bone turnover and osteoporotic fractures in older men and women. *Clin. Endocrinol. (Oxford)* **2007**, *67*, 295–303. [CrossRef] [PubMed]
54. LeBlanc, E.S.; Nielson, C.M.; Marshall, L.M.; Lapidus, J.A.; Barrett-Connor, E.; Ensrud, K.E.; Hoffman, A.R.; Laughlin, G.; Ohlsson, C.; Orwoll, E.S.; et al. The effects of serum testosterone, estradiol, and sex hormone binding globulin levels on fracture risk in older men. *J. Clin. Endocrinol. Metab.* **2009**, *94*, 3337–3346. [CrossRef]
55. Vanderschueren, D.; Pye, S.R.; Venken, K.; Borghs, H.; Gaytant, J.; Huhtaniemi, I.T.; Adams, J.E.; Ward, K.A.; Bartfai, G.; Casanueva, F.F.; et al. EMAS Study Group. Gonadal sex steroid status and bone health in middle-aged and elderly European men. *Osteoporos. Int.* **2010**, *21*, 1331–1339. [CrossRef]
56. Cauley, J.A.; Ewing, S.K.; Taylor, B.C.; Fink, H.A.; Ensrud, K.E.; Bauer, D.C.; Barrett-Connor, E.; Marshall, L.; Orwoll, E.S.; Osteoporotic Fractures in Men Study (MrOS) Research Group. Sex steroid hormones in older men: Longitudinal associations with 4.5-year change in hip bone mineral density–the osteoporotic fractures in men study. *J. Clin. Endocrinol. Metab.* **2010**, *95*, 4314–4323. [CrossRef]
57. Woo, J.; Kwok, T.; Leung, J.C.; Ohlsson, C.; Vandenput, L.; Leung, P.C. Sex steroids and bone health in older Chinese men. *Osteoporos. Int.* **2012**, *23*, 1553–1562. [CrossRef]
58. Hsu, B.; Seibel, M.J.; Cumming, R.G.; Blyth, F.M.; Naganathan, V.; Bleicher, K.; Le Couteur, D.G.; Waite, L.M.; Handelsman, D.J. Progressive temporal change in serum SHBG, but not in serum testosterone or estradiol, is associated with bone loss and incident fractures in older men: The concord health and ageing in men project. *J. Bone Miner. Res.* **2016**, *31*, 2115–2122. [CrossRef]
59. Gennari, L. Aromatase activity and bone homeostasis in men. *J. Clin. Endocrinol. Metab.* **2004**, *89*, 5898–5907. [CrossRef]
60. Catalano, A.; Gaudio, A.; Agostino, R.M.; Morabito, N.; Bellone, F.; Lasco, A. Trabecular bone score and quantitative ultrasound measurements in the assessment of bone health in breast cancer survivors assuming aromatase inhibitors. *J. Endocrinol. Investig.* **2019**, *42*, 1337–1343. [CrossRef]
61. Zitzmann, M.; Brune, M.; Vieth, V.; Nieschlag, E. Monitoring bone density in hypogonadal men by quantitative phalangeal ultrasound. *Bone* **2002**, *31*, 422–429. [CrossRef]
62. Burnett-Bowie, S.-A.M.; McKay, E.A.; Lee, H.; Leder, B.Z. Effects of aromatase inhibition on bone mineral density and bone turnover in older men with low testosterone levels. *J. Clin. Endocrinol. Metab.* **2009**, *94*, 4785–4792. [CrossRef] [PubMed]
63. Vandenput, L.; Labrie, F.; Mellström, D.; Swanson, C.; Knutsson, T.; Peeker, R.; Ljunggren, O.; Orwoll, E.; Eriksson, A.L.; Damber, J.E.; et al. Serum Levels of Specific Glucuronidated Androgen Metabolites Predict BMD and Prostate Volume in Elderly Men. *J. Bone Miner. Res.* **2007**, *22*, 220–227. [CrossRef] [PubMed]
64. Wong, R.M.Y.; Wong, H.; Zhang, N.; Chow, S.K.H.; Chau, W.W.; Wang, J.; Chim, Y.N.; Leung, K.S.; Cheung, W.H. The relationship between sarcopenia and fragility fracture-a systematic review. *Osteoporos. Int.* **2019**, *30*, 541–553. [CrossRef]

65. Tarantino, U.; Piccirilli, E.; Fantini, M.; Baldi, J.; Gasbarra, E.; Bei, R. Sarcopenia and fragility fractures: Molecular and clinical evidence of the bone-muscle interaction. *J. Bone Jt. Surg. Am.* **2015**, *97*, 429–437. [CrossRef]
66. Szulc, P.; Claustrat, B.; Marchand, F.; Delmas, P.D. Increased risk of falls and increased bone resorption in elderly men with partial androgen deficiency: The MINOS study. *J. Clin. Endocrinol. Metab.* **2003**, *88*, 5240–5247. [CrossRef]
67. Kenny, A.M.; Prestwood, K.M.; Marcello, K.M.; Raisz, L.G. Determinants of bone density in healthy older men with low testosterone levels. *J. Gerontol. A Biol. Sci. Med. Sci.* **2000**, *55*, M492–M497. [CrossRef]
68. Tuck, S.P.; Scane, A.C.; Fraser, W.D.; Diver, M.J.; Eastell, R.; Francis, R.M. Sex steroids and bone turnover markers in men with symptomatic vertebral fractures. *Bone* **2008**, *43*, 999–1005. [CrossRef]
69. Mellstrom, D.; Vandenput, L.; Mallmin, H.; Holmberg, A.H.; Lorentzon, M.; Odén, A.; Johansson, H.; Orwoll, E.S.; Labrie, F.; Karlsson, M.K.; et al. Older men with low serum estradiol and high serum SHBG have an increased risk of fractures. *J. Bone Miner. Res.* **2008**, *23*, 1552–1560. [CrossRef]
70. Meier, C.; Nguyen, T.V.; Handelsman, D.J.; Schindler, C.; Kushnir, M.M.; Rockwood, A.L.; Meikle, A.W.; Center, J.R.; Eisman, J.A.; Seibel, M.J. Endogenous sex hormones and incident fracture risk in older men: The Dubbo Osteoporosis Epidemiology Study. *Arch. Intern. Med.* **2008**, *168*, 47–54. [CrossRef]
71. Roddam, A.W.; Appleby, P.; Neale, R.; Dowsett, M.; Folkerd, E.; Tipper, S.; Allen, N.E.; Key, T.J. Association between endogenous plasma hormone concentrations and fracture risk in men and women: The EPIC-Oxford prospective cohort study. *J. Bone Miner. Metab.* **2009**, *27*, 485–493. [CrossRef] [PubMed]
72. Risto, O.; Hammar, E.; Hammar, K.; Fredrikson, M.; Hammar, M.; Wahlström, O. Elderly men with a history of distal radius fracture have significantly lower calcaneal bone density and free androgen index than age-matched controls. *Aging Male* **2012**, *15*, 59–62. [CrossRef] [PubMed]
73. Torremadé-Barreda, J.; Rodríguez-Tolrà, J.; Román-Romera, I.; Padró-Miquel, A.; Rius-Moreno, J.; Franco-Miranda, E. Testosterone-deficiency as a risk factor for hip fracture in elderly men. *Actas Urol. Esp.* **2013**, *37*, 142–146. [CrossRef]
74. Tran, T.S.; Center, J.R.; Seibel, M.J.; Eisman, J.A.; Kushnir, M.M.; Rockwood, A.L.; Nguyen, T.V. Relationship between Serum Testosterone and Fracture Risk in Men: A Comparison of RIA and LC-MS/MS. *Clin. Chem.* **2015**, *61*, 1182–1190. [CrossRef] [PubMed]
75. Vandenput, L.; Ohlsson, C. Estrogens as regulators of bone health in men. *Nat. Rev. Endocrinol.* **2009**, *5*, 437–443. [CrossRef] [PubMed]
76. Kenny, A.M.; Kleppinger, A.; Annis, K.; Rathier, M.; Browner, B.; Judge, J.O.; McGee, D. Effects of transdermal testosterone on bone and muscle in older men with low bioavailable testosterone levels, low bone mass, and physical frailty. *J. Am. Geriatr. Soc.* **2010**, *58*, 1134–1143. [CrossRef]
77. Aversa, A.; Bruzziches, R.; Francomano, D.; Greco, E.A.; Fornari, R.; Di Luigi, L.; Lenzi, A.; Migliaccio, S. Effects of long-acting testosterone undecanoate on bone mineral density in middle-aged men with late-onset hypogonadism and metabolic syndrome: Results from a 36 months controlled study. *Aging Male* **2012**, *15*, 96–102. [CrossRef]
78. Wang, Y.J.; Zhan, J.K.; Huang, W.; Wang, Y.; Liu, Y.; Wang, S.; Tan, P.; Tang, Z.Y.; Liu, Y.S. Effects of low-dose testosterone undecanoate treatment on bone mineral density and bone turnover markers in elderly male osteoporosis with low serum testosterone. *Int. J. Endocrinol.* **2013**, *2013*, 570413. [CrossRef]
79. Bouloux, P.M.; Legros, J.J.; Elbers, J.M.; Geurts, T.B.; Kaspers, M.J.; Meehan, A.G.; Meuleman, E.J.; Study 43203 Investigators. Effects of oral testosterone undecanoate therapy on bone mineral density and body composition in 322 aging men with symptomatic testosterone deficiency: A 1 year, a randomized, placebo-controlled, dose-ranging study. *Aging Male* **2013**, *16*, 38–47. [CrossRef]
80. Rodriguez-Tolrà, J.; Torremadé, J.; di Gregorio, S.; Del Rio, L.; Franco, E. Effects of testosterone treatment on bone mineral density in men with testosterone deficiency syndrome. *Andrology* **2013**, *1*, 570–575. [CrossRef]
81. Permpongkosol, S.; Khupulsup, K.; Leelaphiwat, S.; Pavavattananusorn, S.; Thongpradit, S.; Petchthong, T. Effects of 8-year treatment of long-acting testosterone undecanoate on metabolic parameters, urinary symptoms, bone mineral density, and sexual function in men with late-onset hypogonadism. *J. Sex. Med.* **2016**, *13*, 1199–1211. [CrossRef] [PubMed]
82. Rogol, A.D.; Tkachenko, N.; Bryson, N. Natesto™, a novel testosterone nasal gel, normalizes androgen levels in hypogonadal men. *Andrology* **2016**, *4*, 46–54. [CrossRef] [PubMed]
83. Shigehara, K.; Konaka, H.; Koh, E.; Nakashima, K.; Iijima, M.; Nohara, T.; Izumi, K.; Kitagawa, Y.; Kadono, Y.; Sugimoto, K.; et al. Effects of testosterone replacement therapy on hypogonadal men with osteopenia or osteoporosis: A subanalysis of a prospective randomized controlled study in Japan (EARTH study). *Aging Male* **2017**, *20*, 139–145. [CrossRef] [PubMed]
84. Snyder, P.J.; Kopperdahl, D.L.; Stephens-Shields, A.J.; Ellenberg, S.S.; Cauley, J.A.; Ensrud, K.E.; Lewis, C.E.; Barrett-Connor, E.; Schwartz, A.V.; Lee, D.C.; et al. Effect of Testosterone Treatment on Volumetric Bone Density and Strength in Older Men With Low Testosterone: A Controlled Clinical Trial. *JAMA Intern. Med.* **2017**, *177*, 471–479. [CrossRef]
85. Permpongkosol, S.; Tantirangsee, N.; Ratana-olarn, K. Treatment of 161 men with symptomatic late onset hypogonadism with long-acting parenteral testosterone undecanoate: Effects on body composition, lipids, and psychosexual complaints. *J. Sex. Med.* **2010**, *7*, 3765–3774. [CrossRef]
86. Konaka, H.; Sugimoto, K.; Orikasa, H.; Iwamoto, T.; Takamura, T.; Takeda, Y.; Shigehara, K.; Iijima, M.; Koh, E.; Namiki, M.; et al. Effects of long-term androgen replacement therapy on the physical and mental statuses of aging males with late-onset hypogonadism: A multicenter randomized controlled trial in Japan (EARTH Study). *Asian J. Androl.* **2016**, *18*, 25–34. [CrossRef] [PubMed]

87. Ng Tang Fui, M.; Hoermann, R.; Nolan, B.; Clarke, M.; Zajac, J.D.; Grossmann, M. Effect of testosterone treatment on bone remodelling markers and mineral density in obese dieting men in a randomized clinical trial. *Sci. Rep.* **2018**, *8*, 9099. [CrossRef]
88. Bhasin, S.; Cunningham, G.R.; Hayes, F.J.; Matsumoto, A.M.; Snyder, P.J.; Swerdloff, R.S.; Montori, V.M. Testosterone therapy in men with androgen deficiency syndromes: An Endocrine Society clinical practice guideline. *J. Clin. Endocrinol. Metab.* **2010**, *95*, 2536–2559. [CrossRef]
89. Watts, N.B.; Adler, R.A.; Bilezikian, J.P.; Drake, M.T.; Eastell, R.; Orwoll, E.S.; Finkelstein, J.S. Osteoporosis in men: An Endocrine Society clinical practice guideline. *J. Clin. Endocrinol. Metab.* **2012**, *97*, 1802–1822. [CrossRef] [PubMed]
90. Vescini, F.; Attanasio, R.; Balestrieri, A.; Bandeira, F.; Bonadonna, S.; Camozzi, V.; Cassibba, S.; Cesareo, R.; Chiodini, I.; Francucci, C.M.; et al. Italian association of clinical endocrinologists (AME) position statement: Drug therapy of osteoporosis. *J. Endocrinol. Investig.* **2016**, *39*, 807–834. [CrossRef] [PubMed]
91. Hoppé, E.; Bouvard, B.; Royer, M.; Chappard, D.; Audran, M.; Legrand, E. Is androgen therapy indicated in men with osteoporosis? *Jt. Bone Spine* **2013**, *80*, 459–465. [CrossRef] [PubMed]
92. Gallagher, J.C.; Fowler, S.E.; Detter, J.R.; Sherman, S.S. Combination treatment with estrogen and calcitriol in the prevention of age-related bone loss. *J. Clin. Endocrinol. Metab.* **2001**, *86*, 3618–3628. [CrossRef]
93. Smith, M.R.; Eastham, J.; Gleason, D.M.; Shasha, D.; Tchekmedyian, S.; Zinner, N. Randomized controlled trial of zoledronic acid to prevent bone loss in men receiving androgen deprivation therapy for nonmetastatic prostate cancer. *J. Urol.* **2003**, *169*, 2008–2012. [CrossRef] [PubMed]
94. Smith, M.R.; Egerdie, B.; Hernández Toriz, N.; Feldman, R.; Tammela, T.L.; Saad, F.; Heracek, J.; Szwedowski, M.; Ke, C.; Kupic, A.; et al. Denosumab in men receiving androgen-deprivation therapy for prostate cancer. *N. Engl. J. Med.* **2009**, *361*, 745–755. [CrossRef] [PubMed]
95. Morabito, N.; Gaudio, A.; Lasco, A.; Catalano, A.; Atteritano, M.; Trifiletti, A.; Anastasi, G.; Melloni, D.; Frisina, N. Neridronate prevents bone loss in patients receiving androgen deprivation therapy for prostate cancer. *J. Bone Miner. Res.* **2004**, *19*, 1766–1770. [CrossRef]

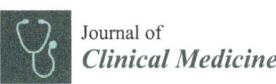

Review

Advances in Osteoporotic Bone Tissue Engineering

Cosmin Iulian Codrea [1,2], Alexa-Maria Croitoru [1], Cosmin Constantin Baciu [3], Alina Melinescu [1,*], Denisa Ficai [4], Victor Fruth [2] and Anton Ficai [1,5]

1. Department of Science and Engineering of Oxide Materials and Nanomaterials, Faculty of Applied Chemistry and Materials Science, University POLITEHNICA of Bucharest, 060042 Bucharest, Romania; codrea.cosmin@yahoo.com (C.I.C.); croitoru.alexa@yahoo.com (A.-M.C.); anton.ficai@upb.ro (A.F.)
2. Department of Oxide Compounds and Materials Science, Institute of Physical Chemistry "Ilie Murgulescu" of the Romanian Academy, 060021 Bucharest, Romania; vfruth@gmail.com
3. Anaesthesia Intensive Care Unit (AICU/ATI), Department of Orthopedics, University of Medicine and Pharmacy "Carol Davila", 020021 Bucharest, Romania; cosminbaciu@hotmail.com
4. Department of Inorganic Chemistry, Physical Chemistry and Electrochemistry, Faculty of Applied Chemistry and Materials Science, University POLITEHNICA of Bucharest, 060042 Bucharest, Romania; denisaficai@yahoo.ro
5. Academy of Romanian Scientists, 050094 Bucharest, Romania
* Correspondence: alina.melinescu@gmail.com

Abstract: The increase in osteoporotic fracture worldwide is urging bone tissue engineering research to find new, improved solutions both for the biomaterials used in designing bone scaffolds and the anti-osteoporotic agents capable of promoting bone regeneration. This review aims to report on the latest advances in biomaterials by discussing the types of biomaterials and their properties, with a special emphasis on polymer-ceramic composites. The use of hydroxyapatite in combination with natural/synthetic polymers can take advantage of each of their components properties and has a great potential in bone tissue engineering, in general. A comparison between the benefits and potential limitations of different scaffold fabrication methods lead to a raised awareness of the challenges research face in dealing with osteoporotic fracture. Advances in 3D printing techniques are providing the ways to manufacture improved, complex, and specialized 3D scaffolds, capable of delivering therapeutic factors directly at the osteoporotic skeletal defect site with predefined rate which is essential in order to optimize the osteointegration/healing rate. Among these factors, strontium has the potential to increase osseointegration, osteogenesis, and healing rate. Strontium ranelate as well as other biological active agents are known to be effective in treating osteoporosis due to both anti-resorptive and anabolic properties but has adverse effects that can be reduced/avoided by local release from biomaterials. In this manner, incorporation of these agents in polymer-ceramic composites bone scaffolds can have significant clinical applications for the recovery of fractured osteoporotic bones limiting or removing the risks associated with systemic administration.

Keywords: bone; biomaterial scaffolds; 3D printing; osteoporosis; strontium ranelate

1. Introduction

Bone grafting is a common surgical method used to improve bone regeneration in orthopedic practice. In the case of considerable diminution of bone mass, bone grafts are essential because the self-healing process would be slow or the could entirely fail [1]. At an estimated total of 2,000,000 bone graft procedures carried out every year, bone repair frameworks remain a promising line of research because of the continuously growing request for it and the reduced stock of bone substitutes [1,2]. Bone tissue engineering aims at delivering novel methods for treating bone tissue deficiencies often resulting from polytrauma, pathological fractures, and osteonecrosis [2] as there is an increasing need to provide functional replacement grafts for the patients [3].

Progresses in medicine have raised both life expectancy globally and age-connected illnesses liable for declining life quality of the elderly [4], with one of the most common and wide-spread skeletal disease being osteoporosis [5], with an increase in osteoporotic fracture in both genders with age [6]. Each year, almost 200,000,000 patients are confirmed as osteoporotic and around 9,000,000 osteoporotic fractures happen globally [5], with a rising number of elderlies being prone to fragility fractures [7]. Bone lesions are difficult for the elderly and can lead to morbidity and substantial socioeconomic costs creating a demand for new and efficient regenerative strategies and better results for patients [4] as the incidence of osteoporosis is predicted to further rise worldwide [5]. This emphasizes the importance and value of preclinical bone repair frameworks capable to transfer into suitable clinical use even more [2].

Bone tissues display inherent regrowth and self-repair features to some extent, but the capacity of the injured bones for the natural process of healing and restore load-bearing function is often insufficient, resulting in fracture nonunion [2]. Larger defects, referred to as critical-size defects, demand clinical interventions in order for the bone to repair or regenerate itself [8]. The ways in which large bone injuries are treated consist of autografts, allografts, and scaffolds [1,4] but currently none of them are adequate because of their specific limitations for instance reduced bioactivity, possible pathogens spreading, inflammation, supplementary surgery, restricted supply, unfit shape and size, and donor site related morbidity [4].

This review reports on the latest advances in biomaterials containing biologically active agents used for their ability to enable osteointegration and osteogenesis in osteoporotic skeletal defect sites. The loco-regional delivery is especially useful because they can assure the desired level of these agents at the bone level, to assure a higher bioavailability and thus to minimize the probability of implant rejection and faster osteointegration and healing. Most of these drug delivery systems are designed to be used as grafting materials to restore the normal ratio between resorption and bone formation and to counteract the effects of osteoporosis.

2. Bone Tissue

Bones are living organs constantly modeling and remodeling throughout life and serve as reservoir for calcium, phosphate and many other bodily elements, thereby, assuring their homeostasis [9]. Bone consists of an organic matrix, mineral components, and water, as presented in Figure 1. The bulk part of the organic matrix consists of type I collagen, but other non-collagenous proteins are also present, mainly extracellular and a small part within the cells [10]. Bone composition, by weight, is approximately 65% mineral (mostly as hydroxyapatite (85%), but also calcium carbonate and calcium fluoride [9]), organic part is approximately 20% to 25%, mostly type I collagen (about 90%) [10], while the water content varies between 10% and 20% depending on several factors including age, species, bone health, etc. [11].

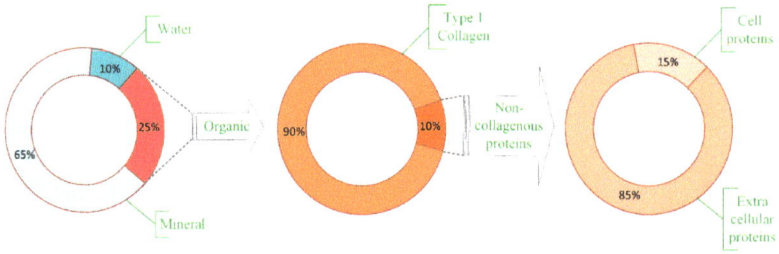

Figure 1. Bone composition. Realized based on [10].

Bone tissue can assume a compact (cortical bone) or trabecular (cancellous bone) structure [12], but indifferently, all experience remodeling throughout life associated with bone resorption, a process performed by osteoclasts subsequent bone formation through the action of osteoblasts [5].

Cortical bone consists of a dense matrix constructed by recurrent osteon units with collagen fibers assembled in a concentric manner around a central canal containing blood vessels [13]. This structure formed by collagen fibers is oriented along with the directions of the loading lines, greatly confirmed with the piezoelectric assistance involved in bone formation [14]. It forms a dense outer shell [9] consisting of well-organized lamellae of hierarchical structures [5] and provides torsion, bending resistance, and compressive strength [9]. They possess remarkable strength but lower capacity to bear loads beyond the elastic deformation range in contrast to trabecular (cancellous) bone, consisting in unparallel fibrillar units of variable porosity (ranging between 50–90%) [5].

Cancellous (trabecular) bone is found in the porous interior [9], possesses a network of interlinked trabeculae containing marrow, organized in a hierarchical manner extended between solid material, trabeculae, lamellae, and collagen-hydroxyapatite composite and having disorganized collagen network [13]. The trabeculae exhibit considerable surface area in which nutrients diffusion and growth factors circulation is easily done, allowing, thus, cancellous bone to play a metabolically active role and permit a more persistent remodeling compared to cortical bone [9]. The mechanical capacity of cancellous bone derives to a great extent from its bone mineral density (BMD), while the stiffness of cortical bone derives to a great extent from its porosity [5].

Bone tissue is distinct due to its capacity to heal free of scar tissue, which determines an unscarred full restoration of bone tissue integrity [15]. Fractured bone repair itself by repeating various steps of endochondral and intramembranous bone formation and healing is devoid of scar tissue. Development of hematoma implies inflammation at the injured site and the action of signaling molecules involved in regulating new bone development (interleukins, tumor necrosis factor-a, fibroblast growth factors, platelet-derived growth factor, vascular endothelial growth factor (VEGF), bone morphogenetic proteins (BMPs), etc.) [9]. Inflammatory cells (macrophages, monocytes, lymphocytes, and polymorphonuclear cells) and fibroblasts infiltrate bone tissue in a process mediated by prostaglandins [11]. Throughout fracture repair, mesenchymal stem cells (MSCs) from the bone marrow are engage at the fracture site in interaction with the local cells influencing the healing efficacy [7]. The emergence of intramembranous bone starts right away at the cortical tissue and periosteum. Later, the fracture stabilization occurs through the action of the outer soft tissues through callus formation. Afterwards, chondrocyte proliferation happens. Ingrowing of blood vessels starts to bring chondroclasts to the site, which reabsorb calcified cartilage, and osteoblastic progenitors, which launch new bone tissue formation [9]. The recruitment of osteoblast on the surface and the emergence of new bone tissue are moreover promoted by the modifications in the ionic dynamics of the microenvironment [16]. Mechanical continuity of the cortical bone tissue is reached through later remodeling of recently formed bone. If the needed regeneration of bone starts due to damage or disease, hematoma building and a quick inflammatory response occurs as a way to facilitate host cell attraction and the discharge of decisive signaling molecules [9]. Hematoma building and inflammation process starts bone healing, which further elapses via the major stages of anti-inflammatory signaling, revascularization, soft callus development, its mineralization and remodeling in the end, macrophages playing an essential role in the process [15], influencing, thus, the success or failure of a bone implant [17]. Macrophages control cell migration to the injured site through the cytokines and growth factors they produce (tumor necrosis factor-a, IL-1, IL-6, IL-8, IL-12, TGF-b, platelet-derived growth factor, and insulin-like growth factor-1), and have effect on cell proliferation, collagen synthesis and angiogenesis [18]. Monocytes, neutrophils, and natural killer cells are also present in the affected site [19]. Inflammatory markers are the following cytokines: TNF-α, IL-1β and iNOS [20]. Osteogenesis, osteoclastogenesis, and angiogenesis are greatly regulated by immune cells and their signaling molecules [21].

Initial inflammatory action is necessary to start the bone healing process but persistent inflammatory action against the implant usually leads to granulation (formation of connective tissue) and formation of a fibrotic capsule around the implant with undesirable results [20] or increased healing time [22].

Bone tissue extracellular matrix is formed out of a non-mineralized organic constituent, largely type-1 collagen with numerous post-translational modifications, but also non-collagenous proteins particularly involved in improved fusion between the mineral crystals and the organic matter [5], and a mineralized inorganic constituent (made up of carbonated apatite mineral particles in the form of 4-nm-thick plates) [8,12]. The nano-composite structure (collagen fibers reinforced by hydroxyapatite) is necessary for compressive strength and toughness towards fracture [12], thus, bearing an impact without cracking [5]. The toughness and flexibility of the collagen fibers adjust bone ductility.

The metaphyseal component of bone is largely made up of cancellous tissue, which is metabolically more active compared to cortical tissue. As a consequence of this attribute, osteoporosis can impact its mass and structural integrity at a higher rate [23], mainly because diffusion is much higher as surface to volume ratio is superior in contrast to the cortical one.

Healing rates are age dependent, as in young people fractures usually heal about the weight-bearing level in approximately six weeks, and about complete mechanical integrity level after approximately one year, and in the elderly individuals the healing rates can be much lower [24]. In pathological or large fractures and defects, the processes of healing and repair can be unsuccessful, due to deficient blood delivery, bone cells or bone forming minerals, but also due to infection in the bone or its adjacent tissues, and systemic affections causing delay or even lack of union [25]. Important factors that affect the process of bone tissue healing are also mechanical stability, proportions of the affected site, severity and incidence of adjacent tissue injuries [11].

After implantation of bone scaffolds in the body, injured blood vessels quickly lead to protein adsorption on scaffold surface and formation of fibrin-rich clot with the role of a transitory surface matrix at the tissue-scaffold interface occurs. It emits various pro-inflammatory cytokines and chemokines, triggering the mobilization of inflammatory and osteoprogenitor cells towards the infixed scaffold. The scaffold is recognized as a foreign body by the immune system, inducing specific immune reactions. The scaffold active regulates the kind and extent of immune system reactions during bone regeneration [17]. To counteract chronic inflammatory action against implants, anti-inflammatory factors such as corticosteroids and prostaglandins were investigated but adverse effects such as hepatotoxicity, cardiotoxicity, and immunological impairment in long-term use were reported. Extended inflammation may cause fibrosis, granuloma formation and further encapsulation and failure of the implant [20].

3. Bone Healing and Types of Bone Grafts

Bone grafts are made of biomaterial implanted in order to assist healing alone or with the aid of other materials, because of the expected properties of osteogenesis, osteoinduction, and osteoconduction either alone or combined [25]. Bone grafts are especially needed if a larger bone lost is recorded. It is worth to mention that in fact, only the need of blood is higher than the need of bone grafts. It is also important to mention that synthetic bone grafts have some advantages against autografts, and this is why many synthetic grafts are studied worldwide [26].

Autografts are obtained by taking bone from another part of the patient's own body [11] and still serves as a point of reference to which other grafts may be compared [1,8,11,27] because of their histocompatibility, absence of immunogenic reactions and all other properties demanded of a bone graft material, respectively osteoinduction (growth factors to drive the regeneration process, i.e., bone morphogenetic proteins), osteogenesis (i.e., osteoprogenitor cells, functionally active osteoblastic cells to produce new bone matrix) and osteoconduction (i.e., three-dimensional, porous matrix) [2,12]. Autografts integrate into the host bone faster [1] and are the most effective method for bone regeneration [11], unfortunately donor site morbidity is a problematic consideration [3,8].

Important health risks such as major vessel or visceral injuries during harvesting are also among the limitations in using autografts [25].

Allografts consist of taking bone from the donor and has a lower rate of incorporation within the bone [11]. They are linked to risks of immune reactions and infection carrying, have low osteoinductive capacity and have no bone cells, since donor grafts are devitalized and processed through irradiation or freeze-drying [12]. The handicap of restricted donor supply and the need for immunosuppressive therapy [3] and batch to batch variation [28] add to the ones previously mentioned.

Xenografts are derived from species other than the recipient, are osteoconductive, relatively inexpensive, do not lengthen the healing time, and the need for a second surgical site for bone harvesting is eliminated [29]. They carry a rare risk of transmission of zoonotic diseases [25], causing an immune reaction, and are unable to gain adequate height and width for large defects [29]. Remains of bovine bone from xenografts can still be unresorbed even after three years as some histological analyses have proved. They are osteoconductive rather than osteoinductive [30] and are considered to be more liable to rejection, even in an aggressive manner [25].

Biomaterial scaffolds (engineered scaffolds) address the limits of autografts, allografts and xenografts. Novel approaches offered by tissue engineering have been conducted with the aim to create grafts for repairing and regenerating damaged tissues [4] through the use of a provisional biomaterial scaffold at the injured site in order to stimulate healing and ensure certain recovery of functionality [3] and harness bone innate regenerative capacity, as bone has a natural potential to repair, remodel, and regenerate itself [24].

Scaffolds need to be engineered with features that provide cells with signals for regeneration in order to cancel the need for extended in vitro culture anterior to implantation. Hence, considerable efforts are committed to advance biomimetic biomaterials to a more complex stage, making them able to incorporate multi-functionality and possess bioinstructive and stimuli-responsive properties [24].

Scaffolds should possess cytocompatibility and imitate biochemical and mechanical properties of the veritable bone, furthering similar biological functions in order to prevail limitations such as donor deficit, immunogenic reaction, and infection carrying, with the main strategies considering the admixture of cells, biologically active molecules, and impermanent 3D fine-tuned porous design [4]. Degradation capability is necessary to integrate the scaffold and should progress at a rate capable of maintaining mechanical support in implantation sites. Apart of that, it plays a critical role in not only in ensuring the means for metabolite diffusion and the development of new blood vessels, but also in releasing the agents loaded into the biomaterial [3]. Scaffolds enable osteogenic cells adhesion of and provide a suitable microenvironment for them in order to secrete osteoid, the matrix of recently formed tissue and deliver signaling molecules to the bone regeneration space (osteoconduction) [2].

4. Biomaterial Scaffolds

Scaffold development usually starts by choosing the scaffold material [3] as chemical composition of the biomaterial plays an essential part in the favorable outcome of the process [9,12]. We distinguish three classes of scaffolds in line with their material composition: metals, polymers, and bio-ceramics, but they may consist also of a combination of these three material types as composites [2,9,27]. Common materials used and approved, such as stainless steel, poly(lactic-co-glycolic acid), and hydroxyapatite can be appealing as they are already safely used as components in existing products [3]. However, they still have their disadvantages such as the necessity for several surgical intervention, stress shielding, wear particle osteolysis [28] and no potential for drug delivery in the case of biocompatible metals and their alloys [16] and inferior mechanical properties that limit its use in load bearing bone parts in the case of bioactive glasses [28]. A further classification is made by considering the origin of the material (natural or synthetic) and its degradation potential under physiologic conditions (resorbable versus non-resorbable) [2].

Other characteristics to take into account is the heterogeneousness of the scaffold, that bone is biologically and biomechanically variable, the ease to handle it as a one-step procedure, its ability to reach suitable mechanical properties in order to bear the load of normal movements, and its ability to allow vascularization in order to obtain a normal bone structure [11], which can thus prevent the scaffold to undergo ischemia and cell death [25].

Scaffold material aims to support the viability of the adequate cell category and simultaneously operate as a nonpermanent replacement of the bone extracellular matrix, as a substitute matrix that will preferably be displaced by newly functional bone tissue [31], while reproducing the properties of normal bone tissue formation [9]. Scaffolds designed to aid regeneration need to encourage migration, cell adhesion, proliferation, and differentiation [8] and ideally some essential features and functions should be certainly considered: architecture, cytocompatibility, bioactivity, biodegradability, and mechanical characteristics [9].

Material characteristics, such as biomaterial porosity and its surface properties, for instance nano/micro topography, play a decisive role in osteoinduction [9,12] and the expected histogenesis [31]. The architectural features consider a controlled porous microstructure and high porous interconnectivity, a controlled degradation rate, mechanical stability, and osteoconductive properties [8]. In addition, for an effective interaction between scaffolds and the cellular component, other design parameters are necessarily acknowledged, such as surface properties, permeability, geometric properties, and mechanical strength, all of which influence nutrients and oxygen transport throughout the scaffolds [32] and influence cell-material interactions [33] controlling, thus, bone regeneration.

Host reactions to the implanted scaffold are greatly influenced by the physical (Figure 2) and chemical properties of the scaffold and design strategies should consider and evaluate this impact [17].

The ability of cells to penetrate, proliferate and differentiate are greatly influenced by pore size, distribution and scaffold geometry, and also the rate of scaffold degradation [34].

Porosity: interconnection between pores promotes the loading of cells into biomaterials due to large internal surface area, which ensures attachment and spreading sites. Because the biomaterial is designed as an open network structure, diffusion of oxygen, metabolites, and growth factors is possible, thus, enabling cells viability and proliferation, and the space needed for the deposition of proteins secreted by the cells. Porosity of the bone tissue facilitate the penetration of host cells and the growth of blood vessels that provide the means to feed the emerging tissue [31]. This microstructure permits the ingrowth of cells, which lead to tissue regeneration. Uniform cell seeding and nutrient exchange are dependent on the interconnectivity of pores [8]. By raising the available surface inside a pore to which cells can adhere on the implant, known as the specific surface area (SSA), a quicker growth of hydroxyapatite appears and thus bone bonding will be more quickly as well [35].

Scaffold architecture needs to consider, in order to assure well-adjusted biological and physical properties of scaffolds, the following key parameters: total porosity, pore morphology, distribution, and size [34]. Given the size of the bone cells of about 20 to 35 µm, materials with a porosity of about 50 to 150 µm seem to be the optimal for bone grafting because, in this case, the bone cells can easily penetrate inside, and can assure an in depth osteointegration of these synthetic grafts. If the pore size increases, it means that the mechanical properties decrease and also the time requested for the feeling of these pores with new bone increase, which overall means a slower healing and a higher risk of secondary failure [36–38].

Interaction between cells and scaffolds is done mostly through the chemical groups (ligands) present on the biomaterial surface. Using materials found naturally in the extracellular matrix (e.g., collagen) have the advantage of initially possessing ligands in the scaffold shaped as Arg-Gly-Asp (RGD) binding sequences, in contrast with synthetic materials, which may need a planned addition of ligands via, for example, protein adsorption. Ligand density is influenced by the specific surface area which is conditional on the mean pore size in the implanted scaffold. Cells migrate into the scaffold if the pores are sufficiently large for them to penetrate, but pores need to be sufficiently small to reach a satisfactory specific surface, with a ligand density high enough to permit adherence of a substantial number of cells to ligands within the scaffold [24].

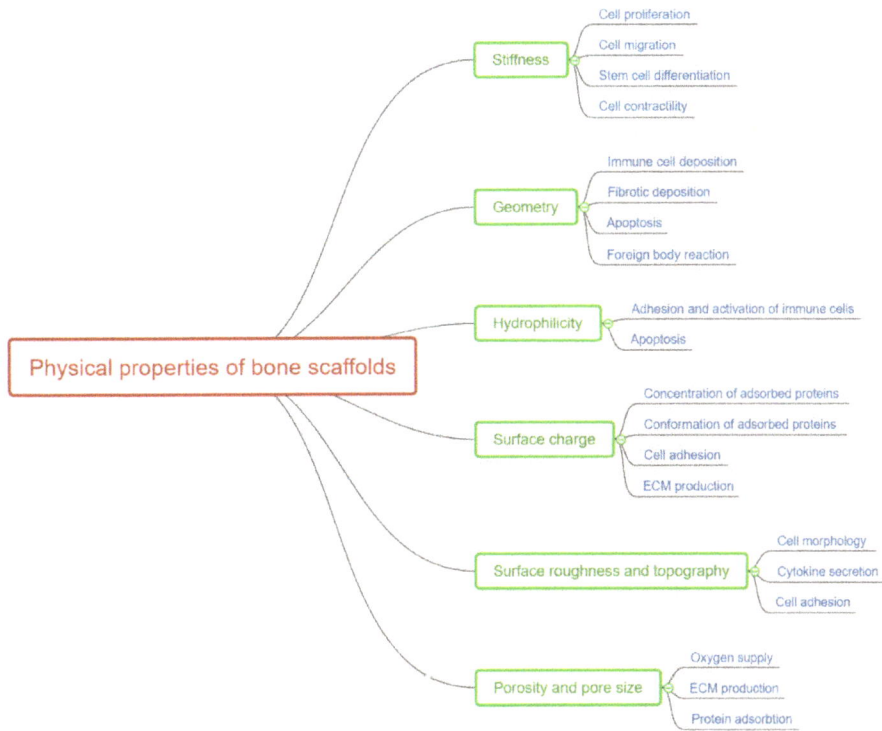

Figure 2. Physical properties of bone scaffolds and their effects on host and bone regeneration. Realized based on [17].

Macroporous scaffolds (ranging between 100 and 600 μm) permit superior integration in the host bone, further angiogenesis, and bone distribution. A higher pore size determines an enhancement in permeability, which leads to better bone ingrowth, while small pores have better results for soft tissue ingrowth [34]. For tissue ingrowth, a minimum pore size about 50 μm is necessary [4] while, in most cases, surpassing a pore size limit of 150 μm determines the abrupt decrease of mechanical properties. It is also important to mention that pore size and porosity play an important role in drug delivery, as will be later discussed. Porosity can influence the scaffolds' ability to induce new blood vessel formation [19].

To create pores or increase porosity of biomaterials used in scaffolds, the following methods are used: freeze-drying, salt leaching, gas foaming, controlled air drying, the use of additional polymers, electrospinning, and inclusion of degradable hydrogel microparticles [31,39,40]. Research is still ongoing regarding whether uniform pore distribution and similar size is a better choice than scaffolds designed with irregular pore size distribution [34]. In 3D printing, two kind of pores can be developed, one induced by printing larger pores, which are larger than the intrinsic porosity of the strands and are essential in a faster cell penetration deep inside the graft. The strands can also have pores suitable for the penetration of the osteoblasts or, at least, to assure the attachment of these cells on the scaffold [41].

Degradation: chronic foreign body responses generate complications for non-degradable biomaterials, so the ideal scaffold is ultimately replaced by new native bone tissues [31] as scaffolds are not intended to be perpetual implants [32].

Degradation rates depend not just on the chemical composition, but also on pore morphology, although this factor is less significant but should still receive attention in some cases [42]. The degradation rate of the implanted construct is an essential factor in its success. Material degradation should be in accordance to tissue synthesis to ensure appropriate mechanical stability in the course of bone tissue hystogenesis. The required residence time of the scaffold is specific to every tissue and need to be sufficient for cells to populate the scaffold appropriately and produce an enduring bone extracellular matrix. If a scaffold degrades faster than enough production of bone extracellular matrix can happen, cells will lose key physiochemical factors for bone tissue regeneration and repair, leading to scar formation. If residence time is prolonged, bone extracellular matrix production and cell proliferation will be suppressed [31].

Degradation rates are supposed by design to match the rate of new tissue development and maturation after transplantation in vivo [34]. The structure and microenvironment of scaffolds should ensure an increase in cell population, particularly for osteoblasts, which have bone-forming properties [43], leading to differentiation of precursor cells into osteoblasts and being supportive towards osteoblasts regenerative actions [8].

The key considerations for designing a scaffold or determining its effectiveness are as seen also in Figure 3 [24]:

1. Biocompatibility: it must trigger a reduced immune reaction to hinder it from causing a severe inflammatory response that might reduce healing or cause rejection by the body. Cells must adhere, function normally, and migrate onto the surface and eventually through the scaffold and begin to proliferate before laying down new matrix.
2. Biodegradability: it must degrade while new tissue is forming, and cells deposit their extracellular matrix. Secondary degradation products must be of low or absent toxicity and able to exit the body easily.
3. Mechanical properties: it should possess enough mechanical integrity to operate from implantation to the completion of the remodeling process. A balance between mechanical properties and enough porous architecture to allow cell infiltration and vascularization is essential.
4. Scaffold architecture: It should possess a structure of interconnected pores with high porosity to ensure cellular penetration and adequate diffusion of nutrients to cells within the construct and to the extra-cellular matrix formed by these cells. A porous interconnected structure is also required to allow diffusion of waste products out of the scaffold, and the products of scaffold degradation should be able to exit the body without interference with other organs and surrounding tissues. A critical range of pore sizes exists, for any scaffold, which may vary depending on the cell type used and tissue being engineered.
5. Manufacturing technology: It must be financially profitable and feasible to scale-up from research laboratory production to batch production, and thus be clinically and commercially viable. The progress to scalable production needs to comply with good manufacturing practice (GMP) standards for ensuring successful translation to the clinic and determining the way in which the scaffolds will be delivered and made available to the clinician.
6. Delivery capability: It is essential to mention that delivery capability through the releasing biological active agents can induce important properties such as faster healing [44,45], antimicrobial [46–48], and antitumoral activity [49,50].
7. "In depth" osteointegration: This requirement is strongly correlated with the pore size and porosity but also with the nature of the biomaterial. Bone grafting went through progressive improvement from the use of first-generation bone grafts (metals and alloys, i.e., titanium and its alloys, stainless steel, Co–Cr alloys) to second-generation

bone grafts (ceramics and polymers, i.e., calcium phosphates, Al_2O_3, ZrO_2; collagen, gelatin, chitosan, chitin, alginate, PLLA, PLGA), third-generation bone grafts (acellular composites or nanocomposites) and fourth-generation bone grafts (composites or nanocomposites containing cells or derived). The fifth generation in bone grafting is assumed to be "material design", the additive manufacturing methods, along with some classical ones, being used in generating desired morphology to assure deep cell penetration inside the graft as well as to allow a controlled delivery of the biological active agents' activity [50].

Plenty of material types have displayed osteoinductive properties, including natural and synthetic ceramics, especially calcium phosphate-based materials in various forms [9,12]. There is evidence for the osteoinductivity of calcium phosphate-based materials namely in the form of cements, coatings, sintered ceramics, and coral-derived ceramics in numerous animal models, while other ceramics, such as bioglass and alumina ceramic, have been lately confirmed to be osteoconductive [12].

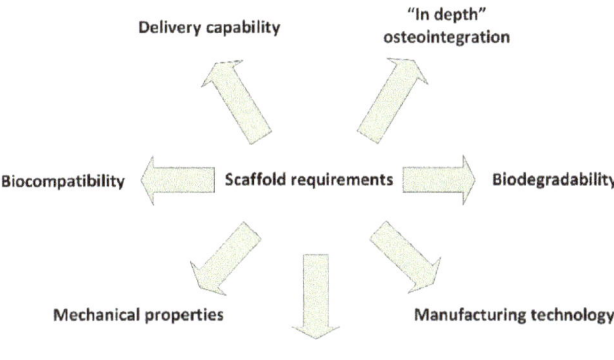

Figure 3. The key considerations for designing a scaffold or determining its effectiveness. Realized based on [24].

Biomaterials effectiveness is assessed in animal metaphyseal osteoporotic models, the ones of critical size being the most clinically relevant ones, as healing occur only with the aid of a graft [51]. In clinical practice, unlike standardized animal models, every fracture is distinct [22]. As clinical studies regarding biomaterials are scarce, due to their classification as medical devices and the strict safety regulations derived from this, clinical data is insufficient to assess performance and research is ongoing [52].

Bioceramics are the basis for porous scaffolds (e.g., bone regeneration), solid scaffolds (e.g., reconstruction of ear ossicles), and powders (e.g., bone filling). Considering the way they interact with the host, bioceramics are classified into resorbable (e.g., some calcium phosphates, calcium sulphate, etc.), bioactive (e.g., bioactive glass), and nearly inert (e.g., zirconia). Bioactive and resorbable ceramics, are considered promising regenerative biomaterials and have been subject of clinical trials [4].

Calcium phosphates ceramics have high potential for bone regeneration applications, due to their injectability, bioactivity, biocompatibility, and ability to deliver stem cells, growth factors and drugs, including anti-resorptive (anti-osteoporotic) drugs [53]. Calcium phosphates have a crystalline structure and chemical composition resembling bone minerals. The widely used hydroxyapatite (HA), having the chemical formula ($Ca_{10}[PO_4]_6[OH]_2$), has a hexagonal structure [27], similar to apatite, the main mineral found in bone, but a low resorption rate [4], being thermodynamically stable at physiological pH and less soluble among other calcium phosphates [35]. HA scaffolds are well-known for being biocompatible, osteoconductive, and osteoinductive and other calcium phosphates, with faster resorption rates, such as β-tricalcium phosphate, have been studied as well [4].

Calcium phosphate scaffolds show the capacity to promote osteogenesis and osteointegration, due to their surface charge, and, also, their chemistry and topography [4]. HA coated implants are proven to promote osteointegration capacity of inert metals [7] but some pioneering works were reported related to COLL/HA composite deposition by using MAPLE [54]. Due to its high biocompatibility, bioactivity, osteoconductive and/or osteoinductive capacity (in certain conditions), nontoxicity, nonimmunogenic properties, and noninflammatory behavior, HA is available and used as a bone filler and as coatings on prostheses, [4].

Calcium phosphate cements also have applicability in osteoporotic fractures in the form of bone void fillers. HA is highly osteoconductive but has no natural osteoinductive capacity and incorporation of cells, growth factors, and also of various ionic substitutions into the crystal lattice such as Mg, Zn, F, Cl, Si, Sr, may prove to be beneficial [7]. The in vivo evaluation of scaffolds, loaded with growth factors and without them, indicated superior new bone development in previous variant compared to the other [4]. Therefore, a more efficient HA scaffold for osteoporotic applications can be made by the addition of bone regulatory agents/biologics with osteogenic and anti-resorptive capacities [7]. There is evidence that the body's hard tissues contain substituting ions such as strontium (Sr) and fluorine (F) and incorporating them into HA can lead to improved material properties such as crystallinity and dissolution rate in physiological conditions [55] and various ions (Ca, Sr, Mg, Co, Cu, and Zn) can influence the implant generated immune response through the effect on immune cells and their cytokine releasing activity [21]. Bone formation is dependent on the extracellular microenvironment and its calcium ion gradient, both influenced by implant proprieties. Calcium ions dynamic and their concentration affect the recruitment and differentiation of mesenchymal stem cells (MSCs). Calcium phosphates ceramic adsorb firmly proteins from bodily fluids which further affect cell behavior and osteogenesis [56].

Natural marine sources for calcium phosphates are fish bones, seashells, corals, and algae. Phylum Porifera (Sponges) and Phylum Cnidaria (Corals) attracted attention due to their skeleton composed of bioceramics of which HA has been obtained. In addition, eggshells are an easily obtained, low-cost source for this material since they are considered food waste and calcium phosphates can be readily obtained by treating with phosphate, calcination and milling [4].

Synthetic HA can be obtained by different methods, as seen in Figure 4. Parameters such as temperature, pH, reaction time, and concentration of reagents during synthesis can affect the properties of the obtained HA [4].

As the biological HA is formed from plate-like crystals with nanoscale thickness, it is considered that nanoparticles of synthetic HA such as bone apatite is the adequate choice to utilize for bone substitution and regeneration. Particle diminution to nano-size level may hinder demineralization. Nanoscale HA have advanced densification and sintering properties as a result of its increased surface energy preventing micro-cracks. Improved surface functional features in HA nanoparticles, compared to micro-size particles, may determine superior cell proliferation and differentiation [55].

However, the drawbacks for this material are still the brittleness, their high deformation rates [19] and lack a fine-tuning biodegrading capacity [4].

Natural polymers are expected to be suitable biomaterial scaffolds for bone tissue engineering, the most common being collagen/gelatin, chitosan, alginate, silk, hyaluronic acid, and peptides [9], the benefits being their capacity to resorb in vivo and their natural biocompatibility and reduced adverse immunological effects [2].

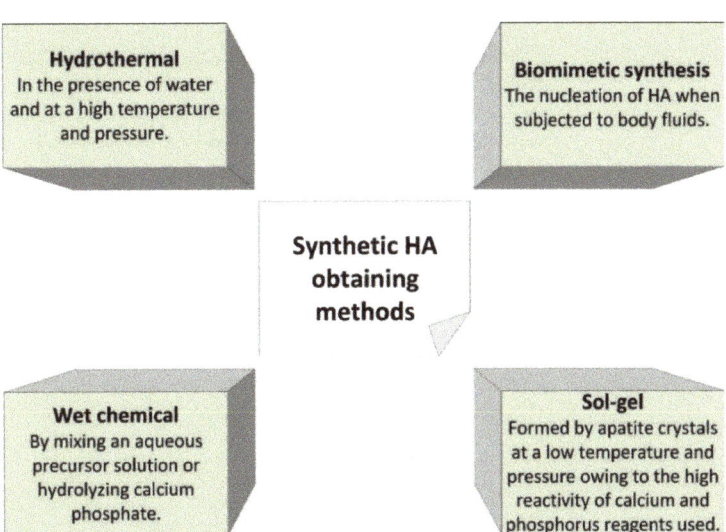

Figure 4. Synthetic HA obtaining methods. Realized based on [4].

Synthetic polymers widely used for tissue engineering are aliphatic polyesters such as polyglycolic acid, polylactic acid, and polycaprolactone [9] and their copolymers [57]. Synthetic polymers scaffolds possess the advantages of versatile fabrication with a broad range of degradation rates and mechanical properties in contrast with natural polymers due to their composition, the copolymer ratio, and the interactions of their polymeric side chains. The options regarding chemical composition and 3D configuration can influence its cell adhesion capacity to incorporate and deliver bioactive molecules in a controlled manner [2]. They are used for scaffolds due to their good biocompatibility and suitability as drug delivery materials for desired molecules in tissue regeneration [31]. These polymers are already used in orthopedic applications for low mechanically loaded implantable devices such as screws and plates for fixing fractured bone fragments, but widespread use is still limited by their low mechanical performances [58].

PGA is highly hydrophilic, and its mechanical strength weakens in two to four weeks after implantation. PLA is more hydrophobic, and degradation can take from months to years after implantation. The degradation rates of these materials can be customized by copolymer blends (PLGA) utilization. Acid-catalyzed hydrolysis and large erosion of these scaffolds is a drawback, which can lead to structural instability and even stopped regeneration [31]. The PLGA scaffolds degradation rate varies, as the ones with wider pore size and reduced porosity degrade faster compared to those with reduced pore size and increased porosity due to higher surface area in the scaffolds with higher pore size, which increase the diffusion of acidic degradation products during the incubation period and lead to accentuated acid-catalyzed hydrolysis [42].

Long-term exposure to PLGA acidic by-products upon degradation may cause tissue necrosis and implant failure. An array of polyphosphazenes has been incorporated in PLGA scaffolds, in order to control degradation rates and create more efficient scaffolds. Polyphosphazenes have nontoxic and neutral pH or basic products upon degradation and can be fine-tuned according to the degradation rates aimed [9]. pH is an important factor to take in account as the calcium phosphate precipitates start appearing with a rise in the pH and the sequential cross linkage of collagen chains depends on pH for bone regeneration [35]. The majority of polymer materials do not have osteoconductive properties and can lead to stress relaxation behavior and creep [16]. Figure 5 present some of the most important biomaterials used in bone tissue engineering: metals and alloys, polymers, and ceramics, but also derived composite materials.

Polymer-ceramic composites represent attractive options for bone substitution and regeneration as it is hard for a single category of biomaterial to fulfill all the requirements of artificial bone scaffolds [27] and fully replicate the properties of bone [59]. Composites take advantage of each of its constituents, organic and inorganic (i.e., biodegradable polymer and ceramic materials), and prove to be more successfully strategy than the separate use of these materials [12]. In fact, this approach is a biomimetic approach which compositionally mimic the nature of the bone, which is also a polymer-ceramic composite material.

Scaffolds fabricated from polymer-ceramic composites biomaterials possess the higher biocompatibility and biodegradability of organic materials and the higher mechanical properties and biological activity of inorganic materials [27]. Because natural bone structure is, indeed, that of a composite biomaterial with an inorganic component—HA crystals and an organic component—collagen fibers [12], the combination of those two components for scaffold material can reproduce the chemical composition of the genuine bone extracellular matrix [27]. Evaluation of scaffolds is generally devised through evaluation of cellular interactions, the scaffold microstructure and mechanical properties [4].

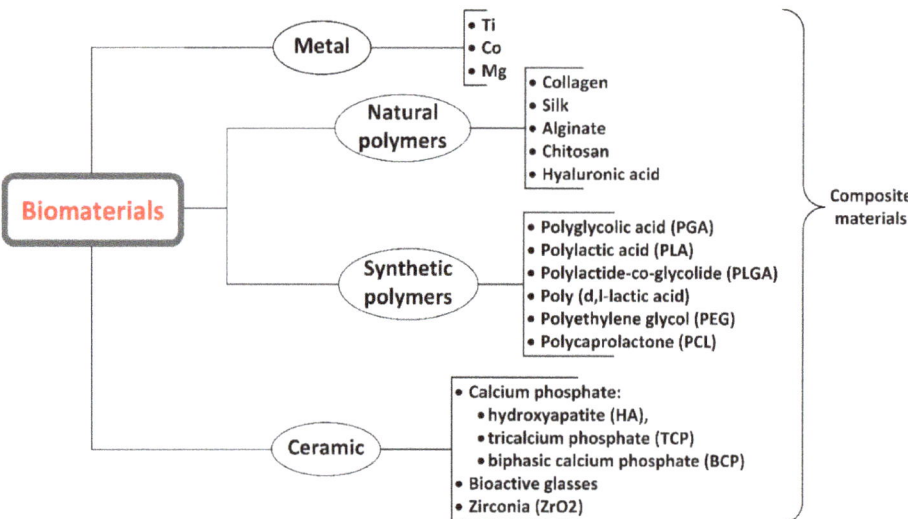

Figure 5. Different biomaterials for bone defect treatment. Realized based on [19,59].

The scaffold microstructure (e.g., pore size, shape, and interconnectivity) allows cell migration, nutrient and waste interchange, angiogenesis, and bone ingrowth and mechanical features ensure the formation of bone tissue after implantation while maintaining its structural integrity [4,9], while porous structures improve mechanical performance [4]. The mechanism of bone fixation is through the deposition of a surface layer of apatite, a process known as bioactivity of biomaterials [60]. This deposition arises from the merging of calcium derived from the bioactive material matrix or the biological fluids and phosphate present in the biological fluids [35]. Physiological fluids such as blood are supersaturated with these ions, but the deposition of the apatite layer is not happening on every surface. In vitro physicochemical analyses showed quite the opposite as faster deposition of apatite layer occurs on more reactive surfaces [16].

Polymer-HA composites containing PLA, PLGA, collagen, gelatin, and chitosan have been realized and proved to be osteoinductive, enhancing bone development in vitro and/or in vivo [12] and ectopically [9]. Combining HA and natural polymer has been proved to enhance mechanical properties and bioactivity of scaffolds in contrast to simple polymer scaffolds and to increase hydrophilicity, in case of PLLA-matrix [58], and potentially reduces adverse effects resulting from degradation of various synthetic polymers, [12] thus making polymer-ceramic composite biomaterial the most promising option for bone scaffolds [27].

A scaffold combining collagen, calcium phosphate, and HA, showed higher mechanical strength compared to scaffolds fabricated only from calcium phosphate, with proper biocompatibility, increased osteoinductivity and bone formation in vivo compared with calcium phosphate scaffolds and collagen-calcium phosphate scaffolds [4]. HA is one of the most promising fillers for the reinforcement of PLLA due to its high hardness and Young's modulus [58].

These biomimetic materials are capable of simulating the formation, precipitation and deposition of apatite from simulated body fluid (SBF), leading to increased bone-matrix interface strength through better osteoblastic cell survival, proliferation and expression of bone-specific markers (i.e., bone sialoprotein and osteocalcin) [12].

Surface modification and functionalization of scaffolds with biologically active molecules can increase the effectiveness of bone regeneration. A specific molecule (i.e., peptide) chosen to initiate attachment of cells and their proliferation or directly their differentiation, can be deposited on scaffold surface or integrated within [8].

To overcome the challenge caused by the relatively low compatibility at the interface between bioceramic and biopolymer, the use of coupling agents has been proposed in the form of a chemical moderating agent with two different functional groups, the first being able to react with polymer molecules, while the second being able to adsorb with the ceramic surface to create a strong bond. There is substantial difference in chemical and physical properties between the two phases, which results in poor bonding strength. Interface interaction are important in determining mechanical properties that need more consideration, as research focused mainly on the reinforcement effect that bioceramics have on biopolymer matrix. The use of a coupling agent can enhance the efficiency of interfacial stress transfer between the two components, thereby improving the mechanical properties of the composite scaffold [27].

As a result of the different properties of bioceramic and biopolymer, it is improbable for bioceramics to disperse equally in the organic component and their low compatibility and interface bonding strength may lead to shrinking and deformation of the polymer on the ceramic surface and cause micro-cracks at their interface throughout processing, further leading to depreciated mechanical properties. After transplantation into the human body of a composite scaffold, the interface layer between the two components is rapidly damaged, and the ceramic is separated soon from the matrix, causing decreased mechanical property in the preliminary usage stage, unsuitable for a successful repairing process. In order to construct a successful bioceramic/biopolymer composite and use it as a bone scaffold is necessary to improve adhesion at the bioceramic and biopolymer interface [27].

5. Material Design by 3D Printing Technology

An innovative area of research concerning scaffold designing and fabrication is the use of additive manufacturing technologies (3D printing) [8] which guides the path in developing 3D structures trough cutting edge methods utilizing various biomaterials [61]. Advances in this field of research are providing the methods to produce complex and highly specialized 3D structures [31] serving as templates in providing a suitable environment for bone tissue regeneration [9]. This is why additive manufacturing techniques open new opportunities and there are premises to consider a fifth revolution in bone grafting materials due to the advanced "materials design". Three-dimensional (3D) printing is realized through adding materials to obtain scaffolds using 3D model data, layer-by-layer, in contrast to subtractive manufacturing methods [62]. These methods have a great flexibility in producing scaffolds of different structural complexity [2]. A concise comparison between different scaffold fabrication methods can be seen in Figure 6.

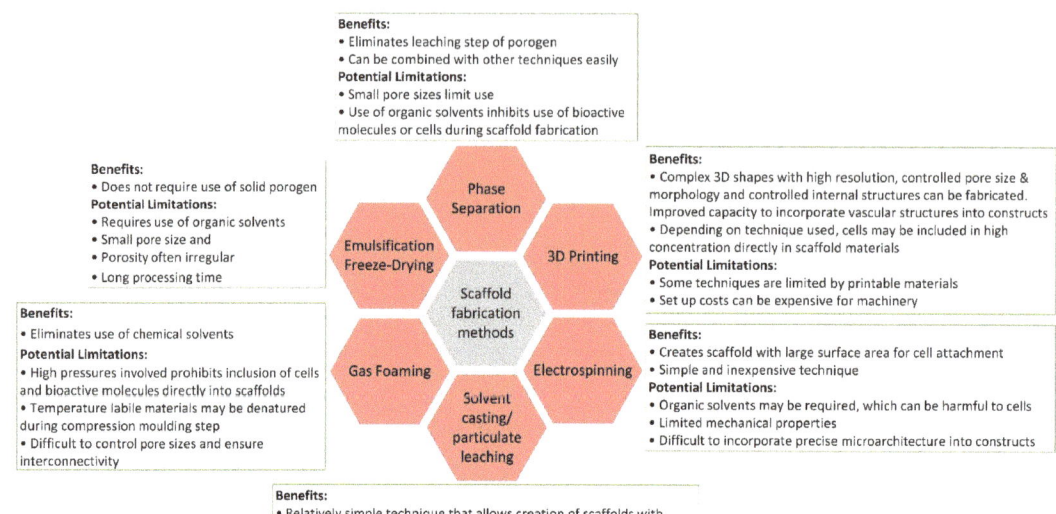

Figure 6. Benefits and potential limitations of different scaffold fabrication methods. Realized based on [59].

The 3D printed scaffolds are advantageous because of their customized shape, porosity/pore size, and mechanical characteristics [62]. This high customization permits a high control regarding the scaffold architecture, flexibility in scaling up fabrication, technically precise reproducibility—which is not always the case in subtractive fabrication techniques [2]—and a precise morphology [4]. The usage of 3D printing for bone tissue engineering possesses an essential advantage, such as the increased spatial control over the deposition of cells and materials that permits design control of complex tissue interfaces [13]. The capacity to precisely shape mechanical and biological properties, and degradation kinetics is linked with control of the scaffold architecture. Additionally, these methods allow the development of dimensionally precise prototypes of bone [4]. The development of 3D printing through computer-aided design (CAD) modelling further increases manufacturing precision and repeatability of scaffolds, and highly controlled porosity at both micro and macro levels [59]. Relevant to mention, is that the macroporosity is important in allowing for a fast cell penetration, fast bone ingrowth, but also in allowing vascularization oxygen and nutrients exchange, etc., while the microporosity is essential in designing the release profile, for instance.

Fused deposition modeling (FDM) 3D printing technology allows printing with polymer and polymer-based composite filaments by extrusion with a resolution of up to 200 microns. Such high printing precision allows designing and manufacturing with high accuracy personified highly porous scaffolds possessing an interconnected system of open pores, thus prompting osteointegration of scaffold [58].

Suitable polyesters for 3D printing of polymer scaffolds, possessing biodegradable and biocompatible properties, like poly(L-lactic acid) (PLLA), poly(vinyl alcohol) (PVA), poly-β-hydroxybutyrate (PHB), polyurethane elastomers, poly(3- hydroxybutyrate-co-3-hydroxyvalerate) (PHBV), poly(D,L-lactic acid) (PDLLA), poly(lactic-co-glycolic acid) (PLGA) and polycaprolactone (PCL) and polyurethanes, can be processed into wires, pellets and powders with the help of high temperature melting-extrusion and sintering, or by dissolution in organic/aqueous solvents to allow micro extrusion-based 3D printing at room/low temperature [62].

Microporous PLGA scaffolds were produced through rapid printing technique by precisely directing solvent streams onto polymer granules or by drilling with dies of a specific size. Reproducibility precision of these cylindrical scaffolds went to millimeter dimensions and the materials supported in vivo bone regeneration in defect models [31]. Due to its properties of thermoplasticity and extremely low thermal shrinkage, 3D printing technologies have also become widespread in PLLA molding [58].

Scaffolds obtained by 3D printing techniques represent an efficient approach for providing local delivery and sustained release of drugs, by mixing them with the synthetic/natural polymer solution, which can be 3D printed into scaffolds [62].

3D methods have precise control over scaffold microarchitecture and spatial content. Together with the wide variety of available bioactive materials, growth factors, functionalization techniques and biomimetic designs, increases the possibility to create complex scaffolds fine-tuned to individual needs, offering chances of treatment to difficult conditions, such as osteonecorosis, critical defects, and osteoporosis [59].

3D printing is a complex process with multiple engineering aspects to consider, due to the material type and 3D structure fabrication method when choosing the most suitable for specific damage or defect [61] and due to facing competition from injectable scaffolds in the form of hydrogels, micro or nanospheres [8]. In certain situations, when direct printing is problematic, such as for instance for the direct printing of the COLL/HA composite gel, the use of a precursor gel based on collagen and calcium hydroxide can be used and the printed microstructured patterns are simultaneously cross-linked with glutaraldehyde and calcium hydroxide are transformed into hydroxyapatite, both processes occurring as a consequence of dipping them into glutaraldehyde solution in phosphate buffer saline or SBF [41].

The following challenges are expected to be overcome in the near future [62]:

1. Imitating exactly the structure of natural bone tissue, as the majority of extrusion-based 3D printed structures have a reduced printing resolution and are capable of imitating the hierarchical structure at a rather reduced level. Superior micro-extrusion nozzle is expected to be capable of producing considerably higher resolution scaffolds;
2. Enabling the manufacturing of customized structures with complex characteristics, adapted to the heterogeneousness and gradient mechanical properties of defected bone tissue;
3. Controlled delivery of angiogenic factors and development of vascular-like duct in the structures are necessary to allow enhanced vascularization able to transport sufficient oxygen/nutrient to the regeneration site;
4. Obtaining both scaffold fabrication and cell incorporation concomitant, as 3D printed scaffolds loaded with cells are considered more effective in healing bone conditions, compared to recruiting host cells into scaffolds after implantation. Subsequent adhesion of cells on scaffolds in vivo usually induces variable cell distribution and low cell density, compared to in situ incorporation of cells through 3D printing, which is preferable. Besides 3D bioprinting, which fabricates cell-loaded hydrogel structure, no other 3D printing technique can sustain cell incorporation during the process;
5. Incorporating anti-bacterial or anti-cancer capabilities in order to treat infection/bone tumor resection-induced defects.

All these challenges can be considered part of the fifth generation of materials which will be obtained by "material design" and developed by using additive manufacturing.

6. Drug Delivery

Scaffolds made from biomaterials loaded with biologically active therapeutic agents (ions, vitamins, drugs) may become the preferable manner in which delivery of these agents at the defect site is realized in order to promote healing and integration [7]. Scaffolds act as reservoirs for delivery of bioactive agents including ions, such as, especially Ca^{2+}, Zn^{2+}, PO_4^{3-}; peptides and proteins, vitamins, genes but even cells and nanoparticles [3], aiding functional restoration of the fractured bone or to treat different diseases, especially infections, osteoporosis, or cancer [7] and their loco-regional delivery in order to minimize side effects at systemic level [41]. In case of osteoporotic fractures, convenient local drug delivery approaches are implant coatings, injectable bone cements and gels, while scaffolds are preferred for large bone defects [22]. The use of these biological active agents is especially welcome, as seen in Figure 7, because they can replace the normal bone resorption/formation ratio by enhancing the formation rate. Figure 7a represents the evolution of bone mass, highlighting the active growth period (formation rate (F) > resorption rate (R)) while, after 25 to 30 years the bone mass usually slightly starts to decrease, and this decrease will be more important after 45 years, especially if this is overlapping with menopause. Once the mass loss is starting, an important imbalance appears between formation and resorption and, in the case of fractures, the healing process will be significantly affected, and the bone density will be lower compared to normal, healthy bone tissue. Figure 7b schematically highlights the influence of the use of biological active agents in the healing of the osteoporotic, fractured bone. Therefore, especially in the case of fractures associated with osteoporosis, the healing could be slow, and the mechanical performances of these regions will be inferior and subsequently, secondary fractures can appear.

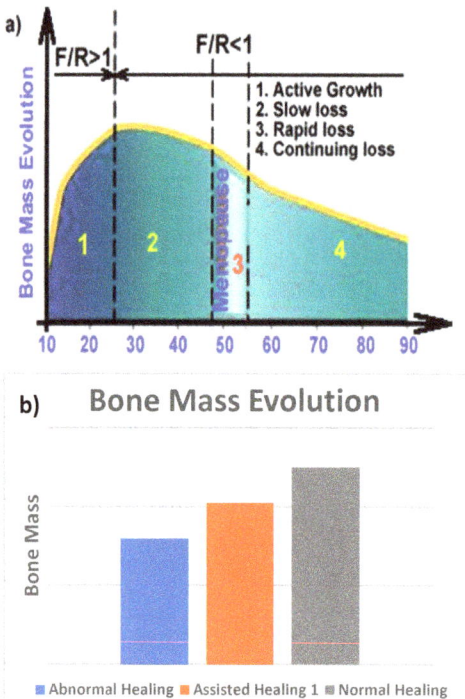

Figure 7. (a) Bone mass evolution during life; (b) bone mass evolution in normal versus assisted healing of bone defects.

The incorporation of several types of ions in the chemical composition of the scaffold is proved to promote the osteoconductivity of CPC [53]. HA can be an outstanding drug delivery carrier for numerous therapeutic agents as a result of its high stability, bioactivity, biocompatibility, and lack of toxicity [63]. In addition, biodegradable polymers have wide usage as drug delivery systems due to their biodegradability and biocompatibility, and, among them, aliphatic polyester (PLA), proteins (collagen, gelatin) or polysaccharides (alginate, chitosan) have the ability to extend the releasing of drugs from some days till some months [57,64–66].

The absence of an exothermic effect in the setting reaction and the natural porosity of CPCs permit the incorporation of therapeutic agents with reduced risk of thermal denaturalization and possible activity loss during preparation or implantation. Incorporation of drugs is realized by simply mixing it with one of the solid or liquid cement components. Drugs can also be added by adsorption onto the scaffold or incorporated into polymeric microfibers or microspheres prior to mixing with the cement paste. Features that impact loading and release of therapeutic agents include the microstructure, porosity and surface area of the cements, drug incorporation method, and the interaction between the agent and the pre-set matrix [53].

Ion substitution of HA is widely researched lately due to its capacity to allow simultaneously both the stabilization of bone defect sites and locally delivering therapeutic ions [63], thus improving bioactivity or mechanical properties of the graft [67]. Ionically modified CPCs (i.e., with Sr^{2+}, $(SiO_4)^{4-}$, Zn^{2+}, Mg^{2+}) were investigated for their capability to influence bone modeling and remodeling processes [53], Sr^{2+} receiving attention for its particular prospects for stimulating new bone formation, hindering cell driven bone resorption and raising BMD, and thus having large acceptance and usage in systemic osteoporosis therapy [63].

Interest is rising regarding the potential of carbonate substituted HA as a way to improve the bioactivity of the composites, adhesion and differentiation of osteoblast cells, collagen and osteocalcin expression and mineral deposition [60]. During an evaluation of the apatite formation capacity of biomaterials in SBF, there were reported visible differences in calcium uptake, the thickness of the freshly precipitated apatite layer and a confirmation of higher degradation rate of carbonate HA [60].

Fluorine can enhance HA crystallization and mineralization during bone formation, as fluorine containing HA, $Ca_{10}(PO_4)_6(OH)_{2-x}F_x$ is reported to manifest the lowest solubility and higher biocompatibility and bioactivity comparing with HA, leading to an increase in the differentiation and proliferation of osteoblasts, inducing, thus, bone regeneration [55].

7. Osteoporosis

Sustaining bone mass depends on bone remodeling processes, which imply the equilibrium between the activity of bone resorbing osteoclasts and bone forming osteoblasts. Unbalanced resorption activity leads to decreased bone mass, altered bone quality, and higher fracture risk in osteoporosis [68]. The same equilibrium of bone remodeling can be affected because of skeletal senescence, which alter the integrity and biomechanical properties of both types of bone tissue [5].

Osteoporosis is a chronic condition [69], characterized by decreasing bone mass and quality [6], making elderly patients, both men and women with the general increase in life expectancy, susceptible to osteoporotic fracture, also known as fragility fracture, due to low-energy trauma [5] and delayed [43] or impaired bone regeneration potential, as such fractures usually do not heal and increase the incidence of subsequent fractures by two to three times in the proximity of the site [7].

Osteoporotic bones have a low BMD [70], because of a low capacity of bone regeneration, excessive activation of osteoclasts [5] and the increased osteoclast induced bone turnover, leading to high crystallinity of the HA in the bone and lower level of acid phosphate [7]. These changes in the microarchitecture cause a reduction in both the cross-linking efficiency and tolerance of the bone towards mechanical stress [7] and increased risk of bone fractures [70]. Osteoporotic fractures are the visible effect of the micro-alterations that raise the susceptibility of bone to the applied load [5].

Surgery is the main treatment strategy, but poor results are obtained because of various biological and surgical factors, which makes it hard to achieve a stable fixation and the failure risk (refracturation) following surgery is significant [5,20]. Treating osteoporotic fractures is difficult because of the reduced healing capacity, which correlates for osteoporotic patients with a far higher (~50%) failure rate of implant fixation than against non-osteoporotic patients [67], making their implants prone to pull out and failure [7], as osseointegration is inhibited by osteoporosis [71]. Decreased bone mass [69], porous structure and low strength are linked to a reduced supporting ability of an implant [20].

Delayed regeneration potential is influenced by compositional difference in vitamin D, non-availability of growth factors, while estrogen is important in stimulating RANK ligand secretion, leading, thus, to osteoclasts activation and bone resorption. For men, testosterone is key for maintaining BMD. Decrease of the parathyroid hormone (PTH) determines reduced calcium absorption and, consequently, a reduction in BMD [7]. The bone fragility specific to osteoporosis subsequent to menopause is caused by an imbalance at the cellular level between exceeding bone resorption and lower bone formation, and from an increase in the rate of remodeling at the tissue level [72]. Although bone turnover is a normal physiological process involved in microfractures repairing, its acceleration determines bone loss [73].

Throughout the evolution of osteoporosis, osteocyte numbers per unit of bone area are constantly declining, and consequently trabecular thickness lowers and intracortical porosity heightens. These significant modifications in the matrix composition and structure cause deteriorated bone quality and lower resistance to mechanical loading [5]. Red marrow starts to accumulate adipose cells, turning into white marrow. Simultaneously with the beginning of osteoporosis, other changes were reported, namely, decreased number, proliferation and osteogenic differentiation potential of MSCs present in the bone marrow micro-environment [7].

Osteoporosis causes inadequate conditions for fracture healing [43], and the simple treatment of the acute fracture is unable to lower the risk of repeated fractures, thus, being necessary to be followed up by appropriate osteoporosis treatment [70]. In these cases, the loco-regional delivery could be an efficient solution because the delivered agents can counteract the bone density decrease and thus can assure an assisted healing where the formation rate is enhanced, the formation/resorption will be improved or even normal bone density can be obtained in the new bone as well as in the neighboring region where these agents are diffusing. In normal conditions, these biological active agents will diffuse during and after the healing process (Figure 8b,c) and the distribution of the bone density in this area will be similar with the one presented in Figure 8c. Similar approaches were also proposed in the patent application RO129822 (A2) [74] which use zinc as the active ion enhancing bone formation, but this approach can be applied also for developing anti-osteoporotic agents such as strontium ranelate. These drug delivery systems can be in solid or gel form, the solids will be implanted after surgical intervention as presented in Figure 8b and, if necessary, metallic supports can be used to take over the mechanical loadings while gels can be injected into the defect.

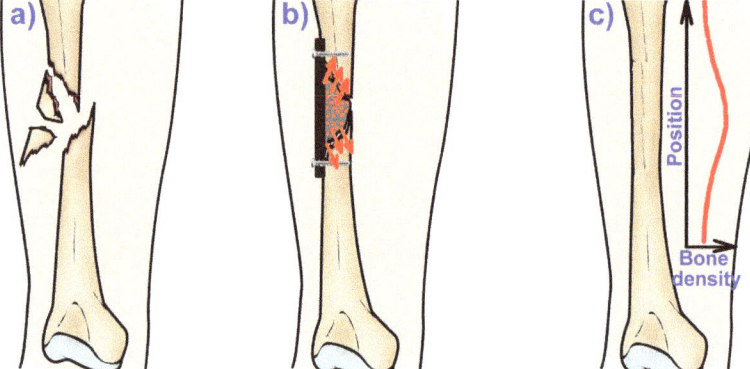

Figure 8. Schematic representation of bone grafting, healing and bone density distribution: (**a**) fracture; (**b**) bone grafting and healing; (**c**) bone density distribution.

Osteoporosis is classified into primary and secondary [6]:

Primary osteoporosis or postmenopausal osteoporosis appears after menopause. Type 1 affects more trabecular than cortical bone, as seen mainly in vertebral and distal radius fractures. It can affect men also, arising in midlife with vertebral fractures or low BMD by DXA. In men, genetic causes may involve genes for IGF-I18 or estrogen metabolism. Type 2 is found in both genders after age 70. Both types of bone are affected, commonly resulting in fractures of the proximal femur, in addition to vertebrae and radii. There are differences in aging-associated changes between genders, as women lose trabeculae and have greater spacing between trabeculae, and men only have thinning of trabeculae as they age. Quantitative computed tomography with finite element analysis have shown that women lose more cortical bone in vertebrae. Men have larger bones at peak bone mass; and with aging, more periosteal bone is deposited in long bones. These differences may explain why men fracture later in life than women [6].

Secondary osteoporosis affects both genders. The initiation of corticosteroid therapy is usually the cause of secondary osteoporosis, namely glucocorticoid-induced osteoporosis, which increase fracture risk as early as three months following oral glucocorticoid treatment [6].

Typical osteoporotic drugs act by either inhibiting bone resorption or favoring bone formation [7]. Currently, therapy for osteoporosis utilize anti-resorptive or anabolic drugs, which determine inconsistent effects on bone mass and fracture incidence [68]. Authorized treatment by FDA for osteoporosis includes the bisphosphonates (alendronate, risedronate and zoledronic acid), the more recent anti-resorptive antibody denosumab and the anabolic agent teriparatide. Bisphosphonates have been connected to bone osteonecrosis [71]. Ibandronate is also available, while strontium ranelate is approved to be used in over 70 countries but not approved by the FDA [6].

Bisphosphonates are a class of drugs that adjust the increased activity of the osteoclasts, and along selective estrogen receptor modulators (SERMs), calcitonin, denosumab and strontium ranelate, are included in the wider group of anti-resorbers. Differently from the catabolic drugs, anabolic drugs favor bone formation and include teriparatide and PTH analog [7].

Delivering a pair of drugs, with a complimentary action on bone dynamics has been considered, mostly with BPs and BMP-2—BPs and PTH being another combination. Simultaneous use of pro-anabolic and anti-catabolic drugs aims to aid impaired healing in osteoporotic patients [52].

New drugs against osteoporosis such as denosumab (targeting RANKL/RANK/OPG pathway) and romosozumab (targeting Wnt signaling cascades), are monitored for cardiovascular outcomes. One meta-analysis indicates that denosumab usage did not increase the risk of major adverse cardiovascular events among patients with primary osteoporosis over a period of 12 to 36 months but romosozumab might raise concerns [75], but after a re-analysis was performed, both Denosumab and Romosozumab association with cardiovascular outcomes was dismissed [76].

Romosozumab is a monoclonal antibody that inhibits sclerostin, an extracellular Wnt inhibitor secreted mainly by osteocytes [77], with a double effect of enhancing bone formation and diminishing bone resorption [75].

Clinical trials of romosozumab show that it is well tolerated and effective in fracture risk reduction, possessing great therapeutical potential for osteoporosis but still has some limitations by the fact that its anabolic potency is restricted to a few months of therapy, after which the large bone mass gaining is diminished. A possible strategy might be the usage of other drugs as well to sustain the bone mass gaining [78].

Odanacatib is an inhibitor of cathepsin K (CatK), and is very active, selective and sensitive, capable increasing bone formation and implant osseointegration and hinder bone loss in osteoporotic conditions. Osteoclasts perform bone degradation trough acid secretion in order to demineralize HA and lysosomal cysteine protease secretion (CatK) in order to degrade the bone matrix proteins. Odanacatib does not alter normal differentiation, migration and polarization of osteoclasts [71].

Increased risk of cardiovascular events, such as stroke, made odanacatib less attractive for future use against osteoporosis [75,79], even though it was proved beneficial for risk reductions of fractures in postmenopausal osteoporosis [75]. Other similar drugs such as balicatib, relacatib and dual cathepsin S/K inhibitor SAR114137 were discarded after adverse effects were observed [79].

Statins are not specific for treating osteoporosis but their capacity to inhibit the HMG-CoA reductase pathway determine an increased bone metabolism [22] and by increasing BMP-2 expression determine healing [52], but their efficiency is still debated.

Clinical reports indicate intrinsic weak bone architecture and impaired osteointegrative ability as the lead cause of implant non-union and ejection. Worrying is also the negative effect osteoporosis has on previously osteointegrated implants [7], including degradable bone graft substitutes [43]. Implants used in osteoporotic fractures need to sustain, alongside mechanical support, a way to counteract the pathology of osteoporosis, thus, aiding bone regeneration. Consequently, local delivering of therapeutic agents that can increase osteointegration, osteogenesis while simultaneously regulate bone remodeling may prove advantageous [7].

8. Strontium Ranelate

Strontium (Sr) is an alkaline earth metal, present in the human body as a trace element, with chemical and physical properties comparable to those of calcium [23]. It is stored in the bone [33] where is stimulates cell growth, hindering bone resorption, opposing osteoporosis [55] and improving both cortical and trabecular bone structures [23]. It has been reported as a key factor in bone remodeling, being linked to both the stimulation of bone formation and hindering of bone resorption [80]. This beneficial double effect it has on bone turnover has been so far used to some extent against osteoporosis [43]. It has the capability to promote bone regeneration while reducing the frequency of fractures in animal models [23] even in small doses [43]. Sr ions have strong bone-seeking properties and often act in the human body similarly to calcium [69] but due to its higher atomic weight, incorporation of Sr ions reinforces the bone through increasing its mass and density [35]. Sr has attracted attention for potential use against osteoporosis as Sr ions increase osteoblast proliferation and reduce osteoclast activity, respectively [7].

Strontium ions have demonstrated effects both in vitro and in vivo studies [43], and is believed to lie in the Sr^{2+} capability to enhance osteoblast-related gene expression and the alkaline phosphatase (ALP) activity of mesenchymal stem cells (MSCs) [55], together with inhibiting the differentiation of osteoclasts [3]. ALP is considered a marker of osteogenic differentiation [28].

Sr hinders the formation of a ruffled border by the pre-osteoclast cells, thus hindering its maturation and resorption ability. Sr controls calcium sensing receptor activity by increasing calcium concentration in the microenvironment, resulting in an enhanced osteogenesis by osteoblast cells. Advanced osteogenic ability (ALP activity) of Sr doped CPCs is indicated by rat OB sarcoma cells model [7]. Sr doped HA/chitosan nanohybrid scaffolds display increased ALP activity, extracellular matrix mineralization, and osteoinductivity [63].

Sr ions promote protein synthesis for both collagen and non-collagen and osteoblastic growth [35] together with the inhibition of osteoclast differentiation and resorption activity, causing a denser and larger bone [23]. Considering this, Sr is believed to be effective in improving the properties of materials, especially bioactivity and biocompatibility, stimulating bone regeneration [80] and being effective against osteoporosis. Through increased expression of angiogenic factors such as VEGF and Ang-1, Sr promotes neovascularization [21].

Strontium ranelate is considered effective in fighting fragility fractures through improving the biomechanical properties of bone [5] reducing the risk of fractures in osteoporotic patients [69]. In contrast to other anti-osteoporotic drugs, Sr has a beneficial effect on the cortical bone, as its mass and thickness increase the following treatment with Sr in animal and clinical studies [23]. It was indicated to consequently reduce the chances of vertebral and hip fracture in elderly woman [35]. Sr has been proved effective in vitro in reducing osteoclast differentiation, activity and bone resorption and increasing osteoblast differentiation [70]. The metabolic activity of osteoblasts is enhanced in the presence of strontium ions, while the activity of the osteoclasts is reduced depending on the concentration of strontium in the microenvironment [43]. Inhibited activity of osteoclast in the presence of Sr is due to reduced synthesis of matrix metalloproteinase coupled with control of osteoprotegerin-RANKL pathway [81].

The mechanisms through which Sr can stimulate new bone formation are the CaR/ERK1/2 and Wnt signaling pathways. Wnt/β-catenin signaling is essential in the bone development and homeostasis. Wnt/β-catenin signaling is activated by Sr^{2+}, which promotes new bone formation by inhibiting the osteoclasts and stimulating osteoblasts through nuclear factor NFATC1. Sr^{2+} concentration levels may lead to different results of new bone formation and side effects, meaning that accumulation of Sr^{2+} should be considered when applied to humans [33].

Cn-NFAT signaling is identified as a mechanism involved in strontium ranelate (SrRan) in vitro displayed osteoblastic stimulatory effects. This involves the activation of Cn-NFATc1 and components of canonical and non-canonical Wnt signaling, making this molecular mechanism the novelty through which SrRan enhanced osteoblastogenesis is explained [68].

Drugs containing strontium show significant effects in the prevention and treatment of osteoporosis [7]. Sr administered as SrRan is a known remedy against primary osteoporosis and difficult fracture healing, being approved for treatment many countries [43]. SrRan influences bone formation through a dual mechanism, by signaling osteoblasts to produce bone and inhibition of osteoclast mediated bone resorption [28]. SrRan in vitro results confirm its dual mechanism and in vivo was shown to determine an advantageous bone balance in experimental osteopenic models. In clinical usage it was also shown to decrease in patients with primary osteoporosis the risk of vertebral and non-vertebral fractures [68], femoral bone fractures also being positively impacted [63]. SrRan remains the main option for cases of severe osteoporosis [81].

SrRan is used for its gastric tolerability, physicochemical characteristics, bioavailability of Sr [82] and to decrease Sr side effects [83].

As SrRan rebalance bone remodeling by increasing bone formation and decreasing bone resorption [5,23,72], it is considered conducive to new bone formation and studies indicate a beneficial effect of SrRan on all parameters related to bone quality and strength [5]. Profiting of its both antiresorptive and anabolic properties, it can increase and stabilize BMD [70]. Its dual mechanism of action is favorable to osteoporotic fracture repair, in contrast with other drugs such as bisphosphonates, which have no effects on bone growth and repair of resorption sites of osteoporotic bone and can cause secondary effects such as inflammatory disease and osteonecrosis [28]. Osteoclasts might not be inhibited as in regular solely anti-resorptive treatment with bisphosphonates [43].

SrRan administrated orally in a daily dose of 2 g seems to be a safe approach and effective in decreasing the risk of vertebral fractures in postmenopausal osteoporosis patients [33,72] and documented to improve BMD, similar to other anti-osteoporotic drugs such as bisphosphonates, selective estrogen receptor modulators (SERMs), parathyroid hormone (PTH), and denosumab [23]. Among them, only Sr has a dual mechanism of action: stimulating new bone formation and reducing bone resorption [8,9], while increasing bone strength and decreasing fracture incidence [23]. Strontium ranelate increased BMD similar in both genders, both having fewer fractures after Sr administration [6]. Due to its anti-osteoporotic effect, ongoing treatment after the fracture occurs has a beneficial effect [23].

Despite all the shown benefits, systemic administration requires a high dose and prolonged drug administration period [7] and can lead to serious adverse effects in osteoporotic patients such as myocardial infarction, venous thromboembolism [43], and skin rashes [7]. The bioavailability of Sr via oral administration is about 25%, making local delivery with the aid of a biomaterial more effective [83]. The safety of SrRan has been questioned after the EMA found that its use increases the risk of heart problems in postmenopausal osteoporotic patients [84].

The Sr treatment is of particular concern because of its cardiovascular risk [84] and is restricted although it is still prescribed to patients who have no other suitable treatment [23], therefore the controlled local release of Sr is decisive as it has a great impact on biological processes [80]. It is not recommended in patients suffering the following conditions: peripheral vascular disease, ischemic heart, cerebrovascular disease, or uncontrolled hypertension [6]. Local release from scaffolds can prevent the side effects [43] as long-term administration is required for Sr to be effective. Research proved that local delivery at the injured site of a low dose of Sr is beneficial for osteoporotic bone healing and has clinical therapeutic importance [7]. In order to decrease the administered drug dose and bypass the adverse side effects, the design of a durable local SrRan delivery system would be clinically important [70]. The use of a low dose is not anticipated to induce persisting adverse side effects and delivering SrRan locally at the defect site through implanted scaffolds, may be a better strategy comparing to oral treatment [7].

In induced osteoporosis models of supercritical rat bone defects, Sr released from SrRan loaded bioactive glass, CPCs, calcium silicate and collagen sponges implanted had a visible accelerated bone regeneration effect depending on concentration [43]. Other osteoporotic models using rats and sheep proved the safety and efficacy of low dose Sr loaded implants (10%) [7]. Sr-containing CPCs has been described to improve bioactivity and biocompatibility, promote osteoblast proliferation and differentiation, and enable deposition of apatite, resulting an increased mechanical strength of the bone–scaffold interface, in both types of bone [80]. Chemical resemblance of Ca and Sr contribute in the development of Sr containing HA (SrHA) scaffolds [7].

Sr substituted calcium phosphates can impact in vitro the differentiation and activity of osteoclasts and osteoblasts [43] and SrHA demonstrates osteoinduction and high solubility, making the incorporation of Sr into HA beneficial for improving bioactivity [55].

Improved Sr and Ca release was noticed for SrHA in comparison to stoichiometric HA granules, which is expected to further healing in vivo through the anabolic and anti-catabolic properties of Sr [67]. When SrHA was added to an allograft it aided the healing of the area around the implant, a fact proved by the extended volume of new bone formed in the respective area, and delayed resorption [85]. Released Sr ions from the biomaterial should stimulate genesis of osteoblasts through ion release or indirectly by increased presence and activity of osteoclasts after material resorption, leading afterwards to osteoblasts stimulation [43].

SrHA coatings at Sr concentrations of 5%, 10%, and 20% showed increased implant osteointegration, improved trabecular microstructure around the implant, and better fixation based on the molar ratio of Sr ions. The results for Ti implants show that Sr could enhance new bone formation on implant surfaces, thus, improve osteointegration with the aid of SrHA and the 20% Sr loaded coating, and proved to be the most beneficial for implant osteointegration among the tested variant in osteoporotic rats [69].

Strontium was added into CPCs to augment their osteoconductivity and accelerate their degradation. Studies indicated that in vitro the rates of osteoblastic cell proliferation are enhanced and in vivo degradation is faster and osteoconductivity is better [53]. Beneficial effects of SrHA on bone mass at interface between implant and bone has been observed in healthy rabbit segmental bone defect model. Some sources indicate a daily dose of 2 mg/per body weight of SrRan in treating osteoporosis systemically [7].

Studies suggest that Sr loaded CPCs induce faster hydroxyapatite growth, high percentage in vitro cell viability and superior durability than the Sr free samples, in the case of Sr replacement of Ca, up to 5% in sol-gel bioactive ceramics with improvements on the proliferation rate of the cell line of human osteosarcoma [35]. It is much harder in vivo to trace and monitor the release, distribution, and accumulations of drugs. High concentrations can be monitored with magnetic resonance imaging (MRI) shortly after implantation, but postmortem examinations remain the most precise approach [83].

In the SrHA coating, Sr ions replace a part of Ca ions leading to an improved dissolution of the SrHA coating, thus, increasing the concentration of Sr, Ca, and phosphorus ions near implant surfaces. Their presence in the microenvironment improve osteoblast activity and new bone development into the implant surfaces [69]. While Sr can prove beneficial, high concentrations can have a negative impact [80]. Recommended concentrations range between 1% and 10% for osteoporotic applications. Using 10% SrHA scaffold to enhance in vitro osteoblast differentiation means a release of 0.11 mM Sr ions/mg is expected, enough to sustain a therapeutic effect in osteoporotic bone healing [7]. The reported minimum dose for in vitro conditions was 0.1 mM for osteoblast activation and 1 mM for osteoclast inhibition [83]. In addition, material properties such as strength, degradability, handling, and component release can be modified by loading with Sr compounds and these properties frequently have non-linear dependence on Sr concentration [43].

SrRan can be encapsulated, also, in PLA matrix using s/o/w and s/w1/o/w2 techniques, the latter being used in order to create sustainable SrRan delivery systems up to 24 wt% SrRan content, with observed precipitation of biomimetic calcium phosphate on the surface and in the pores of the delivery systems [70].

9. Conclusions

Osteointegration of implants and weakened regeneration potential of the host bone remain challenges to be overcome in osteoporotic fracture healing. Functionalized scaffolds capable of improving osteointegration and fast healing are of great importance for osteoporotic patients who have a lower number of osteoprogenitor cells. Loco-regional delivery of anti-resorptive and/or osteogenic factors at the defect site may have significant clinical applications for the recovery of fractured osteoporotic bones. Throughout this review, we have tried to resume the current state of research and the strategies for bone healing scaffolds and the future perspectives in the case of osteoporotic fractures by incorporation of biological active agents such as strontium ranelate in bioceramic/biopolymer composite bone scaffolds. The loco-regional delivery of SrRan can be suitable for administration because the systemic toxicity and especially the cardiovascular adverse effects can be reduced/removed but additional research will be necessary to evaluate the in vivo, short and long-term toxicity. According to the literature it is evident that, even if many researches were already done, many additional studies are necessary to reach optimal formulations. Along with the strontium-based formulations, some other biological active agents are usually used in the therapy of the osteoporosis and thus can be loaded in grafting materials to control the ratio between formation and resorption.

Funding: The financial contribution received from the national project "Innovative biomaterials for treatment and diagnosis", (PN-IIIP1-1.2-PCCDI2017-0629) is highly acknowledged.

Conflicts of Interest: The authors declare no conflict of interest.

References

1. Wang, W.; Yeung, K.W.K. Bone grafts and biomaterials substitutes for bone defect repair: A review. *Bioact. Mater.* **2017**, *2*, 224–247. [CrossRef] [PubMed]
2. Francois, E.L.; Yaszemski, M.J. Chapter 43—Preclinical bone repair models in regenerative medicine. In *Principles of Regenerative Medicine*, 3rd ed.; Atala, A., Lanza, R., Mikos, A.G., Nerem, R., Eds.; Academic Press: Boston, MA, USA, 2019; pp. 761–767. [CrossRef]
3. Zhu, Y.; Wagner, W.R. Chapter 30—Design principles in biomaterials and scaffolds. In *Principles of Regenerative Medicine*, 3rd ed.; Atala, A., Lanza, R., Mikos, A.G., Nerem, R., Eds.; Academic Press: Boston, MA, USA, 2019; pp. 505–522. [CrossRef]
4. Maia, F.R.; Correlo, V.M.; Oliveira, J.M.; Reis, R.L. Chapter 32—Natural origin materials for bone tissue engineering: Properties, processing, and performance. In *Principles of Regenerative Medicine*, 3rd ed.; Atala, A., Lanza, R., Mikos, A.G., Nerem, R., Eds.; Academic Press: Boston, MA, USA, 2019; pp. 535–558. [CrossRef]
5. Xie, Y.; Zhang, L.; Xiong, Q.; Gao, Y.; Ge, W.; Tang, P. Bench-to-bedside strategies for osteoporotic fracture: From osteoimmunology to mechanosensation. *Bone Res.* **2019**, *7*, 25. [CrossRef] [PubMed]

6. Adler, R.A. Osteoporosis in men: A review. *Bone Res.* **2014**, *2*, 14001. [CrossRef] [PubMed]
7. Chandran, S.; John, A. Osseointegration of osteoporotic bone implants: Role of stem cells, Silica and Strontium—A concise review. *J. Clin. Orthop. Trauma* **2019**, *10*, S32–S36. [CrossRef] [PubMed]
8. Rambhia, K.J.; Ma, P.X. Chapter 48—Biomineralization and bone regeneration. In *Principles of Regenerative Medicine*, 3rd ed.; Atala, A., Lanza, R., Mikos, A.G., Nerem, R., Eds.; Academic Press: Boston, MA, USA, 2019; pp. 853–866. [CrossRef]
9. Tripathy, N.; Perumal, E.; Ahmad, R.; Song, J.E.; Khang, G. Chapter 40—Hybrid composite biomaterials. In *Principles of Regenerative Medicine*, 3rd ed.; Atala, A., Lanza, R., Mikos, A.G., Nerem, R., Eds.; Academic Press: Boston, MA, USA, 2019; pp. 695–714. [CrossRef]
10. Burr, D.B.; Akkus, O. Chapter 1—Bone morphology and organization. In *Basic and Applied Bone Biology*; Burr, D.B., Allen, M.R., Eds.; Academic Press: San Diego, CA, USA, 2014; pp. 3–25. [CrossRef]
11. Pereira, H.F.; Cengiz, I.F.; Silva, F.S.; Reis, R.L.; Oliveira, J.M. Scaffolds and coatings for bone regeneration. *J. Mater. Sci. Mater. Med.* **2020**, *31*, 27. [CrossRef] [PubMed]
12. Amini, A.R.; Laurencin, C.T.; Nukavarapu, S.P. Bone tissue engineering: Recent advances and challenges. *Crit. Rev. Biomed. Eng.* **2012**, *40*, 363–408. [CrossRef]
13. Gonzalez-Fernandez, T.; Sikorski, P.; Leach, J.K. Bio-instructive materials for musculoskeletal regeneration. *Acta Biomater.* **2019**, *96*, 20–34. [CrossRef]
14. Silva, C.C.; Thomazini, D.; Pinheiro, A.G.; Aranha, N.; Figueiró, S.D.; Góes, J.C.; Sombra, A.S.B. Collagen–hydroxyapatite films: Piezoelectric properties. *Mater. Sci. Eng. B* **2001**, *86*, 210–218. [CrossRef]
15. Schlundt, C.; El Khassawna, T.; Serra, A.; Dienelt, A.; Wendler, S.; Schell, H.; van Rooijen, N.; Radbruch, A.; Lucius, R.; Hartmann, S.; et al. Macrophages in bone fracture healing: Their essential role in endochondral ossification. *Bone* **2018**, *106*, 78–89. [CrossRef]
16. Gil Mur, F.J. 8—Accelerating mineralization of biomimetic surfaces. In *Biomineralization and Biomaterials*; Aparicio, C., Ginebra, M.-P., Eds.; Woodhead Publishing: Boston, MA, USA, 2016; pp. 267–289. [CrossRef]
17. He, J.; Chen, G.; Liu, M.; Xu, Z.; Chen, H.; Yang, L.; Lv, Y. Scaffold strategies for modulating immune microenvironment during bone regeneration. *Mater. Sci. Eng. C* **2020**, *108*, 110411. [CrossRef]
18. Kolar, P.; Schmidt-Bleek, K.; Schell, H.; Gaber, T.; Toben, D.; Schmidmaier, G.; Perka, C.; Buttgereit, F.; Duda, G.N. The Early fracture hematoma and its potential role in fracture healing. *Tissue Eng. Part B Rev.* **2010**, *16*, 427–434. [CrossRef] [PubMed]
19. Lopes, D.; Martins-Cruz, C.; Oliveira, M.B.; Mano, J.F. Bone physiology as inspiration for tissue regenerative therapies. *Biomaterials* **2018**, *185*, 240–275. [CrossRef] [PubMed]
20. Li, L.; Yu, M.; Li, Y.; Li, Q.; Yang, H.; Zheng, M.; Han, Y.; Lu, D.; Lu, S.; Gui, L. Synergistic anti-inflammatory and osteogenic n-HA/resveratrol/chitosan composite microspheres for osteoporotic bone regeneration. *Bioact. Mater.* **2021**, *6*, 1255–1266. [CrossRef] [PubMed]
21. Chang, J.; Zhang, X.; Dai, K. Chapter 2—Biomaterial-induced microenvironment and host reaction in bone regeneration. In *Bioactive Materials for Bone Regeneration*; Chang, J., Zhang, X., Dai, K., Eds.; Academic Press: Cambridge, MA, USA, 2020; pp. 105–181. [CrossRef]
22. Kyllönen, L.; D'Este, M.; Alini, M.; Eglin, D. Local drug delivery for enhancing fracture healing in osteoporotic bone. *Acta Biomater.* **2015**, *11*, 412–434. [CrossRef]
23. Komrakova, M.; Weidemann, A.; Dullin, C.; Ebert, J.; Tezval, M.; Stuermer, K.M.; Sehmisch, S. The impact of strontium ranelate on metaphyseal bone healing in ovariectomized rats. *Calcif. Tissue Int.* **2015**, *97*, 391–401. [CrossRef] [PubMed]
24. O'Brien, F.J. Biomaterials & scaffolds for tissue engineering. *Mater. Today* **2011**, *14*, 88–95. [CrossRef]
25. Oryan, A.; Alidadi, S.; Moshiri, A.; Maffulli, N. Bone regenerative medicine: Classic options, novel strategies, and future directions. *J. Orthop. Surg. Res.* **2014**, *9*, 18. [CrossRef]
26. de Grado, G.F.; Keller, L.; Idoux-Gillet, Y.; Wagner, Q.; Musset, A.-M.; Benkirane-Jessel, N.; Bornert, F.; Offner, D. Bone substitutes: A review of their characteristics, clinical use, and perspectives for large bone defects management. *J. Tissue Eng.* **2018**, *9*. [CrossRef]
27. Shuai, C.; Yu, L.; Feng, P.; Gao, C.; Peng, S. Interfacial reinforcement in bioceramic/biopolymer composite bone scaffold: The role of coupling agent. *Colloids Surf. B Biointerfaces* **2020**, *193*, 111083. [CrossRef]
28. Prabha, R.D.; Ding, M.; Bollen, P.; Ditzel, N.; Varma, H.K.; Nair, P.D.; Kassem, M. Strontium ion reinforced bioceramic scaffold for load bearing bone regeneration. *Mater. Sci. Eng. C* **2020**, *109*, 110427. [CrossRef]
29. Herford, A.S.; Stoffella, E.; Stanford, C.M. Chapter 5—Bone grafts and bone substitute materials. In *Principles and Practice of Single Implant and Restorations*; Torabinejad, M., Sabeti, M.A., Goodacre, C.J., Eds.; W.B. Saunders: Saint Louis, MI, USA, 2014; pp. 75–86. [CrossRef]
30. Arpağ, O.F.; Damlar, I.; Altan, A.; Tatli, U.; Günay, A. To what extent does hyaluronic acid affect healing of xenografts? A histomorphometric study in a rabbit model. *J. Appl. Oral Sci.* **2018**, *26*, e20170004. [CrossRef] [PubMed]
31. McHale, M.K.; Bergmann, N.M.; West, J.L. Chapter 38—Histogenesis in three-dimensional scaffolds. In *Principles of Regenerative Medicine*, 3rd ed.; Atala, A., Lanza, R., Mikos, A.G., Nerem, R., Eds.; Academic Press: Boston, MA, USA, 2019; pp. 661–674. [CrossRef]
32. Bambole, V.; Yakhmi, J.V. Chapter 14—Tissue engineering: Use of electrospinning technique for recreating physiological functions. In *Nanobiomaterials in Soft Tissue Engineering*; Grumezescu, A.M., Ed.; William Andrew Publishing: Norwich, NY, USA, 2016; pp. 387–455. [CrossRef]

33. Liu, W.; Cheng, M.; Wahafu, T.; Zhao, Y.; Qin, H.; Wang, J.; Zhang, X.; Wang, L. The in vitro and in vivo performance of a strontium-containing coating on the low-modulus Ti$_{35}$Nb$_2$Ta$_3$Zr alloy formed by micro-arc oxidation. *J. Mater. Sci. Mater. Med.* **2015**, *26*, 203. [CrossRef] [PubMed]
34. Abbasi, N.; Hamlet, S.; Love, R.M.; Nguyen, N.-T. Porous scaffolds for bone regeneration. *J. Sci. Adv. Mater. Devices* **2020**, *5*, 1–9. [CrossRef]
35. Kaur, P.; Singh, K.J.; Kaur, S.; Kaur, S.; Singh, A.P. Sol-gel derived strontium-doped SiO$_2$–CaO–MgO–P$_2$O$_5$ bioceramics for faster growth of bone like hydroxyapatite and their in vitro study for orthopedic applications. *Mater. Chem. Phys.* **2020**, *245*, 122763. [CrossRef]
36. Chang, M.C.; Tanaka, J. FT-IR study for hydroxyapatite/collagen nanocomposite cross-linked by glutaraldehyde. *Biomaterials* **2002**, *23*, 4811–4818. [CrossRef]
37. Develioğlu, H.; Koptagel, E.; Gedik, R.; Dupoirieux, L. The effect of a biphasic ceramic on calvarial bone regeneration in rats. *J. Oral Implantol.* **2005**, *31*, 309–312. [CrossRef]
38. Ficai, A.; Andronescu, E.; Voicu, G.; Ficai, D. *Advances in Collagen/Hydroxyapatite Composite Materials*; InTech: Rijeka, Croatia, 2011. [CrossRef]
39. Andronescu, E.; Voicu, G.; Ficai, M.; Mohora, I.A.; Trusca, R.; Ficai, A. Collagen/hydroxyapatite composite materials with desired ceramic properties. *J. Electron. Microsc. (Tokyo)* **2011**, *60*, 253–259. [CrossRef]
40. Ficai, M.; Andronescu, E.; Ficai, D.; Voicu, G.; Ficai, A. Synthesis and characterization of COLL-PVA/HA hybrid materials with stratified morphology. *Colloids Surf. B Biointerfaces* **2010**, *81*, 614–619. [CrossRef]
41. Ardelean, I.L.; Gudovan, D.; Ficai, D.; Ficai, A.; Andronescu, E.; Albu-Kaya, M.G.; Neacsu, P.; Ion, R.N.; Cimpean, A.; Mitran, V. Collagen/hydroxyapatite bone grafts manufactured by homogeneous/heterogeneous 3D printing. *Mater. Lett.* **2018**, *231*, 179–182. [CrossRef]
42. Wu, L.; Ding, J. Effects of porosity and pore size on in vitro degradation of three-dimensional porous poly(D,L-lactide-co-glycolide) scaffolds for tissue engineering. *J. Biomedical Mater. Res. Part A* **2005**, *75A*, 767–777. [CrossRef]
43. Kruppke, B.; Wagner, A.-S.; Rohnke, M.; Heinemann, C.; Kreschel, C.; Gebert, A.; Wiesmann, H.-P.; Mazurek, S.; Wenisch, S.; Hanke, T. Biomaterial based treatment of osteoclastic/osteoblastic cell imbalance—Gelatin-modified calcium/strontium phosphates. *Mater. Sci. Eng. C* **2019**, *104*, 109933. [CrossRef] [PubMed]
44. Mahanta, A.K.; Patel, D.K.; Maiti, P. Nanohybrid scaffold of chitosan and functionalized graphene oxide for controlled drug delivery and bone regeneration. *ACS Biomater. Sci. Eng.* **2019**, *5*, 5139–5149. [CrossRef]
45. Zhang, S.; Chen, J.; Yu, Y.; Dai, K.; Wang, J.; Liu, C. Accelerated bone regenerative efficiency by regulating sequential release of BMP-2 and VEGF and Synergism with sulfated chitosan. *ACS Biomater. Sci. Eng.* **2019**, *5*, 1944–1955. [CrossRef] [PubMed]
46. Dalavi, P.A.; Prabhu, A.; Shastry, R.P.; Venkatesan, J. Microspheres containing biosynthesized silver nanoparticles with alginate-nano hydroxyapatite for biomedical applications. *J. Biomater. Sci. Polym. Ed.* **2020**. [CrossRef] [PubMed]
47. Sebastiammal, S.; Fathima, A.S.L.; Devanesan, S.; AlSalhi, M.S.; Henry, J.; Govindarajan, M.; Vaseeharan, B. Curcumin-encased hydroxyapatite nanoparticles as novel biomaterials for antimicrobial, antioxidant and anticancer applications: A perspective of nano-based drug delivery. *J. Drug Deliv. Sci. Technol.* **2020**, *57*, 101752. [CrossRef]
48. Martin, V.; Ribeiro, I.A.; Alves, M.M.; Gonçalves, L.; Claudio, R.A.; Grenho, L.; Fernandes, M.H.; Gomes, P.; Santos, C.F.; Bettencourt, A.F. Engineering a multifunctional 3D-printed PLA-collagen-minocycline-nanoHydroxyapatite scaffold with combined antimicrobial and osteogenic effects for bone regeneration. *Mater. Sci. Eng. C Mater. Biol. Appl.* **2019**, *101*, 15–26. [CrossRef]
49. Ficai, D.; Sonmez, M.; Albu, M.G.; Mihaiescu, D.E.; Ficai, A.; Bleotu, C. Antitumoral materials with regenerative function obtained using a layer-by-layer technique. *Drug Des. Devel. Ther.* **2015**, *9*, 1269–1279. [CrossRef]
50. Marques, C.; Ferreira, J.M.F.; Andronescu, E.; Ficai, D.; Sonmez, M.; Ficai, A. Multifunctional materials for bone cancer treatment. *Int. J. Nanomed.* **2014**, *9*, 2713–2725. [CrossRef]
51. Alt, V.; Thormann, U.; Ray, S.; Zahner, D.; Dürselen, L.; Lips, K.; El Khassawna, T.; Heiss, C.; Riedrich, A.; Schlewitz, G.; et al. A new metaphyseal bone defect model in osteoporotic rats to study biomaterials for the enhancement of bone healing in osteoporotic fractures. *Acta Biomater.* **2013**, *9*, 7035–7042. [CrossRef]
52. Simpson, C.R.; Kelly, H.M.; Murphy, C.M. Synergistic use of biomaterials and licensed therapeutics to manipulate bone remodelling and promote non-union fracture repair. *Adv. Drug Deliv. Rev.* **2020**, *160*, 212–233. [CrossRef]
53. Xu, H.H.K.; Wang, P.; Wang, L.; Bao, C.; Chen, Q.; Weir, M.D.; Chow, L.C.; Zhao, L.; Zhou, X.; Reynolds, M.A. Calcium phosphate cements for bone engineering and their biological properties. *Bone Res.* **2017**, *5*, 17056. [CrossRef] [PubMed]
54. Neacsu, I.A.; Arsenie, L.V.; Trusca, R.; Ardelean, I.L.; Mihailescu, N.; Mihailescu, I.N.; Ristoscu, C.; Bleotu, C.; Ficai, A.; Andronescu, E. Biomimetic Collagen/Zn^{2+}-Substituted calcium phosphate composite coatings on titanium substrates as prospective bioactive layer for implants: A comparative study spin coating vs. MAPLE. *Nanomaterials* **2019**, *9*, 692. [CrossRef] [PubMed]
55. Rajabnejadkeleshteri, A.; Kamyar, A.; Khakbiz, M.; bakalani, Z.L.; Basiri, H. Synthesis and characterization of strontium fluor-hydroxyapatite nanoparticles for dental applications. *Microchem. J.* **2020**, *153*, 104485. [CrossRef]
56. Chang, J.; Zhang, X.; Dai, K. Chapter 1—Material characteristics, surface/interface, and biological effects on the osteogenesis of bioactive materials. In *Bioactive Materials for Bone Regeneration*; Chang, J., Zhang, X., Dai, K., Eds.; Academic Press: Cambridge, MA, USA, 2020; pp. 1–103. [CrossRef]

57. Hakim, S.L.; Kusumasari, F.C.; Budianto, E. Optimization of biodegradable PLA/PCL microspheres preparation as controlled drug delivery carrier. *Mater. Today Proc.* **2020**, *22*, 306–313. [CrossRef]
58. Dubinenko, G.E.; Zinoviev, A.L.; Bolbasov, E.N.; Novikov, V.T.; Tverdokhlebov, S.I. Preparation of Poly(L-lactic acid)/Hydroxyapatite composite scaffolds by fused deposit modeling 3D printing. *Mater. Today Proc.* **2020**, *22*, 228–234. [CrossRef]
59. Turnbull, G.; Clarke, J.; Picard, F.; Riches, P.; Jia, L.; Han, F.; Li, B.; Shu, W. 3D bioactive composite scaffolds for bone tissue engineering. *Bioact. Mater.* **2017**, *3*, 278–314. [CrossRef]
60. Borkowski, L.; Sroka-Bartnicka, A.; Drączkowski, P.; Ptak, A.; Zięba, E.; Ślósarczyk, A.; Ginalska, G. The comparison study of bioactivity between composites containing synthetic non-substituted and carbonate-substituted hydroxyapatite. *Mater. Sci. Eng. C* **2016**, *62*, 260–267. [CrossRef]
61. Mabrouk, M.; Beherei, H.H.; Das, D.B. Recent progress in the fabrication techniques of 3D scaffolds for tissue engineering. *Mater. Sci. Eng. C* **2020**, *110*, 110716. [CrossRef]
62. Wang, C.; Huang, W.; Zhou, Y.; He, L.; He, Z.; Chen, Z.; He, X.; Tian, S.; Liao, J.; Lu, B.; et al. 3D printing of bone tissue engineering scaffolds. *Bioact. Mater.* **2020**, *5*, 82–91. [CrossRef]
63. Sangeetha, K.; Ashok, M.; Girija, E.K.; Vidhya, G.; Vasugi, G. Strontium and ciprofloxacin modified hydroxyapatites as functional grafts for bone prostheses. *Ceram. Int.* **2018**, *44*, 13782–13789. [CrossRef]
64. Vladu, A.; Marin, S.; Neacsu, I.; Trușcă, R.; Kaya, M.; Kaya, D.; Popa, A.-M.; Poiană, C.; Cristescu, I.; Orlov, C.; et al. Spongious fillers based on collagen-hydroxyapatite-eugenol acetate with therapeutic potential in bone cancer. *Farmacia* **2020**, *68*, 313–321. [CrossRef]
65. Ionescu, O.; Ciocîlteu, M.; Manda, V.; Neacsu, I.; Ficai, A.; Amzoiu, E.; Turcu-Stiolica, A.; Croitoru, O.; Neamtu, J. Bone-graft delivery systems of type PLGA-gentamicin and collagen-hydroxyapatite-gentamicine. *Mater. Plast.* **2019**, *56*, 534–537. [CrossRef]
66. Croitoru, A.-M.; Ficai, D.; Ficai, A.; Mihailescu, N.; Andronescu, E.; Turculet, C.F. Nanostructured fibers containing natural or synthetic bioactive compounds in wound dressing applications. *Materials* **2020**, *13*, 2407. [CrossRef] [PubMed]
67. Sterling, J.A.; Guelcher, S.A. Biomaterial scaffolds for treating osteoporotic bone. *Curr. Osteoporos. Rep.* **2014**, *12*, 48–54. [CrossRef] [PubMed]
68. Fromigué, O.; Haÿ, E.; Barbara, A.; Marie, P.J. Essential role of nuclear factor of activated T cells (NFAT)-mediated Wnt signaling in osteoblast differentiation induced by strontium ranelate. *J. Biol. Chem.* **2010**, *285*, 25251–25258. [CrossRef] [PubMed]
69. Tao, Z.-S.; Bai, B.-L.; He, X.-W.; Liu, W.; Li, H.; Zhou, Q.; Sun, T.; Huang, Z.-L.; Tu, K.-k.; Lv, Y.-X.; et al. A comparative study of strontium-substituted hydroxyapatite coating on implant's osseointegration for osteopenic rats. *Med. Biol. Eng. Comput.* **2016**, *54*, 1959–1968. [CrossRef]
70. Loca, D.; Smirnova, A.; Locs, J.; Dubnika, A.; Vecstaudza, J.; Stipniece, L.; Makarova, E.; Dambrova, M. Development of local strontium ranelate delivery systems and long term in vitro drug release studies in osteogenic medium. *Sci. Rep.* **2018**, *8*, 16754. [CrossRef]
71. Yi, C.; Hao, K.Y.; Ma, T.; Lin, Y.; Ge, X.Y.; Zhang, Y. Inhibition of cathepsin K promotes osseointegration of titanium implants in ovariectomised rats. *Sci. Rep.* **2017**, *7*, 44682. [CrossRef]
72. Meunier, P.J.; Roux, C.; Seeman, E.; Ortolani, S.; Badurski, J.E.; Spector, T.D.; Cannata, J.; Balogh, A.; Lemmel, E.M.; Pors-Nielsen, S.; et al. The effects of strontium ranelate on the risk of vertebral fracture in women with postmenopausal osteoporosis. *N. Engl. J. Med.* **2004**, *350*, 459–468. [CrossRef]
73. Cianferotti, L.; D'Asta, F.; Brandi, M.L. A review on strontium ranelate long-term antifracture efficacy in the treatment of postmenopausal osteoporosis. *Ther. Adv. Musculoskelet. Dis.* **2013**, *5*, 127–139. [CrossRef]
74. Ficai, A.; Andronescu, E.; Sonmez, M.; Ficai, D.; Nedelcu, I.A.; Albu, M.G. Bone Grafts Based on Collagen, Calcium Phosphate and Zinc and Process for Preparing the Same/Grefe Osoase pe Bază de Colagen, Fosfat de Calciu și Zinc si Procedeu de Obținere a Acestora; OSIM: Bucharest, Romania, 2013.
75. Lv, F.; Cai, X.; Yang, W.; Gao, L.; Chen, L.; Wu, J.; Ji, L. Denosumab or romosozumab therapy and risk of cardiovascular events in patients with primary osteoporosis: Systematic review and meta-analysis. *Bone* **2020**, *130*, 115121. [CrossRef] [PubMed]
76. Li, L.; Gong, M.; Bao, D.; Sun, J.; Xiang, Z. Denosumab and romosozumab do not increase the risk of cardiovascular events in patients with primary osteoporosis: A reanalysis of the meta-analysis. *Bone* **2020**, *134*, 115270. [CrossRef] [PubMed]
77. Turk, J.R.; Deaton, A.M.; Yin, J.; Stolina, M.; Felx, M.; Boyd, G.; Bienvenu, J.G.; Varela, A.; Guillot, M.; Holdsworth, G.; et al. Nonclinical cardiovascular safety evaluation of romosozumab, an inhibitor of sclerostin for the treatment of osteoporosis in postmenopausal women at high risk of fracture. *Regul. Toxicol. Pharmacol.* **2020**, *115*, 104697. [CrossRef] [PubMed]
78. McClung, M.R. Romosozumab for the treatment of osteoporosis. *Osteoporos. Sarcopenia* **2018**, *4*, 11–15. [CrossRef] [PubMed]
79. Mullard, A. Merck & Co. drops osteoporosis drug odanacatib. *Nat. Rev. Drug Discov.* **2016**, *15*, 669. [CrossRef] [PubMed]
80. Zhang, W.; Shen, Y.; Pan, H.; Lin, K.; Liu, X.; Darvell, B.W.; Lu, W.W.; Chang, J.; Deng, L.; Wang, D.; et al. Effects of strontium in modified biomaterials. *Acta Biomater.* **2011**, *7*, 800–808. [CrossRef]
81. Rodrigues, T.A.; Freire, A.O.; Bonfim, B.F.; Cartágenes, M.S.S.; Garcia, J.B.S. Strontium ranelate as a possible disease-modifying osteoarthritis drug: A systematic review. *Braz. J. Med Biol. Res. Rev. Bras. Pesqui. Med. Biol.* **2018**, *51*, e7440. [CrossRef]
82. Blake, G.M.; Lewiecki, E.M.; Kendler, D.L.; Fogelman, I. A review of strontium ranelate and its effect on DXA scans. *J. Clin. Densitom.* **2007**, *10*, 113–119. [CrossRef]

83. Rohnke, M.; Pfitzenreuter, S.; Mogwitz, B.; Henß, A.; Thomas, J.; Bieberstein, D.; Gemming, T.; Otto, S.K.; Ray, S.; Schumacher, M.; et al. Strontium release from Sr^{2+}-loaded bone cements and dispersion in healthy and osteoporotic rat bone. *J. Control. Release Off. J. Control. Release Soc.* **2017**, *262*, 159–169. [CrossRef]
84. Adami, S.; Idolazzi, L.; Fracassi, E.; Gatti, D.; Rossini, M. Osteoporosis treatment: When to discontinue and when to re-start. *Bone Res.* **2013**, *1*, 323–335. [CrossRef]
85. Vestermark, M.T.; Hauge, E.M.; Soballe, K.; Bechtold, J.E.; Jakobsen, T.; Baas, J. Strontium doping of bone graft extender. *Acta Orthop.* **2011**, *82*, 614–621. [CrossRef] [PubMed]

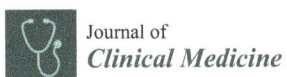

Review

Bone Mineral Density, Osteoporosis, and Fracture Risk in Adult Patients with Psoriasis or Psoriatic Arthritis: A Systematic Review and Meta-Analysis of Observational Studies

Tai-Li Chen [1], Jing-Wun Lu [1], Yu-Wen Huang [2], Jen-Hung Wang [3] and Kuei-Ying Su [4,5,*]

1. Department of Medical Education, Hualien Tzu Chi Hospital, Buddhist Tzu Chi Medical Foundation, Hualien 970, Taiwan; terrychen.a@gmail.com (T.-L.C.); jingwunlu@gmail.com (J.-W.L.)
2. Department of Medical Education, Taipei Tzu Chi Hospital, Buddhist Tzu Chi Medical Foundation, New Taipei City 231, Taiwan; 102311135@gms.tcu.edu.tw
3. Department of Medical Research, Buddhist Tzu Chi General Hospital, Hualien 970, Taiwan; jenhungwang2011@gmail.com
4. Division of Rheumatology and Immunology, Hualien Tzu Chi Hospital, Buddhist Tzu Chi Medical Foundation, Hualien 970, Taiwan
5. School of Medicine, Tzu Chi University, Hualien 970, Taiwan
* Correspondence: kueiying.su@tzuchi.com.tw; Tel.: +886-3-8561825 (ext. 12211)

Received: 19 October 2020; Accepted: 16 November 2020; Published: 19 November 2020

Abstract: Introduction: Awareness of psoriasis-related comorbidities has been established in the current guidelines; however, evidence regarding the association of bone density or bone fragility with psoriatic disease remains inconclusive. Methods: We conducted a systematic review and meta-analysis to assess bone mineral density and the risk of osteoporosis and fractures in patients with psoriatic disease, including those with cutaneous psoriasis and psoriatic arthritis. We searched electronic databases for published observational studies. A meta-analysis was performed using the random-effect model. Pooled estimates and their confidence intervals (CIs) were calculated. Small-study effects were examined using the Doi plot and Luis Furuya–Kanamori index. Results: The analysis of the standardized mean difference in the absolute value of bone mineral density at different measuring sites (lumbar spine, femoral neck, and total hip) revealed no significant difference between patients with psoriatic disease and non-psoriatic controls. The pooled results of the adjusted odds ratios (ORs) demonstrated no increased risk of osteoporosis in patients with psoriatic disease. Notably, patients with psoriatic disease had a higher OR of developing bone fractures (adjusted OR: 1.09; 95% CI: 1.06 to 1.12; I^2: 0%). Conclusion: Patients with psoriatic disease may be more likely to develop fractures compared with non-psoriatic controls. This higher risk for fracture may not necessarily be associated with lower bone mineral density nor a higher risk for osteoporosis.

Keywords: bone mineral density; osteoporosis; fracture; bone fragility; psoriasis; psoriatic arthritis; meta-analysis

---

1. Introduction

Cutaneous psoriasis and psoriatic arthritis (PsA) are chronic inflammatory disorders recognized on the spectrum of psoriatic disease [1–3]. Genetic and immunologic similarities identified in both the affected skin and joints implicate shared mechanisms in psoriatic disease [4–7]. Therefore, it is reasonable to consider combining the management of patients with cutaneous psoriasis and PsA in clinical practice due to the common pathophysiological process [8,9]. With an improvement in molecular biology and immunopathology, abnormal bone remodeling discovered in experimental and clinical research has prompted attention toward bone health in psoriatic disease [10–12]. Although the current guidelines on psoriatic comorbidities do not include bone health [13] recent studies have indicated that patients with psoriatic disease may be at an increased risk of osteoporosis and fractures [14]. However, the evidence regarding the association of psoriatic disease and bone fragility remains inconclusive.

Reduction in bone mineral density (BMD) in patients with psoriatic disease has been reported in a previous systematic review [15]. The prevalence of osteoporosis in patients with psoriatic disease was reported to be 1.4–68.8% in some studies [15–17]. Moreover, patients with psoriatic disease were shown to have a higher risk of developing bone fractures [18,19]. In contrast, other studies reported negative results. Harrison et al., and Busquets et al., revealed no apparent associations between low BMD and psoriatic disease upon clinical observation [20,21]. In several studies, no increased risk of fractures was observed in patients with psoriatic disease than in non-psoriatic controls [22,23]. A complicated and unclear mechanism of bone quality and bone fragility in psoriatic disease may contribute to the controversy above. Additionally, bone fragility and bone strength may be considered beyond bone density alone, making the situation far more complicated [24].

Since the study population, sample sizes, and study designs in individual studies were heterogenous, a comprehensive literature review with meta-analysis is warranted to yield the overall effects. Therefore, in the present study we aimed to perform a systematic review and meta-analysis of observational studies to determine the BMD and fracture risk in adult patients with psoriatic disease.

2. Materials and Methods

We conducted this systematic review and meta-analysis in accordance with the Preferred Reporting Items for Systematic Reviews and Meta-Analyses (PRISMA) statement [25] and the Meta-Analyses of Observational Studies in Epidemiology (MOOSE) guidelines [26]. We registered our protocol at INPLASY.COM(registration number: INPLASY202080106). Two investigators (TL Chen and JW Lu) independently searched for articles, collated data, and evaluated the quality of the qualifying studies. In cases of discrepancies between the investigators, a third author (YW Huang) was consulted to reach a consensus.

2.1. Literature Investigation and Search Strategy

We searched electronic databases (PubMed, Embase, Cochrane Library, and Web of Science) and Chinese medical databases (Airiti Library and Chinese National Knowledge Infrastructure databases) systemically for studies published from the inception of the relevant database until 15 September 2020. In brief, we used the following terms: "psoriasis", "psoriatic arthritis", "bone mineral density", "osteoporosis", and "fracture". The search strategies were modified for the requirements of individual databases, and the details are described in Methods in the Supplementary Materials. Studies in languages other than English or Chinese were excluded. Furthermore, we supplemented our search by examining the reference lists or bibliographies of the available review articles and relevant meta-analyses for additional candidates.

2.2. Study Selection and Eligibility Criteria

Peer-reviewed scientific articles were considered for inclusion. Studies in preprint status and those published in open access journals that were absent on the Directory of Open Access Journals (DOAJ) were considered non-peer-reviewed articles and, thus, were excluded. Studies that fulfilled the following criteria were included: (1) those with observational study design (cross-sectional, case-control, or cohort studies); (2) those in which target participants were adults diagnosed with psoriatic disease (cutaneous psoriasis or PsA) based on clinical or histological information; (3) those in which comparison groups included adult controls without psoriatic disease; (4) those in which the outcomes comprised the absolute value of BMD and/or the effect estimates of osteoporosis or fractures; and (5) those in which BMD was assessed at lower extremities (e.g., lumbar spine, femoral neck, etc.) using dual-energy

X-ray absorptiometry (DXA), ultrasound bone density measurements, or other effective methods. Case reports, case series, review articles, and abstracts from conference proceedings were excluded. We also excluded animal studies or studies performed in laboratory settings.

2.3. Data Extraction and Outcome of Interest

We extracted data regarding the following items: first author, publication year, study design, geographical location, study population (cutaneous psoriasis, PsA, or both), sample size, patient characteristics (age, sex, and body mass index), characteristics of psoriatic disease (disease duration and the usage of potential drugs that may affect bone formation), BMD measurements (device, site, and outcomes), and reported outcomes of osteoporosis and fractures. Systemic corticosteroids, methotrexate, and anti-tumor necrosis factor (TNF)-α agents were considered potential drugs that could be related to bone quality and fragility [27–29]. The conflict of interest study was also listed for each study. The primary endpoint was the absolute value of BMD. The secondary endpoints included effect estimates regarding osteoporosis and fractures.

2.4. Qualitative Systematic Review

A modified Newcastle–Ottawa Scale (NOS) for non-randomized studies was utilized for methodological quality appraisal of the included studies [30,31]; it consists of the following three domains: the selection of study groups, comparability of study groups, and ascertainment of the outcome of interest. Modified NOS for observational studies were demonstrated in Tables S1–S3 in the Supplementary Materials.

2.5. Data Synthesis and Statistical Analysis

Considering the heterogeneity of the study populations, we calculated the pooled estimates and their confidence intervals (CIs) using the DerSimonian and Laird random-effects model [32]. For continuous outcomes (absolute value of BMD), we calculated the standardized mean differences (SMDs) and 95% CIs. SMD was considered because different manufactural modalities were used across studies. For dichotomous outcomes (risk estimates of osteoporosis and fractures), we calculated estimated odds ratios (ORs) and 95% CIs. We focused mainly on the pooled results using maximally-adjusted estimates [33]. However, we still demonstrate the unadjusted ORs for emphasizing the influence of confounding bias [34]. Furthermore, if the enrolled study number of each outcome was less than ten and the pooled effect was statistically significant, modified Hartung–Knapp/Sidik–Jonkman (HKSJ) adjustment was applied to control type I errors and avoid inaccurate CIs [35–37]. We contacted the authors for the desired effect estimates and relevant information for studies that did not report the data available for pooling.

Between-study heterogeneity was quantified using the I^2 statistics [38]. An I^2 value $\geq 50\%$ represents substantial heterogeneity. To explore the potential sources of heterogeneity apart from random error, we conducted several predefined subgroup analyses according to the site of BMD measurement, study population, study design, geographic location, age of participants, body mass index (BMI), disease duration, potential osteoporotic/anti-osteoporotic drugs use, and study quality according to NOS.

We also performed a sensitivity analysis to evaluate the influence of each study on the overall effect by omitting them individually. All statistical tests were two-sided, and p-value < 0.05 was considered statistically significant. The present meta-analysis was performed using Stata v16 (StataCorp, College Station, TX, USA).

2.6. Small-Study Effects

Potential small-study effects, such as publication bias, were examined using Doi plots, a recently developed graphical and alternative method [39]. It has been demonstrated to improve visualized asymmetry with treatment effects on the x-axis and a normal rank-based Z-score on the y-axis. Doi plot asymmetry was quantified using the Luis Furuya–Kanamori (LFK) index, based on the rank-based measure of precision (Z-score) instead of the standard error in funnel plots [39]. LFK indices less than ±1, greater than ±1 but less than ±2, or greater than ±2 were considered to represent no, minor, or major asymmetry, respectively [39]. Moreover, the LFK index has been demonstrated to outperform Egger's regression test for possible small-study effects, especially when the study number is small. We applied the Doi plot and LFK index to detect potential small-study effects in several outcomes of interest, which may be ignored by the inapplicability of funnel plots and quantitative approaches, such as the Egger's p test. MetaXL v5.3 (EpiGear International Pty Ltd., Sunrise Beach, Queensland, Australia) was used to generate the Doi plots and calculate the LFK indices [39].

3. Results

3.1. Search Results

The selection and detailed identification processes are summarized in Figure 1. A total of 3300 unique publications fulfilled the initial screening. We removed 950 duplicates, and the titles and abstracts of the remaining studies were screened for inclusion. The full text of 201 studies was retrieved; of them, 15 met the inclusion criteria. Ultimately, 15 observational studies were included in this quantitative meta-analysis.

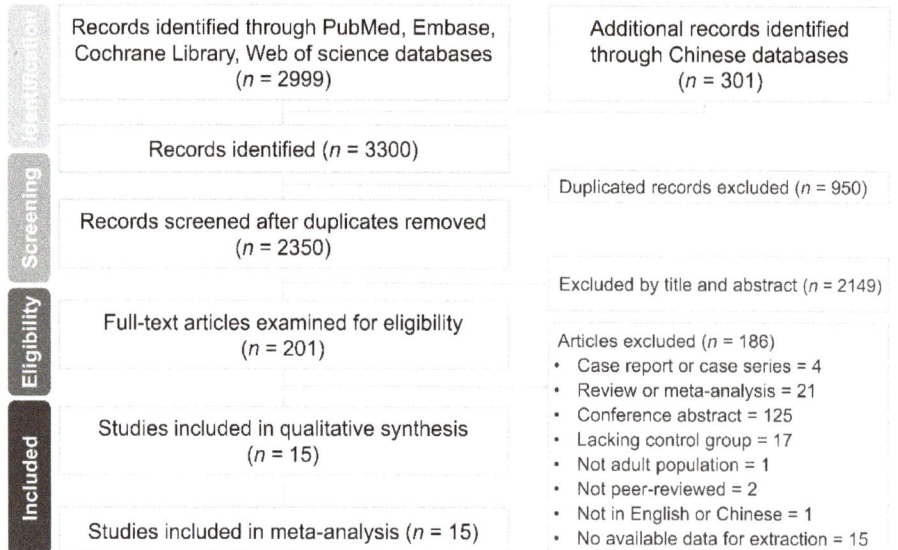

Figure 1. Preferred Reporting Items for Systematic Reviews and Meta-Analyses (PRISMA) flow diagram of the process of screening and including the studies.

3.2. Characteristics of Qualifying Studies

Table S4 outlines the characteristics of the 15 observational studies [16,18,19,22,23,40–49]. A total of 1,277,673 participants, investigated between 2009 and 2020, were evaluated. The demographic data and the reported outcomes of interest were summarized. Female-predominant sex distribution could be observed in most of the studies. The participants were mostly categorized as overweight (25 ≤ BMI < 29.9) or obese (BMI ≥ 30) [50].

After critical appraisal of the studies, eight studies were judged to have "high quality" because they scored ≥7 points on the NOS. Additionally, seven articles were deemed to have "moderate quality (scored 4–6 points)", whereas no studies were considered to have "low quality (scored ≤3 points)". The results of the appraisal are also summarized in Table S4. Two of the enrolled studies declared their conflict of interest with either an institution or company and two studies did not mention their funding source or conflict of interest.

3.3. Pooled Effects of the Primary Outcome

In terms of the overall effect regarding the absolute BMD value, patients with psoriatic disease demonstrated no significantly decreased SMD despite different sites of measurement (SMD in lumbar spine: 0.07; 95% CI: −0.19 to 0.32; I^2: 73.8%; SMD at femoral neck: −0.08; 95% CI: −0.36 to 0.20; I^2: 72.3%; SMD at total hip: −0.05; 95% CI: −0.22 to 0.13; I^2: 34.7%; Figure 2). Subgroup analysis in Table 1 revealed that the age of patients might be a moderator in lumbar spine BMD. After omitting the papers individually for sensitivity analysis, SMD results were similar to the above.

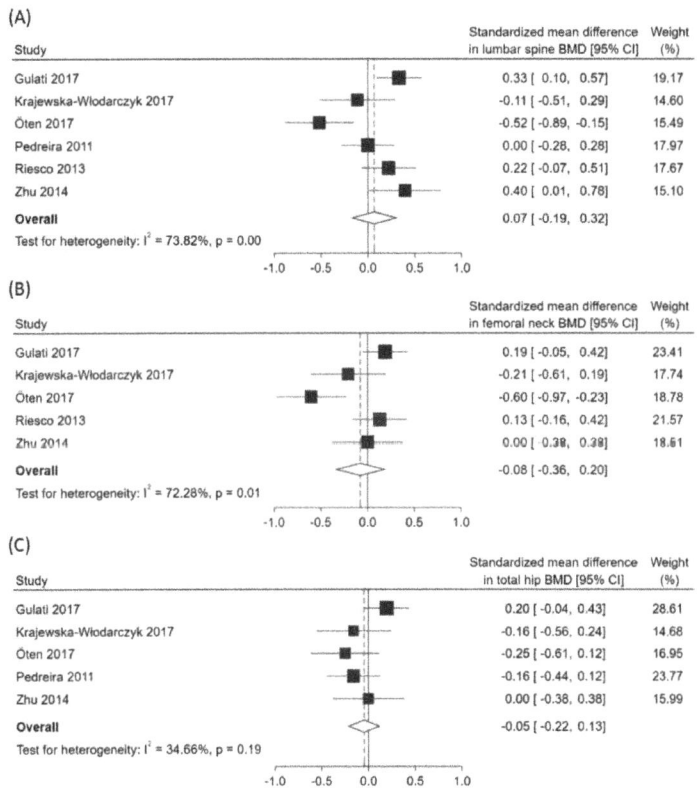

Figure 2. Forest plots of the standardized mean difference (SMD) in absolute bone mineral density. The plots are presented in subgroups of (**A**) lumbar spine, (**B**) femoral neck, and (**C**) total hip. CI, confidence interval.

Table 1. Subgroup analysis of primary outcome.

Subgroups	Lumbar Spine N	SMD (95%CI)	I^2 (%)	Femoral Neck N	SMD (95%CI)	I^2 (%)	Total Hip N	SMD (95%CI)	I^2 (%)
Study population									
Psoriasis	1	−0.07 (−0.40 to 0.27)	NA	0	NA	NA	1	−0.24 (−0.58 to 0.09)	NA
Psoriatic arthritis	6	0.07 (−0.19 to 0.33)	73.5	5	−0.08 (−0.36 to 0.20)	72.3	5	−0.04 (−0.22 to 0.14)	31.0
Study design									
Cross-sectional	5	0.00 (−0.28 to 0.29)	71.9	4	−0.16 (−0.49 to 0.17)	70.0	4	−0.15 (−0.32 to 0.03)	0
Cohort	1	0.33 (0.10 to 0.57) *	NA	1	0.19 (−0.05 to 0.42)	NA	1	0.20 (−0.04 to 0.43)	NA
Geographic location									
America	1	0.00 (−0.28 to 0.28)	NA	0	NA	NA	1	−0.16 (−0.44 to 0.12)	NA
Asia	2	−0.06 (−0.96 to 0.83)	91.3	2	−0.30 (−0.90 to 0.29)	80.1	2	−0.13 (−0.39 to 0.13)	0
Europe	3	0.19 (−0.04 to 0.42)	42.8	3	0.08 (−0.12 to 0.29)	29.5	2	0.06 (−0.28 to 0.40)	54.9
Age (years)									
<50	1	−0.52 (−0.89 to −0.15) *	NA	1	−0.60 (−0.97 to −0.23) *	NA	1	−0.25 (−0.61 to 0.12)	NA
50–59	3	0.31 (0.14 to 0.47) *	0	3	0.13 (−0.03 to 0.30)	0	2	0.14 (−0.06 to 0.34)	0
≥60	2	−0.04 (−0.27 to 0.19)	0	1	−0.21 (−0.61 to 0.19)	NA	2	−0.16 (−0.39 to 0.07)	0
BMI status									
Overweight	4	0.23 (0.06 to 0.40) *	26.2	3	0.13 (−0.03 to 0.30)	0	3	0.02 (−0.20 to 0.25)	45.4
Obesity	2	−0.32 (−0.72 to 0.08)	53.6	2	−0.41 (−0.80 to −0.03) *	50.6	2	−0.21 (−0.48 to 0.06)	0
Disease duration									
≥10 years	5	0.00 (−0.28 to 0.29)	71.9	4	−0.16 (−0.49 to 0.17)	70.0	4	−0.15 (−0.32 to 0.03)	0
<10 years	1	0.33 (0.10 to 0.57) *	NA	1	0.19 (−0.05 to 0.42)	NA	1	0.20 (−0.04 to 0.43)	NA
Medication use									
Yes	5	0.10 (−0.19 to 0.38)	77.6	4	−0.05 (−0.38 to 0.28)	77.7	4	−0.03 (−0.24 to 0.18)	47.0
No	1	−0.11 (−0.51 to 0.29)	NA	1	−0.21 (−0.61 to 0.19)	NA	1	−0.16 (−0.56 to 0.24)	NA
Risk of bias									
NOS ≥ 7	2	0.29 (0.11 to 0.47) *	0	2	0.16 (−0.02 to 0.35)	0	1	0.20 (−0.04 to 0.43)	NA
NOS < 7	4	−0.06 (−0.41 to 0.29)	74.3	3	−0.27 (−0.63 to 0.08)	61.4	4	−0.15 (−0.32 to 0.03)	0

* $p < 0.05$. N, Number of studies; SMD, standardized mean difference; CI, confidence interval; NA, not applicable; BMI, body mass index; DXA, dual-energy X-ray absorptiometry; NOS, Newcastle–Ottawa Scale.

3.4. Pooled Effects of Secondary Outcomes

As presented in Figure 3A, psoriatic patients tended to have a higher risk of developing osteoporosis before adjusting confounding factors (unadjusted OR: 1.35; 95% CI: 1.02–1.78, I^2: 76.4%). However, after adjustment, patients with psoriatic disease were not likely to possess high ORs of developing osteoporosis (adjusted OR: 1.33; 95% CI: 0.78–2.26; I^2: 92.7%) compared with the non-psoriatic controls. In Figure 3B, psoriatic patients were not likely to develop fractures before confounding adjustment (unadjusted OR: 1.16; 95% CI: 0.86–1.57; I^2: 81.0%), but after adjusting for confounding factors, they possessed higher ORs of developing fractures compared with the non-psoriatic controls (adjusted OR: 1.09; 95% CI: 1.06–1.12; I^2: 0%).

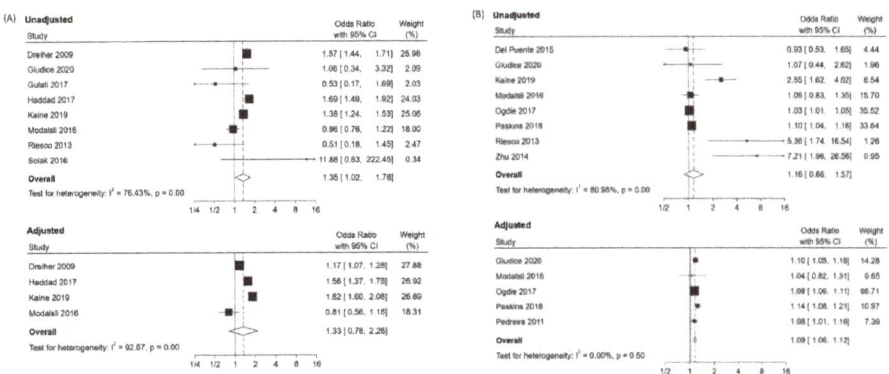

Figure 3. Forest plots of the unadjusted and adjusted odds ratio (OR) of osteoporosis (**A**) and fractures (**B**). CI, confidence interval.

We focused on the adjusted estimates for drawing conclusions and compared them to the unadjusted estimates. The results were opposite before and after confounding adjustment, indicating the substantial role of confounding bias in terms of the overall effect size. Sensitivity analysis yielded similar results, making our pooled effects robust.

3.5. Heterogeneity and Small-Study Effects

Substantial heterogeneity was indicated in nearly all outcomes, except for the group regarding total hip BMD and the adjusted OR of fracture. Subgroup analyses revealed that psoriatic patients' age might serve as a possible moderator in the primary outcome.

Small-study effects were detected using the Doi plot and LFK index. Major asymmetry was indicated in the subgroups of the femoral neck (LFK index: −2.60; Figure S1) in terms of the absolute value of BMD. Minor asymmetry was seen in the lumbar spine group regarding BMD (LFK index: −1.76; Figure S2) and in the adjusted outcome of osteoporosis (LFK index: 1.59; Figure S3). On the other hand, no asymmetry in the Doi plot was observed in the total hip group regarding BMD (LFK index: 0.60) and in the adjusted outcome of fracture (LFK index: −0.13), respectively.4. Discussion

Despite numerous studies concerning bone involvement in the investigative field of psoriatic disease, the findings remain controversial. In this systematic review and meta-analysis, we demonstrated no significant association between psoriatic disease and the absolute value of BMD in the lumbar spine, femoral neck, or total hip. Additionally, patients with psoriatic disease did not have higher risks of developing osteoporosis than the controls; nevertheless, they did have increased OR of sustaining fractures.

A fragility fracture is defined as a pathological fracture that results from low energy insults [51]. It is believed that fractures are associated with decreased bone strength, which reflects the integration of both bone quality and bone density [52]. However, the modalities measuring areal BMD (i.e., DXA) have limited ability to determine bone strength since they have limitations in measuring bone quality, such as microarchitecture, mineralization, collagen cross-links, crystal size, and marrow composition [53,54]. Therefore, osteoporosis defined by DXA may not reflect the actual bone strength reduction and may not serve as an accurate predictor for fractures. This inference may explain why psoriatic patients had increased fracture risk but displayed no association in BMD and osteoporosis in our meta-analysis.

Another explanation for our results is that the increased fracture risk may be attributed to reduced bone quality, namely, the depletion in bone microarchitecture and demineralization. Simon et al. [55] reported that the cortical and trabecular volumetric BMD was significantly decreased in the psoriatic population. Pfeil et al. [56] demonstrated periarticular demineralization in psoriatic disease by measuring the Metacarpal Index at the metacarpal bones. Further in vivo or in vitro experiments and clinical observation are required to clarify the pathogenic process.

Since the pathogenesis of psoriatic disease is complex and multifactorial, potential moderators were identified. Our subgroup analysis found that age may be a potential moderator for the analysis of BMD. Based on previous studies, aging may be related to bone loss with complex interaction between genetic, hormonal, biochemical, and environmental factors [57]. According to the World Health Organization, psoriasis most affects people at the age of 50–69 years [58]. In our study, the lumbar spine BMD increased in this age group, whereas it decreased in patients aged less than 50 years.

Apart from age, several possible confounding factors may affect our results. Previous studies suggested that low bone density in psoriatic disease was identified exclusively in men, usually less affected by bone destruction [16,17]. In contrast, one study reported that there was an increased BMD with postmenopausal women [59]. Hence, the sex of the patients may be a potential confounding factor. Additionally, chronic use of drugs that affect bone formation may also act as a confounding factor in our analysis. Systemic corticosteroids, methotrexate, and anti-TNF-α agents were reported to be either osteoporotic or anti-osteoporotic [27–29]. Finally, the body mass index of patients can also be considered a confounding factor. Epidemiologic research has indicated positive associations between obesity and bone health [60]; while adiposity and weight gain are associated with higher psoriasis risks [61].

Methodological problems regarding the representation of unpublished studies may have a considerable impact on the decision-making in clinical practice [62]. Concerns have been raised about the Egger's asymmetry test and its power to detect asymmetry when the number of studies is small. We then used Doi plot and LFK index to evaluate small-study effects. Compared with the Egger's p test, the LFK index had a superior area under the receiver operating characteristic curve (0.58 to 0.75 vs. 0.74 to 0.88, respectively) as well as higher sensitivity (18.5% to 43.0% vs. 71.3% to 72.1%, respectively) [39]. In contrast, the specificity is higher with the Egger's p test (87.6% to 90.0% vs. 64.7–87.1%, respectively).

To the best of our knowledge, this is the first meta-analysis of observational studies to evaluate the BMD, osteoporosis, and fracture risk in adult patients with psoriatic disease (psoriasis and PsA). This analysis included not only osteoporosis and fracture risks, but also BMD measurements at different sites. This allowed us to estimate the total effect size with large sample size and a higher statistical power. Furthermore, we performed an up-to-date literature search and enrolled in the latest studies in the analysis. We applied sensitivity analyses after omitting each study one at a time, and the pooled results were robust with few changes. We used the novel Doi plot and LFK index to detect small-study effects.

There were some limitations in our studies. First, the inconsistency due to high between-study heterogeneity was observed. We were not able to perform meta-regression due to the availability of <10 studies in each outcome. Although it was a time-consuming effort, we used subgroup analysis to identify moderators in observational studies. Second, our study results could only explain the relationship between psoriatic disease and BMD, osteoporosis, and fractures. Further studies regarding pathogenetic clarification may be necessary. Third, while the LFK index has been demonstrated to discriminate asymmetry better and has higher sensitivity than the Egger's p-value, its specificity is lower than that of the latter. Finally, the opposite results in the secondary outcomes revealed a crucial issue in terms of confounding factors in our enrolled studies, which can introduce bias; therefore, our results should be interpreted with caution.

4. Conclusions

Our results indicate that patients with psoriatic disease may be more likely to develop fractures compared with non-psoriatic controls. This higher risk for fracture may not necessarily associated with lower BMD nor a higher risk of osteoporosis. Future studies are warranted to establish stronger evidence regarding the understanding of bone strength and bone quality in patients with psoriasis or PsA. Based on our findings, we suggest that preventive measures for fractures may be beneficial in current clinical practice for such patients.

Supplementary Materials: The following are available online at http://www.mdpi.com/2077-0383/9/11/3712/s1, Methods: Detailed search strategy modified to accommodate different databases; Table S1: Modified Newcastle–Ottawa Scale for cohort studies; Table S2: Modified Newcastle-Ottawa Scale for case-control studies; Table S3: Modified Newcastle-Ottawa Scale for cross-sectional studies; Table S4: Characteristics of included studies; Figure S1: Doi plot and LFK index of femoral neck BMD; Figure S2: Doi plot and LFK index of lumbar spine BMD; Figure S3: Doi plot and LFK index of osteoporosis.

Author Contributions: Conceptualization: T.-L.C.; methodology, J.-H.W. and K.-Y.S.; software, T.-L.C., J.-W.L., and Y.-W.H.; validation, J.-H.W. and K.-Y.S.; formal analysis, T.-L.C., J.-W.L., and Y.-W.H.; investigation, T.-L.C., J.-W.L., and Y.-W.H; resources, T.-L.C, J.-W.L., and Y.-W.H.; data curation, J.-H.W.; writing—original draft preparation, T.-L.C.; writing—review and editing, J.-W.L., and Y.-W.H.; visualization, J.-H.W. and K.-Y.S.; supervision, K.-Y.S. All authors have read and agreed to the published version of the manuscript.

Funding: No specific funding was received from any bodies in the public, commercial, or not-for-profit sectors to carry out the work described in this article.

Acknowledgments: The authors thank Yu Ru Kou for comments that considerably improved the manuscript. We also thank the Department of Medical Research, Hualien Tzu Chi Hospital, Buddhist Tzu Chi Medical Foundation for the invaluable contribution to the methodological aspects of the present systematic review and meta-analysis.

Conflicts of Interest: The authors declare no conflict of interest.

References

1. Armstrong, A.W.; Read, C. Pathophysiology, Clinical Presentation, and Treatment of Psoriasis. *JAMA* **2020**, *323*, 1945–1960. [CrossRef] [PubMed]
2. Ritchlin, C.T.; Colbert, R.A.; Gladman, D.D. Psoriatic Arthritis. *N. Engl. J. Med.* **2017**, *376*, 957–970. [CrossRef] [PubMed]
3. Bilal, J.; Malik, S.U.; Riaz, I.B.; Kurtzman, D.J. Psoriasis and Psoriatic Spectrum Disease: A Primer for the Primary Care Physician. *Am. J. Med.* **2018**, *131*, 1146–1154. [CrossRef] [PubMed]
4. Li, Q.; Chandran, V.; Tsoi, L.; O'Rielly, D.; Nair, R.P.; Gladman, D.; Elder, J.T.; Rahman, P. Quantifying Differences in Heritability among Psoriatic Arthritis (PsA), Cutaneous Psoriasis (PsC) and Psoriasis vulgaris (PsV). *Sci. Rep.* **2020**, *10*, 1–6. [CrossRef]
5. Stuart, P.E.; Nair, R.P.; Tsoi, L.C.; Tejasvi, T.; Das, S.; Kang, H.M.; Ellinghaus, E.; Chandran, V.; Callis-Duffin, K.; Ike, R.; et al. Genome-wide Association Analysis of Psoriatic Arthritis and Cutaneous Psoriasis Reveals Differences in Their Genetic Architecture. *Am. J. Hum. Genet.* **2015**, *97*, 816–836. [CrossRef]
6. Sakkas, L.I.; Bogdanos, D.P. Are psoriasis and psoriatic arthritis the same disease? The IL-23/IL-17 axis data. *Autoimmun. Rev.* **2017**, *16*, 10–15. [CrossRef]
7. Blauvelt, A.; Chiricozzi, A. The Immunologic Role of IL-17 in Psoriasis and Psoriatic Arthritis Pathogenesis. *Clin. Rev. Allergy Immunol.* **2018**, *55*, 379–390. [CrossRef]
8. Okhovat, J.-P.; Ogdie, A.; Reddy, S.; Rosen, C.F.; Scher, J.U.; Merola, J.F. Psoriasis and Psoriatic Arthritis Clinics Multicenter Advancement Network Consortium (PPACMAN) Survey: Benefits and Challenges of Combined Rheumatology-dermatology Clinics. *J. Rheumatol.* **2017**, *44*, 693–694. [CrossRef]
9. Savage, L.; Tinazzi, I.; Zabotti, A.; Laws, P.M.; Wittmann, M.; McGonagle, D. Defining Pre-Clinical Psoriatic Arthritis in an Integrated Dermato-Rheumatology Environment. *J. Clin. Med.* **2020**, *9*, 3262. [CrossRef]

10. Alivernini, S.; Tolusso, B.; Petricca, L.; Bui, L.; Di Sante, G.; Peluso, G.; Benvenuto, R.; Fedele, A.L.; Federico, F.; Ferraccioli, G.; et al. Synovial features of patients with rheumatoid arthritis and psoriatic arthritis in clinical and ultrasound remission differ under anti-TNF therapy: A clue to interpret different chances of relapse after clinical remission? *Ann. Rheum. Dis.* **2017**, *76*, 1228–1236. [CrossRef]
11. Sirufo, M.M.; De Pietro, F.; Bassino, E.M.; Ginaldi, L.; De Martinis, M. Osteoporosis in Skin Diseases. *Int. J. Mol. Sci.* **2020**, *21*, 4749. [CrossRef] [PubMed]
12. Paine, A.; Ritchlin, C. Altered Bone Remodeling in Psoriatic Disease: New Insights and Future Directions. *Calcif. Tissue Int.* **2018**, *102*, 559–574. [CrossRef] [PubMed]
13. Elmets, C.A.; Leonardi, C.L.; Davis, D.M.; Gelfand, J.M.; Lichten, J.; Mehta, N.N.; Armstrong, A.W.; Connor, C.; Cordoro, K.M.; Elewski, B.E.; et al. Joint AAD-NPF guidelines of care for the management and treatment of psoriasis with awareness and attention to comorbidities. *J. Am. Acad. Dermatol.* **2019**, *80*, 1073–1113. [CrossRef] [PubMed]
14. Oliveira, M.D.F.S.P.D.; Rocha, B.D.O.; Duarte, G.V. Psoriasis: Classical and emerging comorbidities. *An. Bras. Dermatol.* **2015**, *90*, 9–20. [CrossRef] [PubMed]
15. Chandran, S.; Aldei, A.; Johnson, S.R.; Cheung, A.M.; Salonen, D.; Gladman, D.D. Prevalence and risk factors of low bone mineral density in psoriatic arthritis: A systematic review. *Semin. Arthritis Rheum.* **2016**, *46*, 174–182. [CrossRef] [PubMed]
16. Dreiher, J.; Weitzman, D.; Cohen, A.D. Psoriasis and Osteoporosis: A Sex-Specific Association? *J. Investig. Dermatol.* **2009**, *129*, 1643–1649. [CrossRef]
17. Lajevardi, V.; Abedini, R.; Moghaddasi, M.; Nassiri, S.; Goodarzi, A. Bone mineral density is lower in male than female patients with plaque-type psoriasis in Iran. *Int. J. Women's Dermatol.* **2017**, *3*, 201–205. [CrossRef]
18. Ogdie, A.; Harter, L.; Shin, D.; Baker, J.; Takeshita, J.; Choi, H.K.; Love, T.J.; Gelfand, J.M. The risk of fracture among patients with psoriatic arthritis and psoriasis: A population-based study. *Ann. Rheum. Dis.* **2017**, *76*, 882–885. [CrossRef]
19. Paskins, Z.; Whittle, R.; Sultan, A.A.; Müller, S.; Blagojevic-Bucknall, M.; Helliwell, T.; Packham, J.; Hider, S.; Roddy, E.; Mallen, C. Risk of fragility fracture among patients with late-onset psoriasis: A UK population-based study. *Osteoporos. Int.* **2018**, *29*, 1–6. [CrossRef]
20. Harrison, B.J.; Hutchinson, C.E.; Adams, J.; Bruce, I.N.; Herrick, A.L. Assessing periarticular bone mineral density in patients with early psoriatic arthritis or rheumatoid arthritis. *Ann. Rheum. Dis.* **2002**, *61*, 1007–1011. [CrossRef]
21. Busquets, N.; Gómez-Vaquero, C.; Rodríguez-Rodríguez, L.; Vilaseca, D.R.; Narváez, J.; Carmona, L.; Nolla, J.M. Bone mineral density status and frequency of osteoporosis and clinical fractures in 155 patients with psoriatic arthritis followed in a university hospital. *Reumatol. Clin.* **2014**, *10*, 89–93. [CrossRef] [PubMed]
22. Giudice, L.F.L.; Scolnik, M.; Pierini, F.S.; Zucaro, N.M.M.; Gallego, J.F.J.; Soriano, E.R. Fragility fractures in psoriatic arthritis patients: A matched retrospective cohort study. *Clin. Rheumatol.* **2020**, *39*, 3685–3691. [CrossRef] [PubMed]
23. Modalsli, E.; Åsvold, B.; Romundstad, P.; Langhammer, A.; Hoff, M.; Forsmo, S.; Naldi, L.; Saunes, M. Psoriasis, fracture risk and bone mineral density: The HUNT Study, Norway. *Br. J. Dermatol.* **2017**, *176*, 1162–1169. [CrossRef] [PubMed]
24. Paschalis, E.P.; Shane, E.; Lyritis, G.; Skarantavos, G.; Mendelsohn, R.; Boskey, A.L. Bone Fragility and Collagen Cross-Links. *J. Bone Miner. Res.* **2004**, *19*, 2000–2004. [CrossRef]
25. Moher, D.; Liberati, A.; Tetzlaff, J.; Altman, D.G.; PRISMA Group. Preferred reporting items for systematic reviews and meta-analyses: The PRISMA statement. *BMJ* **2009**, *339*, b2535. [CrossRef]
26. Stroup, D.F.; Berlin, J.A.; Morton, S.C.; Olkin, I.; Williamson, G.D.; Rennie, D.; Moher, D.; Becker, B.J.; Sipe, T.A.; Thacker, S.B.; et al. Meta-analysis of Observational Studies in Epidemiology: A Proposal for Reporting. *JAMA* **2000**, *283*, 2008–2012. [CrossRef]
27. Buckley, L.; Humphrey, M.B. Glucocorticoid-Induced Osteoporosis. *N. Engl. J. Med.* **2018**, *379*, 2547–2556. [CrossRef]
28. Orsolini, G.; Fassio, A.; Rossini, M.; Adami, G.; Giollo, A.; Caimmi, C.; Idolazzi, L.; Viapiana, O.; Gatti, D. Effects of biological and targeted synthetic DMARDs on bone loss in rheumatoid arthritis. *Pharmacol. Res.* **2019**, *147*, 104354. [CrossRef]
29. Kawai, V.K.; Stein, C.M.; Perrien, D.S.; Griffin, M.R. Effects of anti-tumor necrosis factor α agents on bone. *Curr. Opin. Rheumatol.* **2012**, *24*, 576–585. [CrossRef]

30. Wells, G.A.; Shea, B.; O'Connell, D.; Robertson, J.; Peterson, J.; Welch, V.; Losos, M.; Tugwell, P. The Newcastle–Ottawa Scale (NOS) for Assessing the Quality of Nonrandomised Studies in Meta-Analyses. Available online: http://www.ohri.ca/programs/clinical_epidemiology/oxford.htm (accessed on 11 October 2020).
31. Anglin, R.E.S.; Samaan, Z.; Walter, S.D.; McDonald, S.D. Vitamin D deficiency and depression in adults: Systematic review and meta-analysis. *Br. J. Psychiatry* **2013**, *202*, 100–107. [CrossRef]
32. Higgins, J.P.T.; Thomas, J.; Chandler, J.; Cumpston, M.; Li, T.; Page, M.J.; Welch, V.A. *Cochrane Handbook for Systematic Reviews of Interventions Version 6.1 [Updated September 2020]*; The Cochrane Collaboration: London, UK, 2020; Available online: www.training.cochrane.org/handbook (accessed on 17 October 2020).
33. Dekkers, O.M.; Vandenbroucke, J.P.; Cevallos, M.; Renehan, A.G.; Altman, D.G.; Egger, M. COSMOS-E: Guidance on conducting systematic reviews and meta-analyses of observational studies of etiology. *PLoS Med.* **2019**, *16*, e1002742. [CrossRef] [PubMed]
34. Metelli, S.; Chaimani, A. Challenges in meta-analyses with observational studies. *Evid. Based Ment. Health* **2020**, *23*, 83–87. [CrossRef] [PubMed]
35. Guolo, A.; Varin, C. Random-effects meta-analysis: The number of studies matters. *Stat. Methods Med. Res.* **2015**, *26*, 1500–1518. [CrossRef] [PubMed]
36. Röver, C.; Knapp, G.; Friede, T. Hartung-Knapp-Sidik-Jonkman approach and its modification for random-effects meta-analysis with few studies. *BMC Med. Res. Methodol.* **2015**, *15*, 99. [CrossRef] [PubMed]
37. Veroniki, A.A.; Jackson, D.; Bender, R.; Kuss, O.; Langan, D.; Higgins, J.P.; Knapp, G.; Salanti, G. Methods to calculate uncertainty in the estimated overall effect size from a random-effects meta-analysis. *Res. Synth. Methods* **2019**, *10*, 23–43. [CrossRef] [PubMed]
38. Higgins, J.P.T.; Thompson, S.G.; Deeks, J.J.; Altman, D.G. Measuring inconsistency in meta-analyses. *BMJ* **2003**, *327*, 557–560. [CrossRef]
39. Furuya-Kanamori, L.; Barendregt, J.J.; Doi, S.A.R. A new improved graphical and quantitative method for detecting bias in meta-analysis. *Int. J. Evid.-Based Heal.* **2018**, *16*, 195–203. [CrossRef]
40. Del Puente, A.; Esposito, A.; Costa, L.; Benigno, C.; Foglia, F.; Oriente, A.; Bottiglieri, P.; Caso, F.; Scarpa, R. Fragility Fractures in Patients with Psoriatic Arthritis. *J. Rheumatol. Suppl.* **2015**, *93*, 36–39. [CrossRef]
41. Gulati, A.M.; Hoff, M.; Salvesen, Ø.; Dhainaut, A.; Semb, A.G.; Kavanaugh, A.; Haugeberg, G. Bone mineral density in patients with psoriatic arthritis: Data from the Nord-Trøndelag Health Study 3. *RMD Open* **2017**, *3*, e000413. [CrossRef]
42. Haddad, A.; Ashkenazi, R.I.; Bitterman, H.; Feldhamer, I.; Greenberg-Dotan, S.; Lavi, I.; Batat, E.; Bergman, I.; Cohen, A.D.; Zisman, D. Endocrine Comorbidities in Patients with Psoriatic Arthritis: A Population-based Case-controlled Study. *J. Rheumatol.* **2017**, *44*, 786–790. [CrossRef]
43. Kaine, J.; Song, X.; Kim, G.; Hur, P.; Palmer, J.B. Higher Incidence Rates of Comorbidities in Patients with Psoriatic Arthritis Compared with the General Population Using U.S. Administrative Claims Data. *J. Manag. Care Spec. Pharm.* **2019**, *25*, 122–132. [CrossRef] [PubMed]
44. Krajewska-Włodarczyk, M.; Owczarczyk-Saczonek, A.; Placek, W. Changes in body composition and bone mineral density n postmenopausal women with psoriatic arthritis. *Reumatologia* **2017**, *5*, 215–221. [CrossRef] [PubMed]
45. Oten, E.; Baskan, B.; Sivas, F.; Bodur, H. Relation Between Osteoporosis and Vitamin D Levels and Disease Activity in Psoriatic Arthritis. *Erciyes Med. J.* **2017**, *39*, 94–100. [CrossRef]
46. Pedreira, P.G.; Pinheiro, M.M.; Szejnfeld, V.L. Bone mineral density and body composition in postmenopausal women with psoriasis and psoriatic arthritis. *Arthritis Res.* **2011**, *13*, R16. [CrossRef]
47. Riesco, M.; Manzano, F.; Font, P.; García, A.; Nolla, J.M. Osteoporosis in psoriatic arthritis: An assessment of densitometry and fragility fractures. *Clin. Rheumatol.* **2013**, *32*, 1799–1804. [CrossRef]
48. Solak, B.; Dikicier, B.S.; Celik, H.D.; Erdem, T. Bone Mineral Density, 25-OH Vitamin D and Inflammation in Patients with Psoriasis. *Photodermatol. Photoimmunol. Photomed.* **2016**, *32*, 153–160. [CrossRef] [PubMed]
49. Zhu, T.Y.; Griffith, J.F.; Qin, L.; Hung, V.W.Y.; Fong, T.-N.; Au, S.-K.; Kwok, A.; Leung, P.-C.; Li, E.K.; Tam, L. Density, structure, and strength of the distal radius in patients with psoriatic arthritis: The role of inflammation and cardiovascular risk factors. *Osteoporos. Int.* **2014**, *26*, 261–272. [CrossRef] [PubMed]
50. Weir, C.B.; Jan, A. *BMI Classification Percentile and Cut Off Points*; StatPearls Publishing: Treasure Island, FL, USA, 2019.

51. Papaioannou, A.; Morin, S.; Cheung, A.M.; Atkinson, S.; Brown, J.P.; Feldman, S.; Hanley, D.A.; Hodsman, A.; Jamal, S.A.; Kaiser, S.M.; et al. 2010 clinical practice guidelines for the diagnosis and management of osteoporosis in Canada: Summary. *Can. Med. Assoc. J.* **2010**, *182*, 1864–1873. [CrossRef]
52. NIH Consensus Development Panel on Osteoporosis Prevention, Diagnosis, and Therapy. Osteoporosis Prevention, Diagnosis, and Therapy. *JAMA* **2001**, *285*, 785–795. [CrossRef]
53. Ott, S.M. Bone strength: More than just bone density. *Kidney Int.* **2016**, *89*, 16–19. [CrossRef]
54. Torres-Del-Pliego, E.; Vilaplana, L.; Güerri-Fernández, R.; Diez-Perez, A. Measuring Bone Quality. *Curr. Rheumatol. Rep.* **2013**, *15*, 373. [CrossRef] [PubMed]
55. Simon, D.; Haschka, J.; Muschitz, C.; Kocijan, A.; Baierl, A.; Kleyer, A.; Schett, G.; Kapiotis, S.; Resch, H.; Sticherling, M.; et al. Bone microstructure and volumetric bone mineral density in patients with hyperuricemia with and without psoriasis. *Osteoporos. Int.* **2020**, *31*, 931–939. [CrossRef] [PubMed]
56. Pfeil, A.; Krojniak, L.; Renz, D.M.; Reinhardt, L.; Franz, M.; Oelzner, P.; Wolf, G.; Böttcher, J. Psoriatic arthritis is associated with bone loss of the metacarpals. *Arthritis Res.* **2016**, *18*, 248. [CrossRef] [PubMed]
57. Demontiero, O.; Vidal, C.; Duque, G. Aging and bone loss: New insights for the clinician. *Ther. Adv. Musculoskelet. Dis.* **2012**, *4*, 61–76. [CrossRef]
58. Global Burden of Disease Collaborative Network. *Global Burden of Disease Study 2010 (GBD 2010) Results by Cause 1990–2010*; Institute for Health Metrics and Evaluation (IHME): Seattle, WA, USA, 2012. [CrossRef]
59. Osmancevic, A.; Landin-Wilhelmsen, K.; Larkö, O.; Mellström, D.; Wennberg, A.-M.; Hulthén, L.; Krogstad, A.-L. Risk factors for osteoporosis and bone status in postmenopausal women with psoriasis treated with UVB therapy. *Acta. Derm. Venereol.* **2008**, *88*, 240–246. [CrossRef]
60. Lee, S.J.; Lee, J.; Sung, J. Obesity and Bone Health Revisited: A Mendelian Randomization Study for Koreans. *J. Bone Miner. Res.* **2019**, *34*, 1058–1067. [CrossRef]
61. Aune, D.; Snekvik, I.; Schlesinger, S.; Norat, T.; Riboli, E.; Vatten, L.J. Body mass index, abdominal fatness, weight gain and the risk of psoriasis: A systematic review and dose–response meta-analysis of prospective studies. *Eur. J. Epidemiol.* **2018**, *33*, 1163–1178. [CrossRef]
62. Atakpo, P.; Vassar, M. Publication bias in dermatology systematic reviews and meta-analyses. *J. Dermatol. Sci.* **2016**, *82*, 69–74. [CrossRef]

Publisher's Note: MDPI stays neutral with regard to jurisdictional claims in published maps and institutional affiliations.

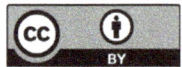

© 2020 by the authors. Licensee MDPI, Basel, Switzerland. This article is an open access article distributed under the terms and conditions of the Creative Commons Attribution (CC BY) license (http://creativecommons.org/licenses/by/4.0/).

MDPI
St. Alban-Anlage 66
4052 Basel
Switzerland
Tel. +41 61 683 77 34
Fax +41 61 302 89 18
www.mdpi.com

Journal of Clinical Medicine Editorial Office
E-mail: jcm@mdpi.com
www.mdpi.com/journal/jcm

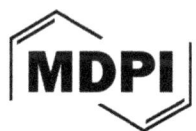

www.ingramcontent.com/pod-product-compliance
Lightning Source LLC
LaVergne TN
LVHW070626100526
838202LV00012B/741